Drug Misuse:
A Practical Handbook for GPs

THE AUTHORS

Dr A. Banks, MB, ChB, is a family doctor in Chelmsford who first started to treat drug users and alcoholics in the early 1970s. From 1980 onwards he felt an acute need for more information for family doctors on drug problems and joined with Dr Waller to write the precursor of this book.

Dr T.A.N. Waller, MB, BS, BSc, DObst RCOG, is a full-time principal in general practice in North London, a trainer and tutor at three London medical schools. He is also a lecturer at University College and the Middlesex Hospital Medical School, London. He was Medical Adviser to City Roads (Crisis Intervention) Ltd from 1978–84 and has represented GPs on the Advisory Council on the Misuse of Drugs since 1983.

Published in association with the
Institute for the Study of Drug Dependence
(ISDD).

First published as a booklet by ISDD in 1983 from
articles which originally appeared in
General Practitioner, 25 March 1983.

Drug Misuse:
A Practical Handbook
for GPs

A. BANKS
MB, ChB
and
T.A.N. WALLER
MB, BS, BSC, DObst RCOG

BLACKWELL SCIENTIFIC PUBLICATIONS

OXFORD LONDON EDINBURGH

BOSTON PALO ALTO MELBOURNE

in association with
The Institute for the Study of Drug Dependence

© 1988 by
Blackwell Scientific Publications
Editorial offices:
Osney Mead, Oxford OX2 0EL
 (*Orders*: Tel. 0865 240201)
8 John Street, London WC1N 2ES
23 Ainslie Place, Edinburgh EH3 6AJ
3 Cambridge Center, Suite 208,
 Cambridge, MA 02142, USA
667 Lytton Avenue, Palo Alto
 California 94301, USA
107 Barry Street, Carlton
 Victoria 3053, Australia

All rights reserved. No part of this
publication may be reproduced, stored
in a retrieval system, or transmitted,
in any form or by any means, electronic,
mechanical, photocopying, recording or
otherwise without the prior permission
of the copyright owner.

First published 1988

Set by DP Photosetting, Aylesbury, Bucks
Printed in Great Britain by
Billing & Sons Ltd, Worcester

DISTRIBUTORS
USA
 Year Book Medical Publishers
 35 East Wacker Drive
 Chicago, Illinois 60601
 (*Orders*: Tel. 312 726-9733)

Canada
 The C.V. Mosby Company
 5240 Finch Avenue East,
 Scarborough, Ontario
 (*Orders*: Tel. 416-298-1588)

Australia
 Blackwell Scientific Publications
 (Australia) Pty Ltd
 107 Barry Street
 Carlton, Victoria 3053
 (*Orders*: Tel. (03) 347 0300)

British Library
Cataloguing in Publication Data

Banks, A.
 Drug misuse.
 1. Great Britain. Drug abuse. Prevention
 & treatment
 I. Title   II. Waller, T.A.N.
 362.2'93'0941

ISBN 0-632-02059-8

Contents

Foreword by Sir Donald Acheson, Chief Medical Officer, DHSS	ix
Preface	xi
Acknowledgements	xiv

Part 1: Theoretical Background by Dr T.A.N. Waller   1

1 Drug Misuse in Perspective   3
- Historical aspects   3
- A medical perspective   5
- The current situation   11
- The development of nomenclature and a system of classification   22
- Communities and drug use   26
- The family and drug use   33
- The aetiology of drug use   33
- The individual and drug use   34

2 Different Drugs of Misuse   41
- Volatile substance misuse   41
- Amyl and butyl nitrite   53
- Cannabis   54
- Opioids   58
- Barbiturates   65
- Benzodiazepines   68
- Amphetamines   74
- Cocaine   79
- Psychedelics   84
- Miscellaneous drugs   90
- Designer drugs   95
- Alcohol and its relationship to drug misuse   97

3 Medical Conditions Arising from Drug Misuse   103
- Overdoses   103
- Hypothermia   103
- Pyrexia   104
- Respiratory complications   104

Cardiovascular complications	105
CNS effects	105
Genito-urinary and sexual effects	107
Psychological effects of drug misuse	109
Psychiatric morbidity and drug misuse	111
Medical hazards of injecting	114
Hepatitis	115
The masking of intercurrent illness	122
AIDS	123
Other infections	141
Drug misuse and its effect on immunity	142
Vitamin and other nutritional deficiencies	143
Mortality and drug use	143
4 Legislation and the GP	**145**
The Misuse of Drugs Regulations	146
5 Prevention	**154**
Education	155
Changing attitudes	156
Restricting supplies and thoughtful prescribing	157
Screening for substance misuse	159
Harm reduction	163
Part 2: Practical Management by Dr A. Banks	**165**
6 Initial Care	**167**
Social care	169
Hospital care	169
Private care	171
General practice care	172
General medical care	173
Referral to other facilities	173
Practical management	174
Treatment of opioid misuse	190
Treatment of non-opioid drug misuse	216
7 Long Term Care	**236**
Where to refer	236
The nature of rehabilitation	240
Therapy possibilities	243
Goal setting for the drugtaker	245
Chronic drug abuse	247
8 Women and Drugs, Pregnancy and Child Care (with Dr T.A.N. Waller)	**251**
Contraception	253
Pre-conception counselling	254

Pregnancy	255
Management of the pregnant drugtaker	262
The management of labour	265
Breast feeding	266
The neonate	266
Treatment of the neonatal withdrawal syndromes	268
Other neonatal problems	270
9 Drugs, the Family and the GP	**274**
On discovering the problem	274
Strategies adopted by concerned non-users	274
A persistant drugtaker in the family	275
Sources of help for the family	276
GP help to family and friends	277
Appendix A: GP Training and Self-awareness	**281**
Appendix B: Sources of Advice and Information	**283**
Appendix C: Resource List	**289**
Appendix D: Drugs Controlled under the Misuse of Drugs Regulations	**293**
Appendix E: A note about Drug Slang	**302**
Appendix F: Advice for People who are HIV antibody positive	**304**
References	315
Index	337

Foreword

The misuse of licit and illicit drugs is a major national problem, which requires a concerted response at every level in the community. The increasing number of injecting drug misusers who are known to be HIV seropositive makes early intervention and treatment of drug misusers all the more important.

The general practitioner with the primary health care team has a key role in early identification of the problem, offering counselling and long-term support to the drug misuser and his family, providing general medical care and in the treatment of drug misuse. Liaison and co-operation with local authority services, community-based drug agencies and secondary health services is essential if we are to develop an effective response.

This book, based on the expertise of two general practitioners who have had long experience in working with drug misusers, provides informative and practical advice on how the general practitioner can address this task.

I hope it will encourage all doctors to play their part fully.

Sir Donald Acheson KBE DM DSc FRCP FFCM FFOM
Chief Medical Officer
Department of Health and Social Security

Preface

Imagine this scenario. You are a family doctor; occasionally you have seen drug users but you have disliked the task and been relieved that you did not have to do more than just refer them on somewhere. Now in your surgery this morning you have a father and mother, long-standing friends of your family, who have made the devastating discovery that their 20-year-old son has been smoking heroin for more than two years. He looks a clean-living lad and has managed to keep the amount low, about 100 milligrams a day, and thus avoided detection. Nevertheless he is solidly hooked and his own efforts to get off have failed. He not only has a steady job but is planning to get married soon, and the news has shattered his fiancée as well as the family. He wants to come off but you know that there is no hospital drug unit in your particular area. The boy does not want to lose his job by going away for treatment. It looks as if you will have to tackle the job yourself but you don't know where to start.

This book is for you. You may never have faced this situation, but in one way or another the problem of drug misuse may present itself in a compelling form at any time. Even if you are experienced in this field you may wish to learn other ways of approaching some of the knottier problems. Our first publication, *Drug Addiction and Polydrug Abuse*, published by ISDD in 1983 was a much briefer and simpler outline of the role of the general practitioner. In this book, it may need a little more digging to find what you are looking for because the subject does require fuller treatment. For once a preface is not apologising for adding one more book to an overcrowded scene. The field is sadly empty. Here is a start.

GPs are generalists working with three-dimensional people; it is appropriate that they become involved 'in the round'. The whole person approach embracing medical, social, psychological, psychiatric and even spiritual aspects is crucial when dealing with drug misuse.

We have attempted to cover most of these facts in the book. There is no other publication in which they are all dealt with comprehensively and brought together as a whole. In this volume we have not attempted to deal with smoking and problem drinking as well, except where one or two aspects of these problems can be helpful in comparison, although we have included a section on problem drinking and its relationship to drug misuse.

We trust there is enough material here to provide a basis for training courses or serious study but we hope it will also be the sort of book you can keep within reach of your surgery chair to dip into when the need arises. We hope, too, that the book will equally be of interest to people other than doctors – the public and workers in the field who wish to know more about the role the GP can play in dealing with drug problems.

The earlier part of this handbook is for those who are interested in learning more of the theoretical side of the subject. At times this earlier section is necessarily technical but we hope this will not put off the interested reader. The section on addiction in pregnancy is written with the practice immediately following theory and since there are few books on the topic we might venture to believe it could have some value for health and social work professionals especially in view of recent legal cases. Thus, apart from pregnancy the book can be seen as divided in two parts: theoretical background and practical care. Family doctors may wonder why some of the medical terms have been defined – e.g. piloerection (gooseflesh) – but we trust that this will be helpful to non-medical readers.

The situation, especially with the advent of AIDS, is changing all the time. We have expanded sections on hepatitis and AIDS, cocaine, designer drugs, drugs and pregnancy, non-prescribing detoxification and family aspects but we know some of this material will become out of date quite soon.

Well, that is where you come in. Once you have become absorbed in this frustrating but fascinating sphere, it will not be difficult to keep up-to-date. Hold on, you say, all this talk is impossibly idealistic. What about the long sessions wasted on someone who lies to you and repeatedly lets you down? What of the kids who, out of rebellion or carelessness, involve themselves in this mess and then expect us to get them out of it? When we have little enough time for the innocent victims of others' actions like road accident victims or sufferers from painful diseases, haemophiliacs, malformed children, and neglected old folk, why should we spend untold hours trying to persuade some ungrateful drug users to change when the results are so disappointing? Why should anyone get involved in this unrewarding field? Yet many family doctors do, without neglecting their more 'deserving' patients. They struggle on, with little guidance from other sources, and are cheered by reaching the occasional target. This book is written particularly for them.

If you start getting involved in the treatment of drug misuse and seek help from others, you will find that those working in the 'drugs' field, whether medical or not, are the most helpful, knowledgeable and likeable of colleagues you could wish to meet. Controversy exists, often heated, but in helping newcomers, foils are laid aside and the advice is generous and frank. In compiling this book, the authors are indebted to many such people, in particular: the Chief Medical Officer and Dr Dorothy Black at the DHSS; Bing Spear and his successor at the Home Office Drugs Branch, Peter Spurgeon; Dr Malcolm Lader, from the Institute of Psychiatry; Dr Peter Tyrer, consultant psychiatrist at Mapperley Hospital, Nottingham; Mr John Ramsay from St George's Hospital Medical School; Dr Jackie Chang who has allowed us to use many ideas from her own booklet; Dr Anthony Pinching at St Mary's Hospital, Paddington; Dr Maurice Lipsedge, Guys Hospital, London; Dr C.C.H. Cook, UCH and Middlesex Hospital Medical Schools, London; Dr Colin Brewer, Director of the Substance Abuse Programme, Stapleford Tawney Essex; Dr Anne MacDonald, Gartnavel Royal Hospital, Glasgow; Dr Roy Robertson; Dr Elizabeth Tylden; Dr John Strang; Dr Herbert Kleber from the Department of Psychiatry, Yale University School of Medicine; Dr Meg Patterson; members of the Association of Independent Doctors in Addiction (AIDA); the staff members of City Roads, Yeldall Manor, the Church House Trust, Lifeline Project, the Standing Conference on Drug Abuse (SCODA) and the Institute for the Study of Drug Dependence (ISDD), particularly Harry Shapiro, our patient and overworked editor, and his assistant Veronique Brooke.

We would also like to thank the colleagues in our respective surgeries for allowing us the time to deal with both the drug users in our care and the demands of preparing this book.

A. Banks
T.A.N. Waller

Acknowledgements

Sections from: *Guidelines of Good Clinical Practice in the Treatment of Drug Misuse* quoted in Chapter 6, courtesy of the Controller of Her Majesty's Stationery Office.

Appendix F: 'Advice for People who are HIV Antibody Positive' courtesy of *Maternal and Child Health* (Barker Publications).

Material quoted from 'Benzodiazepine Withdrawal: an unfinished story' courtesy of the *British Medical Journal*, **288**, 14 April 1984.

Part 1:
Theoretical Background

Dr T.A.N. Waller

Chapter 1

Drug Misuse in Perspective

Historical aspects

1. World events and subsequent legislation

It was the opium smoking epidemic in China during the 18th and 19th centuries which first drew world attention to the devastating effects that drug use can have upon society. Today mainland China is virtually drug-free, but few could fail to see the irony of Britain's present heroin epidemic; for Britain, to her shame, played a major role in promoting China's opium problem during a period that has been described as 'the most protractedly sordid episode of British imperial history'.[1]

For eighty years following the victory of Clive of India against the French at Plessey in 1757, the British East India Company had a monopoly on the opium trade from Bengal to China. This trade was greatly expanded by the use of privateers or 'country ships' licensed by the British East India Company who 'had effective control over every aspect of the chain of distribution, much as today's top heroin traffickers exercise their control ... It was the first time that opium was treated as an international commodity to be marketed on a vast scale'.[2]

Opium smoking increased rapidly throughout the Chinese mainland. In 1839, 40,000 chests of opium were sent to China, but when the Emperor acted to stop the trade in Canton by arresting opium sellers and sending back ships the British responded by 'sending an expeditionary force to punish the Chinese and restore free trade'. This action led to the First Opium War (1839–1842) and was followed by the Second Opium War in 1856. Both of the Opium Wars were lost by the Chinese, who were subsequently forced by the British to legalise the opium trade under the Treaty of Tientsin in 1858.

This 'restoration of free trade' eased the difficulties the British had previously faced when importing the drug and supply and demand both rapidly increased.

In 1859, 60,000 chests of opium were sold to the Chinese and in the space of only 20 years this figure had increased to 105,000 chests. Opium smoking proliferated with opium dens appearing in almost every town in China. The ensuing social disruption and misery was devastating.

Far away in Britain the Oriental Society for the Suppression of Opium worked to prick the public conscience and sway opinion against the opium trade. Indeed, slowly throughout the world there was a growing realisation of the harm that had been engendered in China by the opium trade.

In 1906, China decided to reduce and terminate the domestic cultivation of opium over a period of ten years and negotiated with the newly elected British government to reduce and terminate the importation of opium over the same period.

In 1912, several countries met at the Hague and signed the International Opium Convention, officially consenting to certain fundamental principles for the control of opium and other 'dangerous drugs'. These principles have been retained to the present day and include restrictions on the manufacture and trade of opium, its derivatives, and cocaine and its salts – the trade and manufacture of these drugs being limited to requirements for medical and scientific purposes only. The production and distribution of raw opium was also restricted under the Hague Convention.

Although the United Kingdom was party to the signing of this Convention in 1912, the outbreak of the First World War delayed its implementation. A further eight years went by before Britain was able to introduce domestic legislation controlling opium and cocaine and their derivatives. The Dangerous Drugs Act 1920 was later superseded by further legislation in response to subsequent international treaties. In 1935, cannabis became controlled because of '... the alarming influence of addiction to Indian hemp on the development of criminality'. Subsequently much debate has centred around cannabis', both nationally and internationally, as to its potential to cause social harm with strong disagreement about its dangers.

In 1961, Britain became party to a further international convention, the United Nations Single Convention on Narcotic Drugs (which included cannabis and cannabis resin among the list of prohibited substances). Following this, various drugs which had not previously been controlled in the UK became included within new legislation. Amphetamines became controlled under The Drugs (Prevention of Misuse) Act 1964 and later this was extended to include LSD (1966) and methaqualone (1971). Our present-day legislation, The Misuse of Drugs Act 1971, has also resulted from ratification of the 1961 Single

Convention and consolidates earlier legislation on drug misuse. Several other drugs, including barbiturates and benzodiazepines, are now controlled under the 1971 Act following ratification of another international treaty, the United Nation's Single Convention on Psychotropic Substances, 1971.

Besides being the present legislation by which all drugs of dependence with a potential to cause social harm are controlled in the UK, the Misuse of Drugs Act 1971 also established the formation of a standing committee to advise ministers about current drug problems in Britain. This committee, known as the Advisory Council on the Misuse of Drugs (ACMD) has proved to be extremely useful in helping the government form effective policies in response to both our current drugs problem and the AIDS epidemic, where injecting drug use has been shown to be such an important factor in the spread of this disease.

A medical perspective

2. The 'British System'

The Dangerous Drugs Act 1920 imposed legal controls on British doctors allowing them to use narcotic drugs only for *'bona fide* medical treatment'. This caused considerable confusion amongst the medical profession because there was no clear understanding as to whether or not prescribing controlled drugs to addicted persons constituted *bona fide* medical treatment. To sort out this thorny problem, a Departmental Committee on Morphine and Heroin Addicts (also known as the Rolleston Committee) was set up. In its report [3] published in 1926 the Rolleston Committee distinguished between prescribing drugs to users under proper controls and the supply of drugs merely for their gratification. It outlined indications as to when morphine or heroin could be given, these being:

(a) if the person was being gradually withdrawn; or
(b) if, after attempts at cure had failed, the patient could lead a normal and useful life when provided with a regular supply, but ceased to do so when the supply was withdrawn.

Thus the principle of maintenance treatment was established. It was now considered *bona fide* medical treatment for doctors to maintain drug users on a stable dose of a controlled drug if this enabled them in turn to stabilise their lives (the intention being to withdraw them slowly at a later date). The maintenance treatment method, which became known as the British System or the Rolleston approach, relied on tolerance, the doctor's judgement and was eminently flexible. It was envied by some doctors in other countries with more rigid policies. This approach dominated treatment policy for the next fifty years and it is only recently that there has been a move away from it.

A new wave of drugtakers and the move to specialisation
From the 1926 Rolleston Report until 1960, there were only a few known drug users in the UK, and the number was stable, varying only from 400 to 600 at any one time. These were mainly therapeutic morphine addicts, usually middle-class, middle-aged, and even elderly. Addiction was seen as a chronic relapsing neurotic condition found in those of a nervous disposition. Such individuals were treated mainly by general practitioners.

In 1961, an Interdepartmental Committee on Drug Addiction reported [4] that the drug situation in Britain gave little cause for concern. However in 1965, the Interdepartmental Committee, which had been hurriedly reconvened, issued a second report [5] which reversed the views and proposals of the first. This committee, under the chairmanship of Sir Russell Brain, accepted that a new, young, unstable, non-therapeutic group of drugtakers had emerged and that a handful of London 'junkie doctors' were prescribing dangerous drugs in excessive amounts to this group. Overprescribing by unscrupulous, uninformed or vulnerable doctors open to blackmail was felt to be the main reason why the problem was escalating so rapidly and action was hurriedly taken to make the treatment of drug misuse a specialist service.

The Brain Committee recommended that a number of treatment centres should be set up, run by psychiatrists with a special interest in the problem. GPs were to be allowed to treat drug users if they so wished, but only doctors with a special licence from the Home Office were to be allowed to prescribe heroin and cocaine.

The Drug Dependence Units or Clinics (DDUs or DDCs) were set up in 1968–70 and the treatment of drug misuse became a specialty. To many GPs this was a great relief. They were now officially encouraged to refer to these new specialist services a very difficult and demanding group of patients. There were, of course, not enough specialist services to cover the whole country and GPs were still allowed by law to treat dependence with any drug apart from heroin and cocaine. Nevertheless, most drugtaking in the 1960s and 1970s was concentrated in inner city areas where there was usually access to a DDU, although these clinics usually focused on heroin misusers, to the exclusion of other kinds of drug problems.

The shift of emphasis towards specialisation and the move away from treatment by the primary care services meant that skills were not developed in this field by GPs and other generic professionals (social workers, community psychiatric nurses, probation officers etc). Furthermore the training of this group in the problems and treatment of drug misuse received little attention.

An epidemic of illicit drug use
In the mid-1960s, when it was hoped that the rising drug problem could be contained by the introduction of specialists, no one could have foreseen the extent to which drug misuse was to increase. The graph below gives an indication of the rise of heroin misuse in the UK as shown by the numbers notified to the Home Office as being dependent on opiate drugs, although this rise has recently shown signs of slowing down.

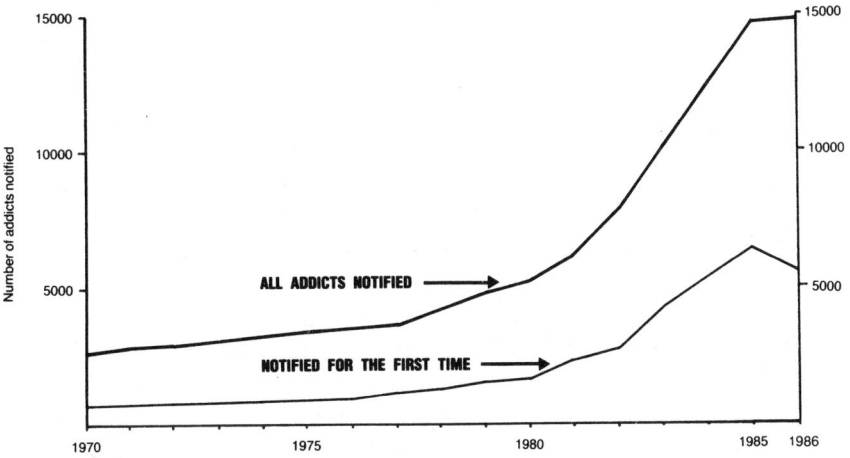

Figure 1.1 Total number of UK addicts notified at any time during the year and the number of these notified for the first time in that year ('new' addicts). (Source: ISDD.)

Research suggests that notifications to the Home Office may give an underestimation of true prevalence by a factor of at least five times, but it is generally accepted that the number of new notifications probably reflects the national prevalence trend better than any other statistic.

There were a number of factors which contributed to the sudden increase in drug use in the late 1970s and 1980s, including cheap supplies of heroin derived from abundant harvests in Pakistan and the Far East; the appeal of high gain, low risk operations for gangs not tradionally involved in drug-dealing; and the widespread introduction of the habit of smoking heroin ('chasing the dragon') obviating the need for needles and making it more attractive to young people.

One result of the increase was a large number of drug-dependent people seeking treatment. At the same time research was published showing that methadone maintenance treatment was not stabilising the new type of drug user. The DDUs, particularly those in the great conurbations, reacted by switching from methadone maintenance to an outpatient detoxification regime. Some clinics prescribed for periods of up to six months, some for shorter periods than this, and others later (mainly in Scotland since 1983) stopped prescribing opioids at all.

The development of a non-substance orientated approach
The move away from the Rolleston approach had been accompanied by an increasing realisation that, on the whole, treatment had previously been too 'substance-orientated'. As one authority [6] put it:

'One major trend has been the move away from a substance preoccupation, so that problem drugtaking may be recognised with a wider range of drugs and drug categories than was previously realised. It is also evident that mere identification of the substance taken does not inevitably identify problematic use.

Thus the physical, psychological, and social problems associated with one person's solvent inhalation may on occasions be greater than those seen with another patient's use of opiates. What is required is a model that permits a more individual assessment of the patient without being blinded by the substance. Just as with alcohol problems, clinicians have come to realise that patients may present with a wide variety of disorders under the mantle of drug dependence or alcoholism. Obviously some disorders may occur more frequently than others, but an approach that catered only for patients with a fixed constellation of signs, symptoms and pathology would not be providing a proper and comprehensive service. It would be demanding that patients fit in with the mould of the service rather than the service responding to the needs of the patient.'

It is now generally accepted that substances and their substitution should not dominate the treatment situation. Nevertheless, substitutes are still commonly prescribed and there is a great variation in opinion as to the type of substance that should be given and the extent to which it should be used, if at all. Indeed, an outside observer might be forgiven for thinking that almost anything goes. For the treatment of problem heroin use, by far the commonest form of drug use leading to help-seeking in present day Britain, the response may vary from a totally flexible approach, including occasional treatment with methadone maintenance, to a rigid outpatient detoxification regime under contract to no detoxification at all. Although oral methadone mixture is most commonly given, injectables are still prescribed by at least one DDU and one professor of general practice. Benzodiazepines are often used to treat heroin withdrawals in the North of England and Scotland. Clonidine is used exclusively by one West Country GP and at least one consultant psychiatrist at a London teaching hospital.

Non-pharmacological treatments also abound and include electroacupuncture, yoga, relaxation techniques, psychoanalysis and psychotheraphy of many different types including cognitive therapy, family therapy and behavioural techniques. Then there are the rehabilitation houses with a wide variety of different approaches varying from the confrontative, highly structured concept houses, to the caring family atmosphere which is found in some of the Christian-based residential projects.

The Treatment and Rehabilitation Report [7] of the Advisory Council on the Misuse of Drugs recommended 'a range of responses ... capable of adapting to the problems presented by each individual's involvement with drugs.' The range of responses that are available for drugtakers would suggest that perhaps this recommendation has been fulfilled. It is regrettable, however, that some of these treatments appear to be given more according to the interests and prejudices of the giver rather than as an adaptation to the needs of the individual drug user.

Moves towards a uniform approach and the decline of maintenance treatment
In an effort to find a more uniform and acceptable approach a medical working group on drug dependence was set up. Its report [8] entitled *Guidelines of Good Clinical Practice in the Treatment of Drug Misuse*, was published in 1984 and sent to every doctor in the country, as *guidelines* of course, rather than rigid rules. Copies are available at the price of £1.00 from DHSS Stores, Government Buildings, Honeypot Lane, Stanmore, Middlesex HA7 1AY. Cheques should be made payable to DHSS.

Methadone maintenance treatment by GPs is forcefully discouraged in the *Guidelines*: 'We strongly recommend that the general practitioner should explain clearly and sympathetically at the first interview that treatment will not necessarily involve prescribing of opioids or barbiturates, and will certainly not involve long-term maintenance prescribing'.

It was easy to see how the conventional, middle-aged, often professional person for whom Rolleston had legitimised maintenance prescribing, could be stabilised on long-term treatment to lead a productive and useful life. It was not so easy to believe that the Rolleston approach could stabilise the 'hedonistic drop-outs' who first appeared in the 1960s. To such people, drugtaking and addiction formed part of a chronic, deviant and often petty criminal lifestyle. The Second Brain Committee [5] recommended that the prescribing clinics to be set up should firstly prepare patients for withdrawal and then admit them for inpatient detoxification. In fact very little inpatient treatment ever took place, and in 1977 it became recognised that there was a 'gradually increasing core of patients on long-term maintenance'. Three out of every four addicts on a prescription at that time were still likely to be on it one year later. Many were maintained for several years.

Interest in the efficacy of methadone maintenance treatment in the new type of user provoked a flurry of research studies [9], [10], [11]. The results were surprisingly similar. An improved, but still very poor, work record was an indication that for a few people greater stability was achieved once they had started on a maintenance programme. For the vast majority, however, there was no evidence of any stabilisation. The death rate and overall crime rate was unaffected and convictions for drug offences actually increased. The latter finding suggests that most people were either using on top of their script or selling methadone in order to buy the drug of their choice. Methadone maintenance was, if anything, contributing to their drug problem. In contrast, the ones who clearly had been stabilised (apart from occasional relapses) were those who had stopped using drugs. Further evidence [12] was obtained by a Home Office researcher, who studied a sample of men notified in 1969 and later treated with an opiate prescription. After five years, more than a third had been almost continuously on a prescription, and three-quarters of these were convicted of criminal offences, mainly arising from continued attempts to obtain opiates by illicit means. Far from a stabilising effect, the researcher commented 'There can be no doubt that the longer men continued to receive prescriptions for opiates, the more likely they were to be convicted of both drug and non-drug, mainly theft, offences'.

In spite of all this evidence methadone maintenance treatment was not abandoned everywhere and even the *Guidelines* did make an exception aimed at those opioid drugtakers with very chaotic lifestyles: 'For some patients it is useful to maintain a stable dose for a month or two months to allow them to make adjustments in their personal life, and to tackle problems related to illicit drug use. This maintenance period should not be prolonged and it should be made clear from the outset that it is only a prelude to a detoxification regime such that prescribing will terminate within a three-to-six month period.'

The current situation

The beginning of the 1980s showed a rapid move away from maintenance regimes throughout the country but particularly in the densely populated urban areas. This was accompanied by a growing movement towards non-substance orientated approaches and a growing realisation that doctors do not hold the only key to treatment.

In 1982 publication of the Treatment and Rehabilitation Report of the ACMD [7] inspired central government funding to pump-prime a number of services for drug users. Similarly, in 1984, publication of another report by the ACMD entitled *Prevention* [13] was also followed by several government-funded initiatives. In response to the Treatment and Rehabilitation Report, £17.5 million was committed to a Central Funding Initiative which provided pump-priming funds for 188 local projects in England. Forty-two per cent of the projects funded were in the voluntary sector and almost half of the funding went to community-based services. Of those projects that were pump-primed for three years, almost all appear to have found continued funding from local sources. Additionally, a few projects have become established in the private sector.

The Welsh Office has not pump-primed projects, but since 1985 has agreed some permanent funding subject to review after three years. Funds totalling £1.064 million had been allocated by 1987 for the development of services for drug misusers in Wales. A further £33,500 per annum was also made available in 1987 for conselling drug misusers in AIDS prevention.

In Scotland, funds have been set aside from 1984 specifically to support drug misuse services. From 1987/88 £1 million per annum is being made available with local Health Boards assuming responsibility for projects previously funded by the Scottish Home and Health Department.

The extent of service provision

Statistics available for 1986 show 11 drug dependence units in England, and 6 joint drug and alcohol units containing 127 and 125 beds respectively. In 1987 there were 36 residential rehabilitation facilities in England including those run by both the voluntary and private sectors. With one exception every District had a Drug Advisory Committee and the majority of these had wide representation. Each of the 14 Health Regions in England provided access to specialist treatment facilities and specialist advice for professionals but residential rehabilitation remained patchy, some Regions (e.g. Wessex) being relatively well provided for but two (West Midlands and North East Thames) without any long-term rehabilitation at all.

In Scotland the situation is rather different; in 1987 there were only two hospital-based services specifically for drug misusers, but neither of these prescribed opioid substitutes to heroin users. Prior to 1983-84, services for drug misusers in Scotland – apart from the two drug dependence units – were almost non-existent. However, by 1987 a number of community-based projects had sprung up and 26 projects received three-year pump-priming grants from either the Scottish Home and Health Department or the Social Work Services Group. Outside of the Strathclyde region, rehabilitation services for drug users were provided mainly by voluntary organisations with support from local authority or NHS personnel. In Strathclyde, the Social Work Department has placed special emphasis on services for drug misusers and has developed a range of community-based services.

In Wales there are also two hospital-based services for drug users and two long-term rehabilitation centres. There are several drop-in advice and counselling centres and an all-Wales Drugline providing 24-hour telephone advice for drug misusers, their families, their friends, and for the professionals working with them.

Northern Ireland appears to have a small drugs problem compared to the rest of the UK. There are six general psychiatric hospitals, each with a consultant with a special interest in dependence. There is also a regional unit in Belfast. Virtually no prescribing with opioid substitutes occurs in Northern Ireland, there is no long-term rehabilitation, nor is there a drugs helpline telephone service. There is, however, an AIDS helpline which receives some requests for help from drug users.

Overall specialist services in the UK have expanded dramatically since the Treatment and Rehabilitation Report in 1982. [7] However, provision remains patchy in places and this is also true of the back-up facilities such as urinalysis.

A new development since 1985 has been the establishment of numerous advice and counselling centres up and down the country and also the establishment of community drug teams in many areas. This expansion of service provision reflects the increasing emphasis that is being placed on community care in Britain.

Community drug teams (CDTs) are usually small and consist of two or three individuals, often a nurse and a social worker, although in districts with a high prevalence of problem drug use they are sometimes larger. Some CDTs contain members from the voluntary sector and thus combine statutory and non-statutory elements. They have a particularly important role in supporting the GP in domiciliary detoxification and are a major development in our treatment services. They function as a catalyst to existing services, offering advice and counselling to drug users, and where necessary helping them find treatment with a chemical substitute such as methadone.

Advice and counselling centres have developed with great rapidity. Originally there were only a handful of such agencies, which were known as 'street agencies', and these were confined to the metropolitan area and concentrated solely on counselling drug users. Most of the agencies that have developed over the last two or three years see their work as being broader based. Many hold regular groups for those dependent on prescribed tranquillisers and most will also see as their remit counselling, or at least giving advice to, the families and close friends of drug misusers.

There is now nowhere in the country that does not have a drug problem for, although illicit drugtaking is particularly prevalent in the urban conurbations, it has permeated everywhere, even the most rural of areas. Indeed, some rural areas that have a good provision of trunk roads, such as North Lincolnshire, now have as high an incidence of drug misuse as some inner city areas. Thus it is important that there is a full and comprehensive service throughout the country.

There is now nowhere in the country that does not have a drug problem for, although illicit drugtaking is particularly prevalent in the urban conurbations, it has permeated everywhere, even the most rural of areas. Indeed, some rural areas that have a good provision of trunk roads, such as North Lincolnshire, now have as high an incidence of drug misuse as some inner city areas. Thus it is important that there is a full and comprehensive service throughout the country.

The Ministerial Working Group

Another development in the 1980s was the setting up of a new group in 1984 with a special remit to look at the work of the police and customs. The Ministerial Working Group, as it became known, was chaired by a minister, originally David Mellor MP, and unlike the

ACMD had an executive rather than an advisory function.

Many international and domestic initiatives came out of the deliberations of this group including two of great importance to the UK. One of these was the fusion of police and customs investigations of drug trafficking in the National Drugs Intelligence Unit (NDIU) in 1985. This replaced the Central Drugs Intelligence Unit (CDIU). At times prior to 1985 there had been occasions when the police and customs appeared to have been working against each other because the police were interested in making arrests, while the customs concentrated on gathering enough intelligence to make large seizures. Before the establishment of the NDIU there had been times, it is said, when the police and customs had both been working independently, observing the same suspect, and a police arrest had prevented the customs from making a large seizure, thwarting several months of painstaking work. To avoid such an occurrence, exchange of information between police and customs had not routinely taken place to the detriment of the work of both in spite of the presence of the CDIU. The NDIU was a very positive move forward to overcome this problem.

A second major initiative of the Ministerial Working Group was to introduce legislation to confiscate the assets of drug traffickers. In doing this the Drug Trafficking Offences Act 1986 not only broke new ground by combining civil and criminal law, but also departed from our system of justice in that a person found guilty of supplying or intending to supply drugs who had a large sum of money in his bank account or elsewhere that he could not immediately account for, had to be able to prove that this was obtained innocently. This is a complete reversal of the principle on which the British system of justice rests: that a person is innocent until he is proved guilty.

One of the more contentious parts of the Act is that anyone, who suspects that a sum of money (anything in excess of £30) has been obtained by drug trafficking, may make a disclosure to the police. In practice it is often a bank manager, but it may be literally anyone who makes such a disclosure. When a disclosure is made the police are then empowered by the Act to investigate it and of the 400 disclosures made in the first nine months following implementation of the Act, approximately 20 per cent were found to relate to either drug trafficking or major crime.

The AIDS epidemic

In the early and mid-1980s the AIDS pandemic first began to make its impact felt in Britain. At first this was through male homosexuals, but evidence from New York and elsewhere soon showed that a second wave of the epidemic would occur in injecting drug users and this was expected to be the main route through which the virus would get into the general heterosexual population. The treatment of drug misuse therefore was not only of value in its own right, but it was also important as the main way of preventing the spread of human immuno-deficiency virus (HIV) into the general population. Furthermore, it was not only those with problem opioid use who needed to come into contact with the treatment agencies, but recreational as well as problem injectors, not only of opioid drugs, but also of amphetamines, cocaine, benzodiazepines, barbiturates and some other drugs as well. Most of the people using drugs in this way were not looking for help and the entire philosophy surrounding the treatment of drugtakers needed to change. No longer was it acceptable to stand back and wait for an injecting drugtaker to be motivated to seek help. Injecting recreational and problem drug users needed to be actively sought out if headway was to be made in reducing the spread of HIV infection. AIDS was seen as a greater danger to both individual and public health than drug misuse and there needed to be a change to a hierarchy of treatment goals, with the achievement of less harmful ways of using drugs being an earlier and more important goal than abstinence. Some drug units had already foreseen this approach and switched back from rigid abstinence-orientated detoxification to more flexible prescribing regimes. The philosophy of the new approach was set out, along with a series of important recommendations, in a report of a working group of the ACMD on AIDS and Drug Misuse [14] which was presented to Ministers in January 1988.

GPs are particularly well placed to intervene with those large numbers of people at the bottom of the pyramid of drug injectors who do not normally come in contact with treatment services, but who need to change both their injecting and sexual behaviours if an impact is to be made in reducing the spread of AIDS. The successful treatment of drug misuse is an important way of preventing HIV spread.

The movement away from specialisation

The recognition that GPs were an important element in the treatment of drug misuse began in a small way in 1982 in the Treatment and Rehabilitation Report of the Advisory Council [7]. This stated: 'Given the widening geographical distribution of problem drug taking and the increased variety of drugs misused, we are aware that it would be unreasonable to expect future hospital services to be developed to the point where they could provide comprehensive cover in all districts, particularly where access to specialist services is poor. We see therefore a possible role for some doctors outside the specialist services to play a part in the treatment of problem drug takers, but with strict safeguards.' A much more positive approach was forthcoming in the 1984 *Guidelines* [8]: 'We wish to encourage as many general practitioners as possible to treat these patients and to help them in every possible way ...' Following this a number of official documents signalled encouragement for GPs to become involved. [15, 16, 17] This was part of a general move away from specialisation and an acceptance that a network of services in the community was also a valuable form of treatment for drug misuse. It was a complete reversal of the policy put forward by the Brain Committee [5] which had dominated thinking in the field for nearly 20 years. Subsequently the first AIDS and Drug Misuse report of the Advisory Council [14] has recommended the establishment of community-based services for drug users in every health district and GPs are seen to play a central role in the treatment of drug misuse. In fact general practitioner involvement in this field had been steadily developing over the previous 15 years although not at a very fast rate.

Since 1972 the proportion of notifications by GPs slowly increased until by 1981 it was over 50 per cent. Other generic workers had also slowly become more involved in helping drug users break free from their dependency. These included probation officers, social workers, community psychiatric nurses, health visitors, teachers, and youth workers. One of the difficulties has been that very few generic workers have had any training on the subject, although this is now changing.

As far as GPs are concerned, training is still haphazard and patchy both at undergraduate and postgraduate level. Clinical teaching, when it occurs, tends to focus more on the medical problems created by drug misuse in the individual (e.g. hepatitis, overdose, septicaemia) rather than upon the social, psychological and environmental aspects of drug misuse, and the prevention, treatment and rehabilitation of drug misusers.

General psychiatrists and drug misuse

Psychiatrists appear to get the most training in drug misuse, but in spite of this some psychiatrists do not view drug misuse as a psychiatric problem and refuse to become involved. Others take a different view and in the North West region a new way of involving the general psychiatric services has been pioneered by Dr John Strang [18]. This has involved the setting-up of satellite clinics at a site away from the central treatment or organisational unit. Satellite clinics provide local bases where the regional specialist and the district general psychiatric services can work together.

Detoxification is given, where appropriate, using pink 'drug clinic' prescriptions (FP10 (HP)(ad)(revised 2/82), which allows the pharmacist to dispense the drug withdrawal regime on a daily basis. The satellite clinics, being locally based, are more accessible and general practitioners are reported as appreciating the relatively easy access to this treatment facility compared with the more remote specialist clinic. Several other health regions have now introduced satellite clinics.

Advantages of GP involvement

It has been suggested that GPs should become more involved in the treatment of drug dependence [8] and, given a free choice, the majority of drug users prefer to be treated by their GP [19]. General practitioner treatment of their drug-dependent patients has the following advantages:

(1) lack of stigma;
(2) accessibility;
(3) help for the whole person;
(4) help for the whole family;
(5) a network of support;
(6) continued care and support after treatment has ceased.

(1) Lack of stigma

Seeing the family doctor is likely to provoke less comment by a passing neighbour than attendance at the local DDU. The lack of stigma of general practice and the opportunity for drug users to have a confidential discussion with a concerned professional who is already known and trusted should not only allow for intervention with those groups who normally find it difficult to come forward, but also should encourage intervention at an earlier stage of drug use. This contention is supported by the findings of a Scottish study [20]. A group of 162 heroin users attending a single group practice was found to be younger and to include more women than previous studies of heroin users attending a consultant clinic. Women are more likely than men to remain in the 'hidden sector' of drug users unknown either to the police or treatment services [21] and it is therefore important that they are more easily able to consult their GP.

(2) Accessibility

GPs are more accessible than most drug clinics. A wait of several weeks to be seen at a drug clinic can be dispiriting. Motivation can be reduced or lost during this period. Many drugtakers will only reach out for help when their drug use has led to a crisis situation (e.g. a court case, break-up of a relationship etc.). GPs, because of their accessibility, are in a position to offer crisis intervention, although this does not imply that they should offer a crisis prescription. With the provision of evening surgeries, GPs are better geared to make treatment accessible to those drug users in employment than many of the drug clinics and thus may see some users earlier in their drugtaking careers.

(3) Help for the whole person

The generalist's approach covering not only straightforward medical and psychiatric illness, but also psychological, social, cultural, spiritual, political, environmental and all the other influences that intertwine to form the complexity of a single human being are of particular relevance when dealing with drug misuse. Drug problems cross all boundaries and affect each one. To say, as some doctors do, that drug misuse is a social problem and should not be the concern of doctors, is a simplistic distortion. It is neither solely a social problem nor solely a medical one. It is both and a lot more besides. It affects the whole person and therefore is clearly the remit of the general practitioner. Some lay people and social workers, who misunderstand the GP's role, resent general practitioners' involvement which they describe as 'medicalising the problem'. Such attitudes are unfortunate as they tend to impair working relationships and consequently may reduce the drug misuser's chances of recovery.

(4) Help for the whole family

GPs are often in a position to help the drug user indirectly by giving help and support to the whole family. Family behaviour frequently becomes deeply disturbed when one member is found to be using drugs. (Families Anonymous describe the whole family as becoming sick.) Furthermore, maximising family involvement in treatment, which the family doctor is well placed to do, has been shown to be associated with a better prognosis for the drug user [22]. Family involvement is not often undertaken by the specialist treatment services who tend to concentrate more on the individual.

(5) A network of support

GPs are also well positioned to involve other members of the primary care team and other workers in the community such as youth workers, probation officers or community drug teams so that there is a network of support for the individual drugtaker. Even where there are no formally structured primary care teams, liaison can and does take place between the different generic workers in the community who are working with drug users.

(6) Continuity of care
GPs have 24-hour responsibility for their patients and one doctor may continue to care for someone, often for several years, sometimes over a person's entire life. This continuity of care became of increased importance following the shift in emphasis in Britain towards abstinence-orientated treatment regimes. Most drug users leave the DDU the moment their detoxification regime has finished and it then becomes the responsibility of the GP to provide care for both the drug user and his family. Regrettably this move is rarely accompanied by a communication from the DDU to the GP. This is a pity as the drug-free period is difficult for the drug user and the family, particularly in the early phases. Relapses are common and GPs are often the first port of call in a relapse. Relapses are in fact so common that drug dependence is often viewed as a relapsing condition. Some recent research has been centring on the prevention of relapse [23] and this may be a fruitful approach that could be applied to a primary care setting.

This description of the advantages of GP care is in no way a statement that GP care is preferential to hospital care. Rather, in order to maximise the advantages of each, the two should work both with each other and with an integrated network of services in the community. However, only too often there is either an absence of a local drug dependence unit or, where this facility exists, GPs and DDUs work in isolation from each other. Most community drug teams recognise the importance of working with GPs and other generic workers but virtually all services, specialist and generic, do at times work in isolation, sometimes as the result of a genuine fear of breaching confidentiality. If this occurs, it invariably weakens an individual's chances of successfully overcoming his or her problem. Whenever possible every effort should be made to obtain a patient's or client's consent to involve a network of support within the community (including other members of the family and close friends).

There is no good reason why the consultant service at the local DDU should not reflect other secondary level care from the acute hospital sector with this service being reserved for the more complicated cases and GPs managing the more straightforward ones. Managing most drug problems is well within the capabilities of the average GP. Detoxification techniques are easily learnt and support from within the community for the drug user from community drug teams, self-help groups, etc. is now more readily available than it has been previously. Successful management is very rewarding. It is not often that a mother will cross the street to thank you for looking after her son with diabetes, but she will if you help him get off heroin.

Current state of involvement of GPs

In a national survey [24] of the extent of contact that general practitioners have with opiate users, a cautious estimate of between 30,000 and 44,000 new cases of opiate misuse presenting to GPs in a year was suggested in 1985. This is of course substantially greater than the 6,409 first time notifications made to the Home Office in that year. Of all first time notifications of drug addicts made by doctors to the Home Office, general practitioners notified 15% in 1970, 29% in 1975, 49% in 1980 and 51% in 1985 reflecting an increasing involvement of GPs with drug misusers. Notification by GPs is known to be low. It was 33% in Glanz's 1985 national survey [25], 34% in a survey of heroin users attending a Scottish general practice [26], and 26% of those referred by GPs to a drug dependency unit. [27]

The 1985 national survey estimated that a typical GP in England and Wales, with a list of 2,000 patients of whom 1,000 are aged 15-44, will have about two new cases of opiate misuse in a year [24]. Clearly, taking into account the fact that there will be many more drugtakers in various stages of remission or relapse already known to the GP, that several others will be misusing non-opioid drugs, and that there are some areas of especially high prevalence, the burden on some GPs must be very considerable.

With regard to the way in which GPs handle drug misusers, the 1985 national survey [25] indicated that only 6% had undertaken or arranged for screening of urine for drugs, although it was stated that this may reflect difficulties of access to appropriate facilities. A substantial proportion of GPs in the survey had prescribed opiate drugs, 18% for a period of less than two weeks and 17% for a period lasting longer than this. (To date there have been no studies published on the effectiveness of such GP interventions.) The extent to which GPs made use of other services was indicated by the following referral rates: DDUs 45%; general psychiatric services 34%; the primary health care team 9%; local authority social services 8%; a voluntary organisation dealing with drug misuse 11%. This showed that referral on to non-medical sources of help tends to be made relatively infrequently

Drug Misuse in Perspective 21

by GPs. This important survey has shown that there is already considerable involvement of some general practitioners in Britain with patients who are using drugs. Responses are variable but this is not surprising given the lack of information and training on the subject for GPs.

Yet in spite of encouraging responses from a few practitioners, it is still only a tiny minority who are involved. It is essential that GPs now become much more involved in the treatment of drug misuse before the AIDS epidemic worsens. Concurrent with this, each GP will need to reassess his or her own attitudes to drug misuse and to educate him or herself as thoroughly as possible in this difficult and demanding subject.

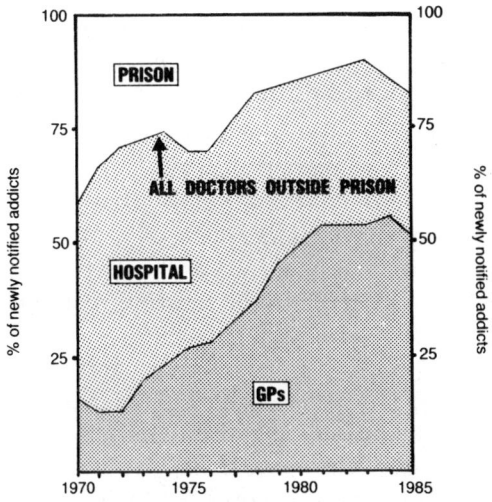

Figure 1.2 Cumulative percentage of addicts notified for the first time by GPs, hospital doctors or prison officers. (Source: ISDD.)

Attitudes of GPs to drug misusers

The problems that result from illicit drug use cross over so many boundaries that some might say generalists are as well, if not better placed than specialists to deal with them. The general practitioner who sees his role as dealing with the whole person, who oversees continuity of care, often in a family setting, and who is prepared to enlist the aid of others, is particularly well placed to help. It is unfortunate that quite often rigidity of views or lack of knowledge and training are obstacles to success.

In the national survey by Glanz of a 5% random sample of GPs in England and Wales [28] almost two-thirds of respondents regarded the treatment required by opiate misusers as beyond the competence of general practitioners, with less than a quarter (23%) disagreeing. This finding may be compared with a similar item in a survey on managing alcohol problems in general practice where 44% of general practitioners felt capable of working with drinkers [29].

The poor response may be a reflection of national policy in the mid-1960s when the Second Brain Committee Report [5] saw the British drug problem as the result of irresponsible prescribing by a few medical practitioners and implemented changes specifically designed to exclude GPs from treating drug users, leaving treatment firmly in the hands of specialist psychiatrists. There has now been a complete turnabout; the British drugs problem is much greater than it was 20 years ago and results almost totally from illicitly imported drugs, rather than from drug-prescribing GPs. Furthermore, the Medical Working Group and the Minister of State with responsibility for policy have both emphasised that GPs now have a responsibility and a 'duty' to provide services to drugtakers [8, 15].

One finding from Glanz's national survey that provides some hope for the future was that newer GPs appeared to be more confident of their ability to deal with drug misusers and indicated that they would probably play a more active part in the treatment of opioid misusers if more back-up resources were available.

A network of supporting services was recommended by the Advisory Council on the Misuse of Drugs (ACMD) in its report on 'Treatment and Rehabilitation' [7] and the Social Services Committee [15], also advocated close liaison with services in hospital and in the community (both statutory and non-statutory). In its more recent report on 'AIDS and Drug Misuse' [14] the ACMD recommended that each health district should have a community-based service with back-up support from the acute hospital sector.

The development of nomenclature and a system of classification

The first attempt to establish nomenclature was made in 1951 when WHO gave a definition of alcoholism [30]. One year later the WHO Expert Committee on Drugs Liable to Produce Addiction also provided a definition for drug addiction [31]. In 1957, the Expert Committee felt a distinction should be made between *drug addiction* (psychological and physical dependence) and *drug habituation* (psychological dependence only), in order to distinguish between different patterns of use [32].

Drug addiction was defined as 'a state of periodic or chronic intoxication produced by the repeated consumption of a drug (natural or synthetic)'. Its characteristics include '(1) an overpowering desire or need (compulsion) to continue taking the drug and to obtain it by any means; (2) a tendency to increase the dose; (3) a psychic (psychological) and generally a physical dependence on the effects of the drug; (4) a detrimental effect on the individual and on society'.

Unfortunately, instead of clarifying matters, this distinction between addiction and habituation to drugs led to a considerable amount of confusion. Furthermore it was felt that the definition of addiction had encouraged the terms 'addiction' and 'addict' to be used in a derogatory sense. The upshot of this was that in 1964, the WHO Expert Committee recommended that 'the misused term drug addiction' should be dropped and the term *drug dependence* should be used to embrace both drug habituation and drug addiction. Drug dependence was defined as '... a state arising from repeated administration of a drug on a periodic or continuing basis'. The following year the Expert Committee reported that it 'was pleased to note the generally favourable reaction to the recommendations'. In spite of this, the words drug addiction and drug addicts are still occasionally to be found in the current literature; they also continue to be used as official legal terms and notifications continue to be made to the Home Office 'Addicts' Index.

Although the terms drug addiction and drug habituation had been shelved, many people still felt that it was important and useful to distinguish between psychological and physical dependence and criticised the 1964 definition of dependence for omitting this. In 1965, Eddy et al. (33) provided an accepted definition of these terms.

Psychic dependence was defined as a condition in which a drug produces '... a feeling of satisfaction and a psychic drive that requires periodic or continuous administration of the drug to produce pleasure or to avoid discomfort'.

Physical dependence was defined as '... an adaptive state that manifests itself by intensive physical disturbances when the administration of the drug is suspended ... These disturbances, i.e. the withdrawal or abstinence syndromes, are made up of specific arrays of symptoms and signs of psychic and physical nature that are characteristic for each drug type.'

Further criticisms of the 1964 definition arose because it gave no way of distinguishing between drug dependence and drug abuse. In 1969, the WHO Expert Committee redefined drug dependence as '... a state psychic and sometimes also physical resulting from the interaction between a living organism and a drug, characterised by behavioural and other responses that always include a compulsion to take the drug on a continuous or periodic basis in order to experience its psychic effects, and sometimes to avoid the discomfort of its absence. Tolerance may or may not be present. A person may be dependent on more than one drug.'

Two years later this definition was criticised for overlooking the social context of drug use [34]. Further discomfort with the definition was felt later as it became apparent that there was no clear dividing line between psychic and physical dependence. It had long been recognised that patients who are prescribed strong opiate drugs for the relief of pain will typically discontinue drug use when the condition is relieved and the pain stops, in spite of developing the opiate abstinence syndrome. Thus it was known that physical dependence could occur in the absence of any apparent psychic dependence. The picture, however, became even more complex when Wikler [35] described ex-smokers and drinkers as reporting the subjective experience of withdrawal effects long after they have given up. He described this as subclinical conditioned withdrawal, which could be invoked as a conditioned response to certain environmental stimuli. A similar phenomenon is evident in drug users who have stopped taking drugs for a period way beyond the normal physical withdrawal phase. Conditional learning can also be used to explain a recent experiment in which animals were taught to associate a ringing bell with receiving a heroin injection. Such animals will have a full-blown withdrawal syndrome if they first hear the bell and then receive an opiate antagonist – even if they have been completely drug-free for months [35].

As investigative and research procedures have become more refined, it has become possible to show that a physical withdrawal reaction can occur after only small quantities of a drug have been given for a short duration of time. All night EEG recordings of sleep will demonstrate a rebound insomnia following the use of short-acting hypnotics for only a few nights [36]. By using the pure opioid antagonist naloxone it is possible to demonstrate the opioid abstinence syndrome in normal human volunteers after a single dose of morphine. Such evidence would indicate that the term physical dependence is a misnomer.

New concepts

(1) Neuroadaptation
Further investigations have shown that there is such a close link

between the physical withdrawal syndrome and acquired tolerance that they are generally believed to be manifestations of the same adaptive process. In view of these findings, Edwards *et al.* [37] have suggested a new term, neuroadaptation, referring to neuronal changes associated with tolerance and withdrawal effects.

(2) The dependence syndrome
The loss of a clear division between psychological and physical dependence led to a shelving of this restrictive dualism. In its place drug dependence is now viewed as 'a socio-psycho-biological syndrome ... a syndrome manifested by a behavioural pattern in which the use of a given psychoactive drug, or class of drugs, is given a much higher priority than other behaviours that once had a higher value ... The intensity of the syndrome can be measured by the behaviours that are elicited in relation to using the drug and by the other behaviours that are secondary to drug use. On the basis of current knowledge, no sharp cut-off point can be identified for distinguishing drug dependence from non-dependent but recurrent drug use. At the extreme, the dependence syndrome is associated with "compulsive drug-using behaviour"' [37]. A method of measuring the severity of opiate dependence has recently been described [38] and may prove to be of importance in determining the treatment needs of patients.

(3) Problem drug use
The concept that problem alcohol use constitutes a separate dimension from dependence on alcohol was originally put forward by a WHO Scientific Group [39]. Later this idea was taken up by experts in the drugs field [7]. *Problem drug use* is one of the key forces behind help-seeking and motivation to change. It is defined as 'social, psychological, physical or legal problems related to intoxication and/or regular excessive consumption and/or dependence as a consequence of the taking of drugs or other chemical substances (excluding tobacco)'. This concept is currently stimulating discussion and research in the drugs field just as it had done previously for those working with drinkers.

Redefinition of drug misuse

Drug abuse and *Drug misuse* are both subjective terms involving value judgements, and, for this reason, it has been impossible to produce a definition which can be interpreted in a standard way. Drug abuse was defined by the WHO Expert Committee [40] as 'persistent or sporadic excessive drug use inconsistent with or unrelated to acceptable medical practice'. It remains an unsatisfactory definition. In addition the term has been so frequently used in a pejorative manner that, like other terms such as addict and alcoholic where this has happened, its use is falling from favour. The slightly broader term drug misuse is preferred. It is less judgmental and also encompasses the taking of legitimately prescribed drugs in an unorthodox way. Edwards et al. [37] have suggested that some clarification of this term can be achieved by subdivision into the following categories.

(a) Unsanctioned use
Use of a drug that is not approved by a society, or a group within that society. When the term is used, it should be made clear who is responsible for the disapproval. The term implies that we accept disapproval as a fact in its own right, without having to determine or justify the basis of the disapproval.

(b) Hazardous use
Use of a drug that will probably lead either to dysfunction or to harm in the user. This concept is similar to the idea of risky behaviour. For instance, smoking twenty cigarettes each day may not be accompanied by any present or actual harm but we know it to be hazardous.

(c) Dysfunctional use
Use of a drug that is leading to impaired psychological or social functioning (e.g. loss of job or marital problems).

(d) Harmful use
Use of a drug that is known to have caused tissue damage or mental illness in the person who took it.

Communities and drug use

(1) Epidemics of drug use

Data has been accumulated indicating that drug misuse follows epidemic rather than endemic patterns, and such epidemics are usually followed by a period when drug misuse is low. The great opium-smoking pandemic which ravaged China in the eighteenth and nineteenth centuries has been followed today by an almost total absence of opioid use in mainland China (although Hong Kong has a major heroin problem). Following World War II there was a notable epidemic of methamphetamine-taking in Japan, which rose and fell again over the ten-year period 1945–55. It is hoped that the current cocaine epidemic of North America, and the heroin epidemic of the UK and other European countries will decline in similar fashion.

Hughes et al. [41] examined epidemiological patterns in local communities and came to the much criticised view that heroin misuse spreads like an infectious disease. Thus on a smaller scale drug misuse also tends to follow epidemic rather than endemic patterns.

(2) Environmental influences on drug use

Social deprivation has been shown to be a factor associated with drug misuse [42]. Adverse environmental influences coupled with the ready availability of a drug can lead to an astonishingly high amount of drug misuse. About 40% of enlisted Americans in Vietnam were considered to use heroin regularly [43]. Twelve months after their return only 7% of those detected as users (by urine tests) remained dependent [44]. Thus environment can have far-reaching effects both in a negative and a positive direction.

(3) Some economic aspects of drug misuse

Some communities depend on illicit drug production for their economic or physical survival. Bolivia, which produces 40% of the world's cocaine, obtains an income from that drug which is two to three times greater than the combined income from its other products [45]. It is claimed that illicit drugs have been used to buy guns and ammunition for the Afghanistan resistance forces [46], making that community politically independent and ensuring its physical survival. In the late 1970s, heroin was used as merchandise to bring money out of Iran by some of the community who fled the country following the deposition of the Shah.

The criminal underworld has increasingly moved into the supply of illicit drugs as profits are so enormous and risks relatively few. One kilo of heroin purchased for £4,000 on the Pakistan/Afghan border may be sold in Britain for £20–25,000. Dilution or 'cutting' with powders of a similar appearance may increase the profits even further. Research has suggested that the British heroin market in 1982 generated net profits of some £48 million [47]. Because of wider recreational demand, cannabis may generate even greater sums.

(4) Drugs and crime

In 1986, 22,982 people in Britain were found guilty of offences under the Misuse of Drugs Act. Of these, 3,463 were given custodial sentences [48]. The number of people in prison for drug offences is currently running at 7–10,000 per year, out of a total of 47,000 prison population [49]. It is likely that a considerably greater number are in prison for offences that have not been recognised as being drug-related. In 1986, cannabis, heroin, cocaine and amphetamine were detected alone or in combination with other controlled drugs and alcohol in 20% of murder and manslaughter cases, 10% of rape cases and in the majority of impaired driving cases submitted to London's Metropolitan Police Forensic Science Laboratory.

There is a well-known link between drug use and crime, exemplified in a report from one rehabilitation centre [50]. This cited 24 residents (14%) who had had convictions for offences under the Misuse of Drugs Act, 133 (76%) who had a record of other convictions, often shoplifting or theft, two (1%) with a record of both and only 15 (9%) with no criminal record. The author, a GP, commented 'while the relationship between illicit drug use and crime may be complicated, many of this group of drug misusers had been in court as a consequence of drug possession or criminal activity to raise money in order to purchase drugs'.

For some time there has been controversy as to whether drug use leads to crime, or crime leads to drug use, or whether both are the result of some other factor such as deviancy.

Mott and Taylor [51] revealed that 54% of the heroin users they studied had a conviction before they started using opioids and posed the question – 'is criminality independent of drug use?'. However, longitudinal studies [52] in America have shown that the amount of crime committed during periods of active drug use far exceeded that committed during drug-free periods, providing very strong evidence that drug use does lead to crime. In a recent study of persons prosecuted in four London and two Merseyside Petty Sessional Divisions, Mott found that 1–15% in Merseyside and 3–11% in London had been notified to the Home Office. She concluded that the presence of relatively large numbers of young male opioid users in a local population may well contribute to an increase in the number of residential burglary offences in the area.

The House of Commons Social Services Committee [15] has said: 'Heroin does not automatically induce criminal or antisocial behaviour. Crime is however often committed by addicts to get money for drugs.

We have indeed been given alarming estimates by some senior police officers of the amount of crime which is drug-related. Addiction too often leads to crime' [para 6].

The scale of drug-related crime in some areas is very high, although statistics of this sort are not often kept. However, around 30% of persons arrested for house-breaking offences in Edinburgh were either 'regular drug users' [53] or 'had links with drug use' [54]. Of course crime is not the only source of money to buy drugs. Goldstein [55] reports one study on this topic which showed that predatory crime accounted for 50% of the total cash income. The rest was derived from selling drugs, legitimate employment, welfare benefit, contributions from friends or family and miscellaneous hustling (e.g. begging). Johnson et al. [56] noted that drug users minimise expenditure on food and often basic necessities, which releases income for the purchase of drugs.

Having shown that drug use does lead to crime, the next question to answer was – does treatment reduce the crime rate? Du Pont [57] showed that the arrest rate for users who remained in a methadone treatment programme in Washington was 2.8% per patient per month compared with 5.7% for those who dropped out of the programme. Schut et al. [58] found that the proportion of users who had been arrested for violence, property crime and drug-related crime decreased significantly after they had started treatment with methadone.

These demonstrations that the treatment of problem opioid use with methadone will reduce criminal activity in the user have encouraged some authors to make speculations. Trebach [59] believes that, if GPs became more involved in prescribing to users, there would be a reduction in the use of black market drugs and a monumental decrease in the number of crimes committed by drugtakers. Ditton and Speirits [60] argue that returning to a policy of unrestricted free prescribing of heroin would lead to the elimination of user-related crime.

Both of these suppositions have been shown to be wrong. Bennett and Wright [61] have demonstrated, in a study of treatment by drug clinics, GPs, and private practitioners (including maintenance and outpatient detoxification treatments by the two drug clinics in the study), that the vast majority of those under treatment continued to use black market sources in addition to receiving a prescription. Additionally, since crimes continued to be committed while treatment was being undertaken, albeit at a reduced rate, the authors commented 'it seems unlikely that an unrestricted prescribing of opioids to addicts would lead to the elimination of addict non-drug crime'.

(5) Drugs and unemployment

There is a known association between problem drug use and unemployment although there has been dispute as to which is cause or effect. Stimson and Ogbourne [62] showed that only 30-40% of drug users in the treatment population are in regular employment. (This compares with a 70-80% full-time employment rate for problem drinkers.) In addition, Parker *et al.* [42] showed that young unemployed people living in areas with higher than average rates of social deprivation were more likely to become known to the medical and social agencies in the Wirral as opioid users.

(6) Drugs and employment

Certain jobs carry a high risk of substance misuse. This comes about as a result of availability of the substance misused and/or socio-cultural factors. Thus doctors and nurses are at special risk of drug dependence just as publicans, servicemen, seamen, actors and journalists seem particularly prone to develop alcoholism. In some cases certain jobs may be attractive to people dependent on drugs or alcohol, e.g. heavy drinkers may be attracted to work as publicans.

(7) Drugs and accidents

The cause of traffic accidents are multifactorial and are affected by the road, the vehicle, and the age, experience, health, and emotional status of the driver. It has now been shown [63] that nearly 200 psychoactive substances are potentially hazardous for drivers and of these, just over 100 are considered especially hazardous [64]. The use of sedatives/hypnotics in therapeutic doses more than doubles the risk factor; stimulants, antidepressants and particularly antihistamines in addition to their own sedative effects also potentiate several other drugs. Opiate users do not seem, according to epidemiological data, to be at special risk of road traffic accidents. However, according to recent studies in North America and Italy, cannabis users constitute a significant proportion of the victims or survivors of traffic accidents, and several laboratory studies have also furnished evidence that cannabis impairs driving performance. Alcohol intake usually potentiates the effects of psychoactive drugs and alcohol itself figures highly in accidents, being an associated factor in 40% of road traffic accidents involving pedestrians, 33% of all domestic accidents, and 30% of drownings.

(8) Socio-cultural factors

Dembo and Shern [65] have put forward a theory of relative deviance and suggest that individuals who deviate from the norms of general behaviour for their particular socio-cultural groups will tend to use psychoactive substances that are also less acceptable to that group.

In contrast to this, a distinct subculture where drugtaking is the norm has been recognised since the mid-1960s. Indeed, different subcultures are often associated with different drugs of misuse. Magic mushrooms and heroin often attract different kinds of people and hence separate subcultures emerge. However, in those places where drugs are particularly prevalent, such as London and Liverpool, drug users deviate less from the norm as it becomes more normal to take drugs. In such areas a distinct subculture associated with illicit drug use may be hardly identifiable.

(9) Violence, drugs and alcohol

15 per cent of all cases of non-accidental injuries to children in the United States have a drugs or alcohol component. Furthermore, about half of the rapes and two-thirds of murders in the UK are committed under the influence of alcohol.

Aggression from intoxication with drugs which are CNS depressants also occurs in a manner similar to alcohol. It is widely believed that this is brought about through disinhibition of aggressive tendencies. Further violence may be induced by ideas of persecution secondary to drug use, particularly with the use of amphetamines. In general, however, it is the experience of most professionals that drug users are not normally given to violence.

(10) Community responses to drug misuse

Donoghoe et al. [66] have described the responses of a community in a number of council estates in a large town in the North West of England. In this community there was a sense of social identity emphasising the strong, communal and collective aspects of working class culture. The main focus of communal activity was in the tenants' associations in that area.

In 1985, heroin dealers and users became noticeable throughout the estates. The problem rapidly escalated and crowds of young people would congregate at set times to pick up single dose bags of heroin from small dealers, and then use drugs in the stairwells of the estates.

The problems that the tenants complained of were:

(1) The mess: no one liked the mixture of matches, foil, and vomit on the stairwells.
(2) Fear: many residents, particularly pensioners felt intimidated by the sheer presence of so many young people.
(3) Violence: in some cases, residents who protested directly to prospective users or to dealers were threatened in no uncertain terms.
(4) Police inaction: police seemed reluctant to act on information received.

The response of the residents was described in the following way:

'Meetings were called, local leaders emerged and were supported, a series of demands were made upon police, health and welfare agencies, and the Council buildings department, and these demands were articulated publicly through local newspapers. Direct action also took place involving confrontation between young people 'hanging around' and groups of residents. Some residents also

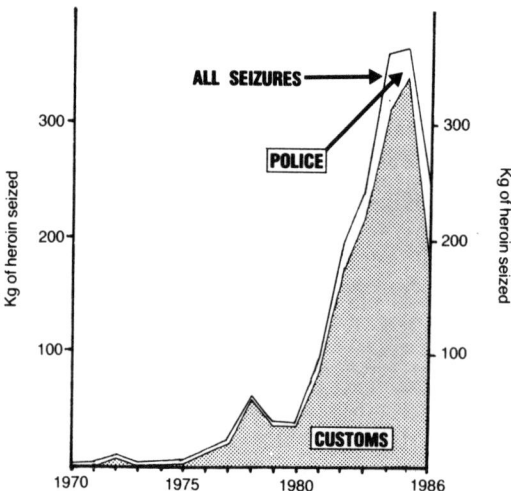

Figure 1.3 Quantity of heroin seized by UK Customs and Excise and police, and cumulative total seizures. (Source: ISDD.)

engaged in quasi-vigilante activity, such as congregating outside the houses of known dealers to harangue them.'

Eventually, the residents' shouting, haranguing, and determined surveillance of their estate, plus eventually some police activity, did help to move the problem on. Their biggest success was undoubtedly to get the Council to knock down and rebuild parts of the estates that gave the greatest opportunities for drug use, and to carry out simple measures, such as the fitting of entry phones to other blocks.

THE AETIOLOGY OF DRUG USE

THE FAMILY AND DRUG USE

(1) Family influences

It is generally accepted that there is no single cause for drugtaking in any individual, and while there is little doubt that a disturbed upbringing increases a person's vulnerability, it is not inevitable that he or she will take drugs. Because of the many factors influencing drug misuse, the extent to which the family unit plays a role in its causation remains unclear.

In his work on the role of the family in schizophrenia, Laing [67] put forward the concept that the nuclear family is inherently psychopathological – an oppressive entity and the source of both the subordination of women and the behavioural and emotional problems we call mental illness. This would imply that the family unit is the root cause of drug misuse. However, in spite of a considerable amount of research, this has never been shown to be so. In fact, no single cause or consistent pattern of multiple causes has ever been identified.

Family disruption may be a factor in an individual case but many observers stress that drug misuse begins at an age when family influences decline and are superseded by other factors, such as peer group pressure.

(2) Genetic influences

There is some evidence that genetic influences may play a part in the causation of alcoholism, but evidence for a genetic factor in the aetiology of drug misuse is more tenuous.

(3) Parental example

There are some grounds for suggesting that drug or alcohol use by a parent may influence the development of drug use in their children. However, most of this work relies on data collected from the children rather than the parents. Vogt [68] comments that, when information is collected from parents on their own behaviour and that of their children, the relationship is less clear and suggests that a child's perception of his parents' drug-using behaviour is more important than their actual pattern of use.

Most commentators would, however, support Edwards' suggestion that 'parental example is generally more important than parental genes' [69]. Studies performed at the New Jersey Medical School between 1969 and 1974 showed that the regular use of mood-altering agents such as tranquillisers by either parent was associated with a two to sevenfold greater likelihood that their children would use some illicit drug. This study found that it did not matter whether such drugs were prescribed by doctors or whether the parents obtained them by other means. There was also found to be a close relationship between parental tobacco use and the use of illicit drugs by their children – heavy cigarette use by either parent was a significant risk factor for their children [70]. Blum showed that, the more liberal parents are in the use of medicines to treat both physical and psychological problems, the more likely it is that their children will engage in illicit drug use [71].

A high frequency of paternal alcoholism has been found among adolescent drugtakers [72]. Children of problem drinkers may often become alcohol dependent themselves. This may be due partly to genetic factors but imitation of parental behaviour is also thought to play a role.

The individual and drug use

Drug dependence occurs by a complex interaction between an individual, a drug, and the environment. Various factors have been examined to try to pinpoint those who may be at risk of developing drug dependence. These include the following:

(1) Personality factors

In the late 1960s a plethora of research projects were undertaken in many centres looking for personality characteristics which might predispose an individual to develop drug dependence. A compilation of the results gives a list of personality traits that is almost endless and there is a singular failure to demonstrate any consistent personality type which is particularly prone to develop dependence on drugs. By and large the search for a pre-addictive personality type has now been abandoned. Indeed, Hoffmann [73] has argued that such a search, if fruitful, would lead to the use of stereotypes and thus limit rather than increase our understanding of the individual.

Variables of personality that have been associated with drug use include anxiety, depression, emotional instability, nonconformity, hypochondriasis, defensiveness, rebelliousness, hostility, and loss of control [74]. It has also been shown that drug users tend to rely on people and institutions to an excessive degree [75].

In many of the studies there have been claims to isolate predisposing personality factors when clearly those factors are merely correlates and could equally well be the result of prolonged drug use on the mind or even pharmacological effects of the drugs themselves.

The work on locus of control is of some interest. Rotter [76] showed that people could be categorised into internal controllers, who tended to explain what happened to them in terms of their own actions, and external controllers, who tended to explain what happened to them as if they had little control over it. Later Wallston and Wallston [77] showed that internal controllers are more successful in giving up smoking than external controllers and devised a scale for the siting of the locus of control. They also showed that the position of this siting could be influenced relatively easily.

(2) Socio-cultural factors

The sociologist Jock Young [78] pointed out that socio-cultural factors have been overlooked in the 1969 WHO definition of drug dependence ('drug dependence is a state, psychic and sometimes also physical, resulting from the interaction between a living organism and a drug ...'). He viewed drug use as the 'interaction between the physiological effects of a drug and the norms of the group of which the drugtaker is a member'. He wrote in support of this claim that 'the role of the Bohemian involves smoking marihuana just as the role of the merchant seaman involved heavy drinking'. Socio-cultural factors are also reflected in the greater male to female ratio among problem drinkers and the fact that this ratio has reduced significantly over the past few decades. Other evidence that socio-cultural factors may change is demonstrated by the fall in the number of doctors who smoke and more recently an apparent decline in the number of doctors who are heavy drinkers, as evidenced by a decline in the relative mortality rate of doctors from cirrhosis of the liver compared to other groups from 310% to 114% of the average (100%) between 1970 and 1982.[79]

(3) Availability

Drug misuse occurring in a higher proportion of doctors and nurses than would normally be expected is usually explained by easy access to drugs rather than vulnerable personalities [80], just as the high rate of alcoholism among publicans is explained by the ready availability of alcohol. However, the misuse of drugs is not well documented among pharmacists or dentists [81].

(4) Other risk factors

A large number of epidemiological studies have also been carried out to attempt to identify other risk factors predisposing an individual to drug misuse. Louria [82] cites three major reasons given when students were asked why they used illicit drugs. These were peer group pressure, pleasure and curiosity. He also identifies the following risk factors:

- Broken family
- Unhappy family relationships
- Not practising any religion
- Regular parental use of mood-altering drugs
- Parental use of one pack or more of cigarettes per day
- Excessive alcohol use by parents
- Poor academic achievement
- Low self-esteem
- Lack of ambition for the future
- Non-participation in extra-curricular activities
- Involvement in political or protest movements
- Drug use among friends
- Regular cigarette use
- Sibling use of illicit drugs

These and other risk factors were examined by multivariate statistical analysis. The results indicated that peer group pressure outweighed all other risk factors that were studied, even if all the other risk factors were considered together.

(5) Deviancy

Drug misuse is not always the outcome of deviancy or maladjustment as illicit drug use does not always break social norms. The social norm for any individual will depend upon the activities of his or her peer group. As drug misuse becomes more widespread in a community, so the individuals participating in it become more normal and are more likely to try it under the influence of peer group pressure.

In those communities where drug use is less prevalent, drugtaking becomes a deviant activity and someone who participates in it is likely to be rejected by his peers, leading him to identify with others who are taking drugs. The theory of deviancy amplification states that further rejection by family, friends and the State (the latter by imposing rigorous controls), leads to intensification of this identification with the drug scene. The deviant person is thus made more deviant by society's rejection of him. This theory may well explain the stereotyping and strong subcultural images that are held about drugtakers.

Does cannabis smoking lead to heroin use?

In the 1930s, when cannabis was first internationally controlled, it was claimed with some insistence that cannabis use led directly on to involvement with more dangerous drugs such as heroin. This claim was based on the finding that about 95% of heroin users had previously smoked cannabis before trying heroin. The fact that at the time there were about 200 million cannabis users worldwide and only a handful of heroin takers did not deter the law-makers.

The sequential use of drugs is of course a well-recognised phenomenon. A typical drug history might reveal under age smoking, followed by cannabis use and progressing on to amphetamines, barbiturates, LSD or magic mushrooms, and finally heroin. Nevertheless it remains true to say that the vast majority of cannabis users do not turn to heroin, a fact confirmed by Plant [83] in his study of drug use in Cheltenham. However, Louria [82] has shown that if there is frequent cannabis use there is more likely to be subsequent use of more dangerous drugs and Dembo *et al.* [84] have shown that in the presence of adverse personal characteristics there is also an increased likelihood of subsequent heroin use in cannabis smokers.

Psycho-social effects of drug misuse

These are best subdivided into:

(a) pharmacological effects of a drug or drugs;
(b) non-pharmacological consequences of drug misuse.

Pharmacological effects of a drug or drugs

Those effects that lead to psychological or social problems are described in detail later in this book. They include elation and euphoria, anxiety, depression, violence, accidents, loss of libido, loss of memory, impairment of conciousness and disturbances of perception.

Non-pharmacological consequences of drug misuse

Because of the complexity of environmental, psychological and physiological interactions that lead to and result from dependency, drugtaking and drugseeking behaviours, it is not always possible to distinguish between cause and effect of drug use in psycho-social terms. Thus, although various psycho-social characteristics are known to be associated with the taking of illicit drugs, it is not yet clear, for example, whether unemployment and a poor self image prompt people to use drugs or whether they are the consequences of drug misuse. Nevertheless, some psycho-social consequences of drugtaking, which are recognised and volunteered by the users themselves, can be seen repeatedly in individual drugtakers and follow a recognisable pattern. These are outlined below.

For dependent drugtakers, the taking of drugs and maintenance of their supply become the first priority. Everything else is secondary to it. Most of the day is spent either thinking about drugs, taking them or making efforts to obtain them, and other responsibilities at home or at work become neglected. Marital discord and family frictions occur, work performance declines and often attendance at work becomes erratic. If this situation continues, it often becomes intolerable for family, friends and employers with the result that the drug user loses his job and/or is asked to leave the family home. The resultant isolation from normal supporting systems may be a crisis for the drugtaker that stimulates him to seek and accept help. However, if it does not, or if help is not forthcoming, it becomes increasingly likely that the drugtaker will turn to his or her drug-using friends for support, making his chances of recovery less likely. Such friends will have already been made in order to ensure a ready supply of drugs.

A regular drug supply requires funding and amounts varying from £5 to more than £200 per day for regular heroin use are not unusual.

As tolerance develops, a larger supply of drugs is needed to give the same psychic effect and a person's 'habit' thus becomes more expensive. When a drugtaker's normal income is no longer sufficient, other devices are used to obtain money. The ones most commonly resorted to are stealing, prostitution and selling drugs. Such activities reinforce identification with the drug subculture but also cause a loss of self-esteem.

Throughout the career of a drugtaker, attempts are usually made at intervals to stop using drugs. Most drugtakers will have experienced 'cold turkey' at least once and some will have bought methadone on the street and given themselves their own detox. Others may have gone abroad in order to get away from the drugs scene, although many relapse from lacking the insight to see that they cannot escape from themselves by changing their geography. Eventually, many drug users do succeed in coming off drugs, at least for a time, but repeated failures to do so are invariably perceived as resulting from personal weakness, reinforcing an already battered self-image.

Feelings of self-hatred soon supervene and are projected onto others. Those who are emotionally closest to the drugtaker will bear the brunt of any verbal or physical aggression. Children may become involved and non-accidental injury occur. Self-esteem is reduced even further by such events and the drugtaker may become recognisably depressed.

It is not unusual for drugtakers to exhibit aggressive behaviour towards themselves, cutting their own forearms with knives or razors. Overdoses, intentional and semi-intentional ('I didn't care whether I died or not') may result from depression or, alternatively, be taken to 'blot things out' and escape from the stark reality of the downhill spiral that is occurring.

As the individual goes further and further downhill he or she accepts appalling happenings as normal events. What would have been a disaster and a crisis a few months previously become part of an accepted pattern. Overdoses are no exception. Sometimes a drugtaker will overdose several times a week, or even several times a day, and accept this as normal behaviour. Homelessness, innumerable court cases, loss of job, family and friends may also occur without the recognition of a crisis. This lack of self-awareness may also extend to failing to recognise any changes within himself. While concerned relatives speak of a drugtaker as having changed into a different person from the one they used to know and love, he himself will often have no conception of any such changes.

The cessation of drug use and reconstruction of a normal life allow the psychic changes that were the consequences of drug use to disappear with eventual reversion back to their original state. Recovery is slow, taking several months or even years and may be aided by the continuing support of a concerned GP.

Chapter 2

Different Drugs of Misuse

Volatile substance misuse

Although solvent misuse is the most commonly used term for this activity, it is inaccurate in that some of the inhaled organic compounds (e.g. aerosol propellants) are not, strictly speaking, solvents. We have therefore decided in this book to use a more correct term – volatile substance misuse (VSM).

Glue sniffing is by far the commonest form of VSM, but all of the volatile compounds seem to have similar effects when inhaled. Initially there is an excitatory effect with feelings of euphoria and exhilaration, similar to that obtained with mild alcohol intoxication. Indeed the sniffer may appear drunk. This stage is commonly followed by one with auditory or visual hallucinations. The person experiencing them is said to be always aware that these are unreal and so they are sometimes called pseudo-hallucinations. As more is inhaled cerebral depressant effects appear with disorientation, blurred vision, dizziness, slurred speech, ataxia and drowsiness. Finally, all volatile substances have a concentration at which they rapidly cause unconsciousness. It is thought that these effects are brought on because all volatile hydrocarbons have the property of marked lipid solubility and this causes changes in neuronal membrane permeability, thereby impairing neural transmission.

Apart from glue, other favourite substances sniffed are Tipp-Ex thinners (trichloroethane), lighter fuel (butane, propane), nail polish remover (acetone), and aerosols (a mixture of volatile compounds). Many ordinary household chemicals contain organic solvents which may be inhaled. Occasional direct sniffing may occur – aerosols sprayed directly into the mouth or, less commonly, petrol sniffing from a can. More often the volatile liquid is placed on a cloth or in an airtight bag such as a polythene bag or empty crisp bag. The latter method allows the fumes to become more concentrated and is often the method of choice of the chronic sniffer.

The volatile compounds commonly encountered are:

- *Adhesives*
  Toluene
  Acetone
  Ethyl acetate
- *Aerosols*
  Propellant 11 ⎫
  Propellant 12 ⎭ halons
  Methylene chloride
  Butane
  Propane
- *Solvents*
  Trichloroethylene
  Trichloroethane
  n-Hexane
  Tetrachloroethylene
- *Fuel gases*
  Butane
  Propane

Other more rarely inhaled volatile compounds include:

- Petrol
- Methyl ethyl ketone (occasionally present in adhesives)
- Chloroform (nowadays a rare solvent)

Incidence

Although nitrous oxide, ether, and chloroform were inhaled recreationally by the Victorians long before they were used for anaesthesia, the modern sniffing phenomenon began in North America in the mid-1950s. In the UK, it was first recognised in 1962 and the practice has grown rapidly since that time, although the true prevalence is unknown. The available information from selected groups may not reflect incidence in the general population. Additionally there may be under-reporting in school surveys.

In 1982, Ramsay [1] reported a point-prevalence of 9.8% for boys aged 13 to 15 attending a Glasgow secondary school. One quarter of these reported regular sniffing, one quarter sporadic sniffing and the rest said that they had only sniffed once. Screening a selected population like this is expected to produce higher figures than attempts to determine incidence in an area by asking the various agencies working in that area to identify the number of sniffers who have come to their attention. In the same year as Ramsay did his survey, Gay et al. [2] identified 304 users from 250,000 individuals at risk in the county of Avon over a six-month period. In this sample, 77% were aged between 14 and 17 years, only 24% had used volatile substances for more than six months, and only 4% had also used other drugs or alcohol.

Social characteristics of volatile substance misusers

Although a few people go on inhaling these substances into their 20s and 30s, the majority are mainly confined to the 10 -16 age bracket. 14-year-olds seem to do it more frequently than anyone else and the incidence in boys is said to be twice that of girls. The male to female ratio among those whose deaths were associated with volatile substance sniffing between 1971–1981 was however 13:1. This difference is not explained but may indicate that boys take more risks than girls while under the influence of these substances.

There is an accepted association between chronic glue sniffing and underachievement at school. Sniffers, however, do not appear to have less potential abilities than other students and their low academic performance is more likely to stem from poor motivation rather than from a direct effect of the substances on the brain.

There seems to be some correlation between volatile substance misuse and parental, particularly maternal, problem alcohol use, but the evidence that parental unemployment, low socio-economic status and family instability are causative factors is conflicting.

There is, however, a seasonal incidence and the summer, particularly the school holiday period, is known to be a time of greater prevalence.

Volatile substance misusers fall into two broad categories:

(1) Experimental/recreational users
This is the largest group and comprises those who as a result of cultural and/or peer group pressure experiment with solvents or other volatile substances. These are essentially normal adolescents who do it for a short period of time, sometimes only once or twice, and almost invariably in a group situation.

(2) Regular users
This second group is smaller and comprises those who are psychologically habituated. These regular sniffers again often sniff as a group activity but the ones who do it alone are much more likely to be

underachievers with family backgrounds of low socio-economic status, family instability and heavy use of alcohol or drugs by parents. These lone sniffers who repeatedly continue the habit are usually those who need the help of a child psychiatrist or family therapist. They are also most at risk of injury or death as they often sniff to the point of unconsciousness in isolated places, without the benefit of friends who can summon help.

Overall, the majority of adolescent sniffers do not continue for more than a year, and those who do, usually stop as soon as they reach the age when they are legally able to purchase alcohol. For these people the practice of inhaling these substances should be considered a normal part of growing up and it is important in this context that doctors do not allow a crisis situation to develop if an adolescent sniffer is brought into the surgery by an anxious parent. Except at the very beginning when a stern warning from some figure of authority may prevent much useless misery and worry, intervention is not usually indicated. Forcibly stopping a child sniffing, even if possible, could cause harm in this adventurous stage of development.

Clinical signs of sniffing

The GP may be summoned urgently by parents or friends while the patient is under the influence of inhaled substances. Although initially there is an excitatory phase with euphoria, disinhibition, exhilaration, tinnitus, dizziness and difficulty in focusing, this is followed by a phase of lethargy and somnolence. In practice it may be difficult to distinguish clinically between these two phases, but the observer will usually be aware of lack of coordination, slurred speech and impaired judgement. Occasionally, additional clinical manifestations may be seen: coughing and sneezing, nausea, vomiting, diarrhoea, diffuse pains, tremor, paraesthesia and epileptic convulsions. Any impairment of consciousness is quickly reversed; in all, the effects last from 30 to 45 minutes and it is rare for misusers to require hospital admission. Furthermore, in a study of 105 patients who did go to different hospitals in the UK, 81% remained in hospital for less than 24 hours, suggesting that severe intoxication was the commonest cause of admission [3]. Another study of 20 consecutive cases admitted showed that all of them had neurological presenting features, including coma, ataxia, dysarthria and epileptic convulsions[4].

Because of the short duration of action of volatile substances it is much more likely for the GP to be involved at a stage after the acute effects have passed.

In the immediate post-sniffing phase, hangovers are unusual, but other clinical signs may be apparent. Many of these signs are temporary but some may persist for as long as three weeks. There may be rhinitis, halitosis, conjunctivitis, and associated personality and behavioural changes. Glue is sometimes seen on the hands and clothing. In the repeated sniffer an acneiform rash may be seen around the nose and mouth. This is usually in the form of a V shape on the chin and an inverted V over the bridge of the nose. After effects vary according to individual constitution, extent of abuse, and the substance inhaled. Additionally there may be tiredness and cough, abdominal pain, vomiting, headache, blurring of vision and paraesthesia of the hands and feet.

Most sniffers enjoy the experience but a few become overwhelmed by feelings of depression. Clinical effects after sniffing are almost instantaneous and usually last from 15 to 45 minutes, although occasionally they may persist for as long as two hours. Because of their short duration of action it is possible for the experienced user to exert some measure of control. Most will inhale only enough to feel euphoric, but some will sniff to unconsciousness and risk death. This type of sniffing may be accidental in the unexperienced sniffer, or purposeful either with the aim of impressing the peer group, or to give relief from unpleasant emotions. The latter is often seen in the lone user and is particularly dangerous.

Tolerance and psychological dependence do occur but a physical withdrawal syndrome, although recognised, appears to be rare. Tolerance is unlikely to occur if the duration of sniffing is less than three months.

Mortality from volatile substance misuse

Deaths from VSM are rare but increasing. By 1981 they accounted for just over 1% of deaths from all causes in 10-19 year olds. Since that time the mortality rate has more than doubled.

There are interesting comparisons between an earlier survey by Anderson et al. for the periods 1971-81, [5] and the 1981- 85 survey (see Table 2.1)[6]. In the first survey, 51% of deaths were caused indirectly (trauma 8%, suffocation from plastic bags 19%, inhalation of stomach contents 14%) and just under half (49%) were attributable to a direct toxic effect of the substance inhaled. In the 1981-85 survey, 53% of cases were attributable to the direct toxic effect of the substance, and there was a significant downward trend in deaths associated with plastic bags from around 20% to 10%.

Table 2.1 Number (%) of deaths associated with misuse of various volatile substances in the UK 1981–1985.

	1981	1982	1983	1984	1985	Total
Gas fuels	15(33)	11(18)	19(24)	31(38)	30(26)	106(28)
Aerosol sprays	1 (2)	8(13)	12(15)	9(11)	20(17)	50(13)
Solvents in glue	16(35)	18(29)	24(30)	15(19)	35(30)	108(28)
Other volatile substances	13(28)	24(39)	25(31)	26(32)	28(24)	116(30)
Substances unknown	1 (2)	1 (2)	0	0	3(3)	5 (1)
Total:	46	62	80	81	116	385

Although glue sniffing is the commonest type of volatile substance misuse, with toluene (the commonest solvent to be found in glue) being present in 73% of samples received at the National Poisons Information Service in 1982. A contribution of Anderson's two surveys has shown that during the period 1971–1985, a minimum figure of 22% of deaths associated with glue sniffing could be attributed to a direct toxic effect of the solvent. Comparable figures for other volatile substances were: aerosols 62%, gas fuels 61%, other substances (including fire extinguishers and cleaning fluids) 62%. Thus from the point of view of mortality glue sniffing is relatively safe. Sudden sniffing deaths from aerosol inhalation were first reported by Bass [7] who considered the cause of death to be cardiac dysrhythmia provoked by catecholamine release during exercise, the myocardium being unduly sensitised by halons used as aerosol propellants. (Halons are fluorinated or chlorinated hydrocarbons, usually substituted methane or ethane derivatives).

Most deaths occur when alone at home and those who inhale these substances repeatedly on their own in isolated places are at far greater risk of injuring themselves as well. Lone sniffers who are misusing volatile hydrocarbons in order to help them cope with, or escape from, difficult emotional problems also appear to be at greater risk of going on to the misuse of alcohol or drugs.

Morbidity from volatile substance misuse

For a long time it was thought that, apart from a few rare deaths, there was little or no physical or neurological damage resulting from the inhalation of volatile substances. A study in Glasgow of 115 patients referred to a doctor for solvent misuse failed to show any abnormality when investigated for haematological indices, ESR, liver and renal function tests and urinary microscopy [8].

In view of this and because many of the deaths were caused by accidents during intoxication, a very reasonable attempt at harm reduction was made by the Institute for the Study of Drug Dependence [9], and the following suggestions were made as part of a strategy for health educators: 'if you are going to sniff glue don't use a polythene bag because you could suffocate; don't do it alone in an isolated place; and don't do it on a roof or other dangerous places, like canal banks'.

With the use of more refined techniques of investigation, e.g. CT scans, and with increasing knowledge, it has become evident that most of the volatile compounds inhaled cause some physical and/or neurological damage if inhaled regularly over long periods of time. Indeed, a few of these substances will induce organ damage even if sniffed only on a few occasions.

Some of our current knowledge on the harmful effects of the commonly misused volatile substances comes from studies of sniffers themselves, but this is often complicated by the fact that most have, at times, inhaled several different volatile substances, and some have used alcohol and drugs as well. Further knowledge has been gleaned from studies in industry where the effect of a substance on the human body can be measured in isolation. Although this is a much more precise measurement of the effect of a single substance, it generally results in studies of low levels of a volatile compound over a prolonged period of time (e.g. 20 years). In VSM, of course, there are generally high levels of these compounds absorbed over a short period of time, and industrial studies, although relevant, are therefore not necessarily comparable. Nevertheless, it is hoped that the following will provide a reference guide for the doctor who wishes to know what harm may have been engendered when presented with a patient who is known to have been misusing a particular volatile compound. It should always be borne in mind that these are rare complications that are usually only seen in the chronic sniffer and that for the vast majority of casual sniffers no harm is engendered.

Toluene

The concentration of toluene sniffed for purposes of intoxication exceeds allowable concentration for industrial operations by about 50 times. As toluene is one of the most commonly misused of all the volatile substances there is a relatively good understanding of the harmful effects of this solvent. Toluene is the usual solvent to be found in glues, but it is also found in a number of other household products. It was widely used to replace benzene, to which it is chemically related, because benzene is well known to have an adverse effect on the bone marrow, causing aplastic anaemia and acute leukaemia.

The complications of toluene misuse include:

(a) The cerebellar syndrome with ataxia, particularly of the gait, but also of the arms, is well recognised. In some of the described cases carbon tetrachloride and n-hexane were also inhaled but there is no doubt that toluene alone can cause this complication. Nystagmus may be present. The severity of cerebellar signs have been significantly correlated with the width both of the cerebellar sulci and the superior cerebellar cisterns on CT scans[10]. The mean age of the subjects involved was 23 years. A degree of recovery after some weeks or months of abstinence is usual and indeed full recovery may take place. King [11] however demonstrated that some signs were still present 18 months after stopping. Transient cerebellar signs are a common result of acute toluene intoxication, but in some cases more persistent cerebellar abnormalities can occur, particularly in cases of severe prolonged misuse of toluene.

(b) A mild peripheral neuropathy has been reported [10] in pure toluene misusers, but this is a rare complication of very prolonged misuse.

(c) Cerebral and cerebellar atrophy as shown by pneumoencephalography and computerised tomography [10] occurs in association with chronic glue sniffing. Although many of those investigated were also abusing alcohol and drugs, it appears from the evidence that chronic severe toluene misuse does play a causative role. The radiological abnormalities described are widening of the cerebellar and cerebral sulci and basal cisterns, with enlargement of the ventricular system. These appearances are similar to those described in chronic alcoholics [12] although cerebellar abnormalities may be more frequent in glue sniffers.

(d) Cognitive impairment has been shown in 16 out of 24 long-term severe toluene misusers, although there was no correlation between duration of toluene misuse and the severity of cognitive deficits [10]. It has also been demonstrated that toluene impairs psychomotor performance [13]. Tests of IQ, memory, and language ability, however, appear to be unaffected by the misuse of any volatile hydrocarbon. Although toluene misuse is often seen in individuals with high psychiatric morbidity, it does not in itself appear to cause psychiatric illness.

(e) Other neurological complications that occasionally occur include epilepsy (status epilepticus has been reported in two cases), optic neuropathy, and sensorial deafness.

(f) Respiratory complications have been shown in one study where 12 out of 18 chronic glue sniffers aged 14–18 had a restrictive defect or reduced diffusion capacity on lung function testing, indicating that toluene affects the alveolus [14].

(g) The Devathasan study [14] showed that the pulmonary vasculature was also affected in several cases and although pulmonary wedge pressures were not done, five had right ventricular dilatation on echocardiography and a raised JVP, suggesting cor pulmonale. This was reversible and all five cases returned to normal two months after abstinence. Taylor and Harris [15] found that toluene produced ECG abnormalities and sensitised the heart to asphyxia-induced atrioventricular block, thereby predisposing to ventricular fibrillation or arrest.

(h) Depression of the bone marrow is extremely rare in toluene misusers. In those cases where it has been described, benzene was almost always also present. However, six cases have been described [16] of aplastic anaemia where toluene alone appears to have been misused. It is interesting to note that five of these were also suffering from sickle cell disease.

(i) Acute hepatorenal failure and dangerous electrolyte disturbances have been described in association with toluene misuse but are rare complications.

Acetone and *ethyl acetate* both have similar clinical effects causing dizziness, lacrimation, mucous membrane and skin irritation.

Halons
These fluorinated or chlorinated hydrocarbons (usually substituted methane or ethane derivatives) are a particularly dangerous group of substances to inhale. Their main effect is on the heart, causing cardiac arrhythmias, depression of myocardial contractility and reduction in cardiac output. Death, which can occur in first-time sniffers, is almost invariably attributed to sensitising the myocardium to circulating catecholamines. Sudden sniffing deaths from aerosol inhalation associated with vigorous exercise has been reported by Bass [7]. There has been considerable pressure recently to ban fluorinated hydrocarbons, but this is because they deplete the ozone layer of the atmosphere rather than because of their toxic effects when sniffed.

Methylene chloride (e.g. in paint stripper)
To date no adverse effects of methylene chloride misuse appear to be

reported in the literature. It is, however, known to be far from harmless, causing hepatic necrosis in animals. Furthermore, massive exposure to any of the other halogenated hydrocarbons, as may occur in people who sniff them, can result in death from cardiac arrhythmia [17].

Butane, propane, and n-hexane (e.g. lighter fuel)
These are all aliphatic hydrocarbons which will sensitise the myocardium to circulating catecholamines. In some circumstances, particularly 'fright or flight' reactions, increased levels of catecholamines in the blood stream can lead to ventricular fibrillation and cardiac arrest, and like halons, this can occur on first time use. n-Hexane inhalation is also well known to cause a severe peripheral neuropathy involving both sensory and motor components, but with sensory loss predominating. It may, in addition, cause hepatorenal toxicity but the position on this is unclear. n-Hexane is not as toxic as other isomers.

Tetrachloroethylene (e.g. dry cleaning fluid)
This is the most common solvent used in dry cleaning. Following inhalation, irritation of the eyes, nose and throat becomes apparent, then nausea and vomiting which may persist for several hours. Hepatic and renal dysfunction may develop while cardiac dysrhythmia and pulmonary oedema (non-cardiogenic) have both been reported.

Trichloroethylene (e.g. as a degreasing agent)
This is another halogenated hydrocarbon and so may induce cardiac arrhythmias. It will cause hepatotoxicity and nephrotoxicity but only at extremely high concentrations. Such concentrations are sometimes achieved in chronic trichloroethylene sniffers and some have been found at autopsy to have hepatic necrosis and nephropathy, while others who have survived have been found to have permanent liver and kidney damage. Chronic trichloroethylene misusers may also develop optic atrophy, cranial nerve palsies, and/or impairment of intellectual functioning. At low doses, however, it was considered harmless enough to be used as a general anaesthetic, although it is mainly used now as a degreasing agent.

Trichloroethane (e.g. Tipp-Ex thinners)
As Tipp-Ex thinners, trichloroethane is widely misused. It is thought to have a low toxicity, although a few deaths have been recorded in the literature. Clinical features include dizziness, nausea, coma and respiratory depression.

Morbidity from rarely encountered volatile substance inhalation

Petrol

Petrol contains a mixture of C4–12 hydrocarbons, including paraffins, olefins, and aromatic hydrocarbons. Most petrols also contain about 3 mls of tetraethyl lead per gallon as an 'anti-knock' agent. Benzene is also present in varying amounts in petrol and this raises the possibility of *myelotoxicity* as benzene has been recognised since 1897 to cause depression of the bone marrow. So far no cases of aplastic anaemia have been reported in petrol sniffers. It is possible that the hydrocarbons in petrol sensitise the myocardium to circulating catecholamines [17], but also high concentrations of gasoline vapour may lead to death from respiratory failure, and sudden death from petrol sniffing has been reported.

Chronic petrol sniffing may also induce lead poisoning. Although tetraethyl lead is non-toxic, it is converted in the liver to triethyl lead. In addition it is possible that further degradation may occur to inorganic lead [17]. Symptoms appear after a latent period of about one week following exposure. Clinical features are said to include:

- nausea, vomiting, diarrhoea;
- insomnia, irritability, restlessness, anxiety;
- hypothermia, relative tachycardia, hypotension;
- muscle weakness, brisk reflexes, extensor plantar responses, tremor, chorea, convulsions, myoclonus, encephalopathy;
- loss of short-term memory, mania and suicidal tendencies [17].

Petrol sniffing is almost the only way in which children contract organic lead poisoning [18].

Chloroform and carbon tetrachloride

Neither carbon tetrachloride nor chloroform are found in domestic products and both are rare. These halogenated hydrocarbons are both hepatotoxic and nephrotoxic. At the high levels of exposure found in volatile substance misusers these compounds will cause fatty liver and centrilobular necrosis. The accumulation of fat in the liver is probably due to inhibition of the transference of triglycerides from liver to plasma [19]. Carbon tetrachloride is metabolised to form a free CCl_3 radical which is the putative toxin. In the kidney the proximal tubule is principally affected causing polyuria, glycosuria and proteinuria. The large doses of chloroform and carbon tetrachloride encountered in sniffers can lead to complete hepatorenal failure. Chloroform appears to be hepatotoxic through its metabolite, phosgene. All halogenated hydrocarbons have the ability to sensitise the heart to circulating catecholamines so that cardiac arrhythmias and even cardiac arrest may occur. In experimental animals both chloroform and carbon tetrachloride will cause hepatic tumors. Carbon tetrachloride will also occasionally cause cerebellar damage and optic neuritis, adrenal cortical necrosis, pancreatitis, pulmonary oedema, aplastic anaemia and haemolytic anaemia in humans.

Methyl ethyl ketone (MEK)
This is occasionally present in a few adhesives. It is a CNS depressant which will cause irritation of mucous membranes. Occupational exposure leads to emphysema of the lungs, congestion of the liver and kidneys, dermatitis and a peripheral neuropathy. Numbness of the fingers and arms has been reported in workers exposed to small quantities of MEK vapour and liquid. It is likely that those who deliberately inhale this solvent will be at risk of developing similar problems.

Other volatile substance inhalation
(a) Salbutamol inhaler misuse is well recognised. This is not only for the halon propellant but also for the central stimulating effects of excessive amounts of salbutamol.
(b) Some substances sniffed contain chemicals or metals which are more toxic than the hydrocarbon intentionally inhaled. Moreover, some of these chemicals or metals, such as vinyl chloride, lead, copper and zinc are not excreted by the body and remain, with the possible future risk of cancer, chronic metal poisoning or gradual brain damage. This is in direct contrast to the observation that neurological damage from inhaling volatile hydrocarbons often slowly improves with time, which may be explained by the fact that although these hydrocarbons disappear quite rapidly from the plasma, they remain in the nervous system and fat deposits and only slowly disappear after several weeks or months.

Legislation

Scotland was the first region of the UK to enact laws on VSM. In May 1983 solvent misuse was added to a number of other conditions which might justify referring a child to a childrens' panel. (The childrens' panel system was created by the Social Work (Scotland) Act 1968 for dealing with young offenders and other young people who might be in need of compulsory measures of care.) Then in November 1983 the Court of Criminal Appeal ruled that selling glue sniffing 'kits' to children was a crime under Scottish common law.

In June 1985 the rest of the UK followed suit with the Intoxicating Substances (Supply) Act 1985, making it an offence for a retailer to supply or offer to supply a substance (other than a controlled drug) to a person under the age of 18, if it is known or believed that the substance is likely to be inhaled for the purposes of intoxication. Similarly, a retailer can be prosecuted for supplying such a substance to a person whom he knows, or believes to be, acting on behalf of another person under the age of 18. A person found guilty of such an offence may be liable to a heavy fine or up to six months' imprisonment.

Amyl and butyl nitrite

The fragrant fumes from the volatile clear yellow liquid, amyl nitrite, are often inhaled by homosexual men for recreational use in the belief that they promote a sense of abandon and intensify sexual experience.

Medicinally, amyl nitrite has been used for over a century in the treatment of angina pectoris for which its vasodilator properties brought almost instant relief. It also has been used in the past for the relief of renal and biliary colic (because of its smooth muscle-relaxant properties) and for the immediate treatment of cyanide poisoning (it induces the formation of methaemoglobin which combines with cyanide to form non-toxic cyanmethaemoglobin). It is the fastest acting of all the nitrites, vasodilatation being evident in the face of the user within ten seconds. However, as its effects last only five minutes, its use in medicine has been superseded by longer acting nitrites.

Butyl nitrite has similar effects to amyl nitrite but has no medicinal uses.

Amyl nitrite used to be marketed in glass capsules known as vitrellae which were opened by crushing between finger and thumb. The vapour was then inhaled. This method of liberating the fumes has earned these compounds the name of 'snappers' or 'poppers'.

Users of both drugs frequently feel dizzy and develop headaches, and there may be fainting, nausea and vomiting. In those with cardiac problems, there is also some risk of over-stimulation and heart failure. In spite of these problems, amyl and butyl nitrite have retained their popularity among the male homosexual community, although for a while the erroneous suggestion that there was a link between the use of these alkyl nitrites and the development of Kaposi's sarcoma as a first symptom of AIDS led to a reduction in their use. One reason for continued use is the action of nitrites in dilating the anal sphincter together with the widespread belief that they lengthen the time and intensity of the pleasurable feeling associated with climax. Amyl nitrite is a pharmacy medicine under the Medicine's Act so it is theoretically available from any chemist without a prescription. However, as it is not a drug, butyl nitrite is free from even this limited control and is easily purchased in certain pubs, bars and sex shops frequented by male homosexuals. This product is generally imported from the USA where it is marketed as a 'room odoriser' to avoid being classed as a drug under American drug legislation. However, the use of such trade names as 'Ram' and 'Thrust' are suggestive of the intended market.

Alkyl nitrites are taken solely for recreational purposes; their use does not appear to lead to drugseeking behaviour nor other hallmarks of dependence, and their ability to cause social harm is limited.

Cannabis

Prevalence

Cannabis is undoubtedly the most widely used illicit drug in this country. However, all British estimates of its prevalence are, to date, of questionable validity. For example, the British Crime Survey [20], although a good representative cross-section of the adult population, was a face-to-face interview and the questions were posed in the context of offences against the law. It is likely, therefore that the figure of 5% ever having used cannabis and 2% admitting to having used it in the previous 14 months is an underestimate.

An indirect method of estimating prevalence was devised by Atha [21] from the sales of Rizla cigarette papers. In 1979, the sales of hand-rolling tobacco were only sufficient to account for about two-thirds of the Rizla cigarette papers sold. Rizla has a virtual monopoly on cigarette papers and Atha estimated that the shortfall would suffice to make 12,000 million 'joints', or roughly 3.5 million 'joints' per day.

Atha's 'Rizla Method' has been criticised on two points. Firstly, it ignores the fact that not all cannabis consumed in the UK is in the form of 'joints' – probably about a third is taken in other ways. Secondly, it fails to take into account the fairly obvious point that 'joints' contain tobacco as well as cannabis resin. Wagstaff and Maynard [22] have suggested that Atha's figures should be approximately doubled to take account of these criticisms, and have estimated that approximately 1,000 tonnes of cannabis were consumed in 1979 by 5.5–6.9 million regular users in the UK (11–14% of the population over the age of 15).

The present figure may be higher as the use of cannabis is thought to be increasing in most developed countries [23].

Cultivation, forms and routes of use

The cannabis plant, *Cannabis sativa*, is relatively easy to grow in Britain, although to do so is illegal. Some plants will reach 15 feet in height. Two surveys sponsored by the Legalise Cannabis Campaign in 1982 [21] showed that although three-quarters of participants had previously tried to grow cannabis plants, only 9% of the cannabis consumed at the time of the survey was homegrown. The rest was imported: 42% was Lebanese hashish, 30% was black hashish from the Indian subcontinent, and 10% was Moroccan hashish. Only 9% was imported herbal cannabis, although the black community which is known to favour this variety was not adequately represented in the survey.

There are three basic preparations of cannabis in common use:

(1) The dried leaves and flowering tops of the uncultivated plant, known as 'bhang' if it is infused and drunk, and 'marijuana' if it is smoked;
(2) The small upper leaves and flowering tops of cultivated female plants, known as 'ganja' and smoked;
(3) Pure resin which is exudated from the flowering tops and leaves of the female plant. Cannabis resin is known as 'hashish' and is usually smoked.

A purer liquid form of cannabis obtained by extracting cannabis from the resin with a non-aqueous solvent, followed by a process of filtration and evaporation, is occasionally encountered. This is known as 'hashish oil'. Tobacco is dipped in it and then smoked.

A variety of other names are used for cannabis (dope, weed, sinsemilia, etc.). Sometimes there is a slight variation in terminology amongst purists depending on whether twigs, stems, and seeds are included.

Pharmacological and clinical effects of cannabis

Cannabis has three times the tar content of ordinary cigarettes and is potentially carcinogenic. Because the inhaled smoke is retained longer than smoke from a normal cigarette, the blood carbon monoxide level is comparatively larger. It is on average five times the level found from smoking ordinary cigarettes. Cannabis is a pharmacologically 'dirty' drug since it contains a number (probably more than 50) of cannabinoids which have a variety of different actions.

Δ-9 tetrahydrocannabinol (THC) is the most potent cannabinoid but THC is rapidly metabolised in the liver to 11-hydroxy-tetrahydrocannabinol which is 20% more active than THC itself. As THC and its metabolites are highly lipophilic they remain for long periods in the fatty tissues of the body from where they are slowly released into the blood stream over a period of days or weeks. Regular cannabis users who take the drug more frequently than every eight-ten days are liable to slowly accumulate it. This is important because the toxic psychotic effects of THC have been clearly demonstrated to be dose-dependent [24] (although there are some idiosyncratic individuals who have psychotic episodes at low doses). For this reason it is also helpful to know in what form, by what route, and how often cannabis is taken. Bhang and marijuana contain about 1-3% THC, ganja has about 6-10% THC, cannabis resin has a THC content of 8-15%, and up to 60% of hashish oil is THC. Taken orally, absorption of the drug is very variable and considerable metabolism occurs during the first pass through the liver. If smoked, about three times as much of the drug gets into the systemic circulation, than when it is taken by mouth. The amount of THC absorbed from one cigarette is in the region of 2.5-5 mg [25].

THC is 97% bound to plasma proteins. This may have important clinical consequences but these do not appear to have been documented [26].

The pharmacological effects of cannabis are confusing not only because of the multiplicity of pharmacologically active cannabinoids, but also because oral THC increases the plasma volume and extends the half-life of several other drugs and alcohol, whereas when cannabis is smoked it reduces the half-life of many drugs.

One of the best known and most striking clinical effects is a persistent tachycardia which is dose-related and can be blocked by propranolol. Cannabinoids also have 'psychotropic, hypnotic, tranquillising, antiemetic, anticonvulsant and analgesic effects, they lower intra-ocular pressure, increase appetite, and affect the cardiovascular, respiratory, reproductive, and immune systems'. [27]

Psychotropic effects

Most users experience euphoria with feelings of self-confidence, wellbeing, and relaxation. They often have an altered perception of time which seems to pass slowly. In addition there may be heightened perceptions of taste, smell, touch and hearing. There may be an associated difficulty in concentration coupled with memory, cognitive and psychomotor impairment. Some people experience a dysphoria which is not pleasurable and they become anxious, agitated and suspicious.

Distortions of time and space estimation, reduced vigilance and incoordination mean that small 'social' doses of the drug are likely to impair car driving, aeroplane flying, and the use of industrial machinery.

Cannabis use is almost certainly a frequent unrecognised cause of road traffic and industrial accidents. Industry is now beginning to take this problem seriously. A recent study [28] of offshore oil and gas rig workers immediately prior to deployment offshore showed that 9.2% had urine that gave positive reactions for cannabis. New employees had their contracts terminated while established workers were disciplined.

An amotivational syndrome has been alleged in cannabis users, characterised by apathy, lack of drive, chronic lethargy and indifference to social values. Whether a 'drop-out' way of life is chosen deliberately by cannabis users or whether it is a drug effect is difficult to ascertain.

Cannabis psychosis
At high levels of use a cannabis psychosis may occur. Occasionally this is evident in some people who have only taken small amounts of cannabis – sometimes after only smoking one 'joint'. The existence of a cannabis psychosis was at one time doubted but the evidence is now overwhelming, and it has also been demonstrated in a clinical setting to be dose-related [29]. It is almost certainly an under-recognised condition in the UK. One report showed that psychosis after cannabis use appeared to be more common among patients discharged from Shenley Hospital than in England and Wales overall [30]. Cannabis psychosis is characterised by confusion, delusions, hallucinations, and emotional lability. It lasts a few hours or days, almost always resolving within a week of withdrawal of the drug. Regular heavy cannabis users may suffer repeated psychotic episodes and some may effectively maintain themselves in a chronic psychotic condition. There is no convincing evidence that cannabis use *per se* leads to any long-lasting or chronic psychosis, although there are several reports of symptoms with an unpleasant feeling of strangeness relating to the self (depersonalisation) or the environment (derealisation). Such feelings may last for several months, a fact which may be related to the slow elimination of cannabinoids from the body. Flashbacks have been

described as a prolonged effect, but, in almost every case, LSD or other psychedelic drugs had also been taken.

A study comparing 25 consecutive cases of cannabis psychosis of the paranoid type with 25 consecutive cases of paranoid schizophrenia has been described by Thacore and Shukla [31]. They defined cannabis psychosis as occurring in 'those in whom a clear temporal relationship between prolonged abuse of cannabis and the development of psychosis has been observed on more than two occasions'. Although the results showed that both groups suffered from hallucinations, visual hallucinations were only present in those using cannabis. There was no clouding of consciousness or evidence of thought disorder (thought block, disturbance of conceptual thinking, etc.) in those with cannabis psychosis. Indeed, many had rapidity of thought and flights of ideas. This finding is supported by Rottanburg et al. [32] who have also shown a significantly high occurrence of hypomanic symptoms associated with cannabis psychosis. Athough cannabis psychosis can be distinguished from schizophrenia, there is evidence to suggest that cannabis use may precipitate schizophrenia and lead to poor control in patients with this condition who have previously been well stabilised on neuroleptics [33].

Dependence and cannabis use

Tolerance to cannabis use is recognised and an abstinence syndrome, similar to that seen after withdrawal of benzodiazepines, is occasionally encountered. Dependence and problem drug use are not, however, major features of cannabis use. Help-seeking is only likely for the psychiatric complications that are a feature of high dose use (or occasionally low dose use in a susceptible person). When help-seeking does occur the diagnosis of cannabis psychosis is likely to be overlooked by both the patient and the doctor.

Opioids

The term opioid not only includes the naturally occurring opiates, which are extracts of the opium poppy, but also their synthetic analogues such as methadone.

Prevalence

Aside from cannabis and amphetamine, heroin is the most prevalent of the illicit drugs in this country. However, the following indicators, taken together, suggest that the prevalence of heroin use may be levelling out:-

(a) Seizures have fallen from 366 kilos in 1985 to 179 kilos in 1986, the first decrease since 1980, although in 1987, the figure was up slightly to 189 kilos.
(b) The price has risen to about £95 a gram while the purity has fallen to about 30%.
(c) There was only a slight increase in the total number of those notified to the Home Office as opiate-dependent throughout the year.

A number of opioid drugs are known to be misused but the frequency with which this occurs in relation to heroin is only known if the drug is notifiable. If it is not notifiable as is the case, for example, with codeine, dihydrocodeine and buprenorphine, there may be little indication as to the extent of misuse.

Hartnoll et al. [34] used a variety of methods to determine prevalence of opioid use in the London boroughs of Camden and Islington. Their results suggested that the prevalence of regular opioid use was about five times the total number of addicts recorded in the Home Office Addicts Index to have been notified during the year. Hartnoll and Lewis [35] using this 'addict' multiplier figure, estimated the number

Table 2.2 Estimated annual UK heroin consumption 1979-1984.

		1979	1980	1981	1982	1983	1984
(1)	No. notified addicts	4,787	5,107	6,157	7,962	10,235	12,489
(2)	Multiplier: Low	4	4	4	4	4	4
	High	10	10	10	10	10	10
(3)	Frequency of use (months/year)	7.5	7.5	7.5	7.5	7.5	7.5
(4)	% receiving opioids on prescription	10%	10%	10%	10%	10%	10%
(5)	Heroin addicts as % new notifications	69.5%	71.9%	73.8%	75.8%	85.0%	91.0%
(6)	No. using illicit heroin at any one time:						
	Low:	7,486	8,262	10,224	13,580	19,575	25,571
	High:	18,714	20,655	25,560	33,948	43,639	63,928
(7)	Average daily intake (g)	0.25	0.25	0.25	0.25	0.25	0.25
(8)	Total annual UK consumption (kg)						
	Low:	720	750	930	1,240	1,790	2,330
	High:	1,710	1,880	2,330	3,100	4,460	5,830

using illicit heroin at any one time in the UK. Wagstaff and Maynard [37] produced the following table using the same methodology, with a low multiplier figure from Hartnoll *et al.* [34] and a high figure from Ditton and Speirits [36]. They also took into account variables such as the frequency of use of the average heroin user per year (Hartnoll and Lewis found this to be about seven and a half months/year), the percentage receiving opioids on prescription and heroin addicts as a percentage of new notifications.

Most experts in the field believe that by 1988 there were approximately 100,000 regular heroin users in the UK.

Mechanism of action

Receptor sites exist in the brain and elsewhere and are the sites of action of opioid drugs, triggering neuropharmacological pathways to produce analgesia and other opioid effects. At least 15 endogenous, biologically active opioid peptides are known to utilise these glycoprotein receptors in the mammalian brain. They are known as endorphins or enkephalins and are stored in three large biologically inactive precursor molecules known respectively as proenkephalin, prodynorphin and propiomelanocortin [38]. Each opioid peptide has a different spectrum of activity and they all have the pentapeptide methionine or leucine enkephalin sequence at their N terminus. It is probable that the opioid peptides function as neurotransmitters or neurohormones, and have ramifications for many aspects of human physiology and behaviour, including regulation of respiration, blood pressure, appetite and hormones. They may also be involved in common mechanisms for:

(1) various compulsive behaviours and 'loss of control';
(2) reinforcement and pleasure or pain;
(3) the complex and intertwined phenomena of tolerance, dependence, and withdrawal [39].

As exogenously administered analgesics produce their effects by fitting onto opioid receptor sites, these sites have until recently been studied by examining the effects of different opioid drugs on the body. Originally, an attempt was made to understand all the opioid drugs by comparing them with morphine. At that time morphine was thought to exert its action through a single receptor, μ (mu). Taking morphine as the standard, and calling it a pure agonist, other drugs may be classified as partial agonists, or pure antagonists, according to their effects. Pure antagonists (e.g. naloxone) will bind with the μ receptor and competitively inhibit binding of other morphine-like drugs. Pure antagonists have no intrinsic activity of their own at this site. Partial agonists (e.g. buprenorphine) also competitively inhibit binding of other morphine-like drugs at the μ receptor but, unlike pure antagonists, do have some limited activity of their own at this site.

This simplistic theory did not, however, explain the actions of some opioids. For example, nalorphine in low doses competitively antagonises the analgesic effects of morphine, but at higher doses it becomes less effective. It also provokes a different abstinence syndrome from morphine. These findings led Martin in 1967 to propose a second receptor responsible for some analgesic effect that was the site of action of nalorphine but not of morphine. Nalorphine was thus thought to act at two sites – a concept he called receptor dualism. It had antagonist effects at the μ receptor and partial agonist effects at the new receptor site. It was thus put in a new class of agonist – antagonist drugs.

The new receptor became known as kappa (κ) and later it became clear that a third receptor was needed to explain the dysphoric side effects including unpleasant hallucinations, of nalorphine, side effects which limited the clinical application of this drug. The hypothesis of three opioid receptors μ, κ, and σ (sigma) was categorised in the following way:

The μ receptor was said to mediate supraspinal analgesia, respiratory depression, euphoria, and physical dependence.
The κ receptor: spinal analgesia, miosis, and sedation.
The σ receptor: dysphoria, hallucinations, and respiratory and vasomotor stimulation [40], (morphine, it was realised did have some activity at the κ receptor).

Martin's hypothesis of three different types of receptor, μ, κ, and σ has been widely accepted. However, on the basis of the pharmacological effects of different opioid drugs, nearly a dozen receptor sites, each with its own biological effects, have now been suggested. Perhaps in the future this work will be correlated with the biological effects of the 15 known opioid peptides to give us a clearer understanding of the way our bodies work and a deeper knowledge of the pharmacological actions of the opioid group of drugs.

The recognition that several different receptors account for the mechanism of action of the opioid drugs has been accompanied by the knowledge that it should be possible to develop opioids with highly specific activity. Consequently there has been a flurry of activity in the research laboratories over the last 20 years searching for the ideal analgesic, antidiarrhoeal agent, and antitussive, free from problems of dependence and toxic side effects. This has resulted in a very large number of opioid drugs on the market. Unfortunately, all of them have, at least to some degree, a potential to induce dependence.

Most opioid users will, if they are unable to obtain the opioid of their choice, use any other opioid drug in its place. For example, a heroin user unable to obtain his usual supply may take codeine linctus, dextromoramide or buprenorphine. Not all these drugs have the same pharmacological effects and in addition they may compete with and antagonise each other at some receptor sites. Additionally, recent work with long-acting opioid antagonists (e.g. naltrexone) is proving to be an interesting new approach that may well in the future be a beneficial supplement to existing treatments of opioid dependence. A good understanding of the underlying pharmacological mechanisms of action of the opioid drugs is therefore important. In gaining such knowledge, however, the importance of the psycho-social aspects of dependence must not be neglected. In his 1985 Dent Memorial Lecture Dr Philip Connell said '... If one could produce a perfect antagonist which did not produce dysphoria; which had no adverse side effects; which could not be neutralised by merely increasing the dose of opioid and which could still allow of adequate pain relief during physical painful crises unrelated to drug misuse, there would still be a very large population of addicts who would not comply with its use ...'

Illicit heroin

Illicit heroin comes in powder form and may be sniffed, smoked, or injected. It is not taken orally as metabolism on the first pass through the liver means that little is left for the systemic circulation. Heroin does not bind to opioid receptors and so is not itself biologically active. It is, however, metabolised to active metabolites, 6-acetyl morphine and morphine. The reason for its popularity among the drug-using fraternity lies in its greater lipid solubility. It crosses the blood-brain barrier faster than morphine, so that the onset of its effect is faster and the euphoria more intense.

Smoking heroin or 'chasing the dragon' is a method of taking the drug that has made recreational heroin use more popular and has contributed to the scale of our current drug problem in this country. The powder is placed on tin foil and heated underneath with a lighted match. As the heroin heats up, it blackens and wriggles like a snake

Different Drugs of Misuse 63

(hence the name). The rising fumes are then sucked up through a tube.

Problems associated with opioid use

(1) Dependence
The overall liability for misuse of any opioid is not established by any one single factor; rather it is a composite based on a number of factors. These include:

(1) The capacity of the drug to produce the kind of physical dependence in which drug withdrawal causes sufficient distress to bring about drug-seeking behaviour.
(2) Its ability to suppress withdrawal symptoms caused by withdrawal of other agents.
(3) The degree to which it induces a state of euphoria similar to that produced by morphine and other opioids.
(4) Its duration of action and thus the frequency with which it is taken.
(5) The patterns of toxicity that occur when the dose is increased beyond the useful therapeutic range.
(6) Physical characteristics of the drug, such as water solubility, that may determine whether it is likely to be used by the parenteral route.

Dependence is a characteristic feature of all opioid drugs and this has been one of the major limiting factors in their clinical use.

(2) Problems arising from injecting opioids
The other problems associated with opioids, and in particular heroin, are generally those arising from injection practices. These are either through:

(i) the substance or substances used to 'cut' (i.e. dilute) the heroin powder. Lactose powder is commonly used to 'cut' illicit heroin and is relatively harmless. However, any substance that looks like street heroin may be used. Sometimes, in the past, baking powder, Vim and brick dust have been added. In past years small amounts of phenobarbitone have been present in consignments of heroin imported from Pakistan. However, recent consignments from Pakistan have been found to contain as much as 10–30% phenobarbitone and/or methaqualone, probably added at source. This amount is enough to lead to dependence on these drugs and could theoretically precipitate withdrawal convulsions, although this has yet to be reported. Users are rarely aware of these contaminants, although they may show up in a routine urinalysis. (Being in a base form, heroin powder is fairly insoluble. Solubility can be enhanced for the purposes of injecting by adding citric acid, or more often lemon juice).

or

(ii) from the use of unsterile injection techniques, in particular the sharing of needles and syringes. The British Pharmaceutical Society has recently changed its ruling that pharmacists should not dispense syringes and needles to anyone whom they believe to be drug users and now leave it to the individual pharmacist's discretion. Most of the medical problems from opioid use are derived from unsterile injecting practices (e.g. hepatitis, septicaemia, abscesses, HIV infection) and these will be covered more fully later in the book.

(3) Overdoses

Overdoses on heroin may be purposeful or due to an intentional or accidental summation effect with other CNS depressant drugs such as alcohol. Unintentional overdose may occur following a period of prolonged abstinence when tolerance has unknowingly been lost. About 10% of all user deaths occur within the first few days of leaving prison.

(4) Amenorrhoea

Amenorrhoea, often prolonged, is common among women opioid users, particularly those using $\frac{1}{4}$ gram or more of street heroin per day or its opioid equivalent. This is due to a direct effect of the drug on opioid receptors in the median eminence of the brain, affecting the release of anterior pituitary-regulating substances from the hypothalamus. Both luteinising hormone (LH) and follicle stimulating hormone (FSH) are inhibited by this mechanism.

(5) Loss of libido

For both sexes, prolonged opioid use causes loss of libido. Often the relationship of a heroin-using couple is based almost exclusively around drug-seeking and drug-using behaviour and the recovery of one or both partners may be more than that relationship can stand. Couples who go into rehabilitation together usually do badly.

(6) Social problems

With the exception of HIV infection, although medical problems from drug use are often serious and sometimes life-threatening, in the mind of the user they become dwarfed by associated social problems and it is these that generally motivate a drug user to reach out for help. The GP must be alive to this issue and be prepared to treat the whole person – social problems and all.

Barbiturates

Barbiturates were first made available to clinicians in 1903. They are said to have been named after a barmaid called Barbara who worked in a Munich beer hall! [41]

Prevalence

At one time treatment with barbiturates was accepted and indeed encouraged for anyone suffering from anxiety or insomnia. They became widely prescribed. Slowly, the problems associated with their use came to the attention of the medical profession – not least the problem of dependence. Very large numbers of people became dependent on prescribed barbiturates, largely as a result of over-generous prescribing by general practitioners. In a 1973 survey of mental hospital admissions where the diagnosis was drug dependence, barbiturates were easily the commonest group of drugs identified in both teenagers and the over-forties. Overdoses were common at that time accounting for about 10,000 hospital admissions and between 1,500 and 2,000 deaths each year – between a third and a half of all drug overdose fatalities [42]. A Campaign on the Use and Restriction of Barbiturates (CURB) was set up by a group of concerned doctors and ran from 1975–77. However, it was launched at a time when the prescribing of barbiturates was already declining and did not appear to have markedly influenced the prescribing of these drugs in general practice. Today there are very few therapeutic barbiturate misusers. Prescriptions have fallen from 6.8 million in 1976 to 1.3 million in 1986.

From the mid-1960s, for about 15 years, barbiturates, particularly those that were relatively short-acting such as Tuinal, Nembutal, Seconal and Amytal, were readily available on the black market and widely misused by the drugtaking population. By 1980, this degree of misuse was falling off as many 'barb freaks' changed to heroin which had suddenly become cheap and plentiful. Although the misuse of barbiturates is not as common now as it was in the early and mid-1970s, it is still frequently encountered. Moreover, some drug users take barbiturate unsuspectingly as it is commonly added to heroin either by suppliers or at source to make the heroin appear to be more potent. The incidence of barbiturate misuse is unknown as no attempt has ever been made to assess it on a national basis.

Actions of barbiturates

Barbiturates act by depressing the activity of the entire central nervous system. It is thought that they probably do this by stabilising nerve membranes and reducing the easy transfer of ions across them. By this means the neural action potential is prevented from reaching the level required to initiate or transmit a nerve impulse.

At therapeutic doses there is sedation with some impairment of memory and cognitive processes, a reduction in the level of any concurrent anxiety and sleep is facilitated. If the dose is increased, the person may begin to behave as though he or she is drunk. Increasing impairment of consciousness causes the speed of thought and speech to be slowed down; reaction time is also delayed and there is a progressive impairment of muscle coordination – movements become clumsy and gait increasingly unsteady. At higher doses coma ensues and the respiratory centre may become depressed with a potentially fatal outcome.

One of the main problems of barbiturates is their narrow margin of safety. There is only a small gap between the therapeutic and lethal doses. For this reason accidental overdoses in the barbiturate user are common, particularly when tolerance is established and the user increases the dose. Some regular barbiturate users are frequently taken to Accident and Emergency Departments in a comatose state, discharging themselves on return to consciousness only to come back again in a coma a few hours later. Such patients are a source of frustration to those working in A & E Departments.

Barbiturate injecting

Barbiturate users may take their drugs orally or they may inject the powder contained in the capsules after dissolving it in water. Barbiturates are highly irritant to tissues. If injected outside a vein, they will cause local tissue damage and often subsequent ulceration (a 'barb burn'). If they are injected by mistake into an artery rather than a vein, they will cause intense vasospasm with resultant ischaemia or gangrene of the tissues supplied by that artery. This is particularly seen with the femoral artery which lies adjacent to the femoral vein (the usual preferred site of injection when thrombophlebitis prevents intravenous injection into the superficial veins of the arms and legs). Several barbiturate users have had to have a leg amputated as a result.

Tolerance and the withdrawal syndrome

Metabolic tolerance occurs relatively quickly due to enzyme induction by the P450 cytochrome system of the liver. This enzyme induction will also increase the speed of metabolic degradation of a number of other drugs including warfarin, phenytoin, and steroids (e.g. the contraceptive pill). Tolerance also occurs from adaptation of the neurones themselves to the effects of barbiturates. Cross-tolerance with other CNS depressants such as alcohol occurs as well, but barbiturates and alcohol when used together summate in their effects.

The physical withdrawal syndrome leads, as do all abstinence syndromes, to the opposite clinical effect from that engendered by the drug itself. Its features start within 24 hours and reach a peak within two days of cessation of drug use. There is anxiety and restlessness, tachycardia, tremor and insomnia. When sleep occurs, it is fitful and accompanied by frequent and vivid dreaming. Associated with this is an increased REM sleep pattern which is also evident for five weeks after the withdrawal of therapeutic doses of barbiturates [43]. Delirium tremens may occur. Blood pressure, respiration rate and temperature may all be mildly elevated. Convulsions may occur and should be considered to be imminent if there is a persistent tachycardia of more than 100 beats/minute. Status epilepticus may supervene in extreme cases, and death has been recorded both from cardiovascular collapse and from inhalation of vomit during a convulsion.

Regular heavy barbiturate misusers requesting help present a major problem for the GP. Clearly it is dangerous for them either to continue or suddenly to stop using drugs. If prescribing is to be undertaken, then it must be recognised that most such people are so chaotic that they would find it difficult on an outpatient basis to take their drugs as they have been prescribed. In addition, others would abuse any drugs given, which could in itself be life-threatening. Ideally, an immediate inpatient supervised withdrawal should be available but this is rarely possible. A withdrawal regime which is possible to use on an outpatient basis with relative safety is given in the treatment section of this book.

The frequent label of 'soft drugs' given to barbiturates belies their real nature. Along with a few of the so-called designer drugs (which have yet to surface in this country), they are the most dangerous of all the drugs of misuse.

Benzodiazepines

Originally, benzodiazepines were successfully marketed as safe alternatives to barbiturates although at that time it was not well understood that, although benzodiazepines are relatively safe in overdosage (when not in combination with other drugs), they are neither free of side effects nor of the problem of dependence. During the 1960s and 1970s, as prescriptions for barbiturates fell, there was a rise in the prescribing of benzodiazepines.

However this was not a straightforward substitution of benzodiazepine for barbiturate by GPs; when reviewing prescription data for England and Wales for the period 1965–70, Parish found a 19% increase in the prescribing of psychotropic drugs with prescriptions for non-barbiturate hypnotics and tranquillisers increasing by 145% and

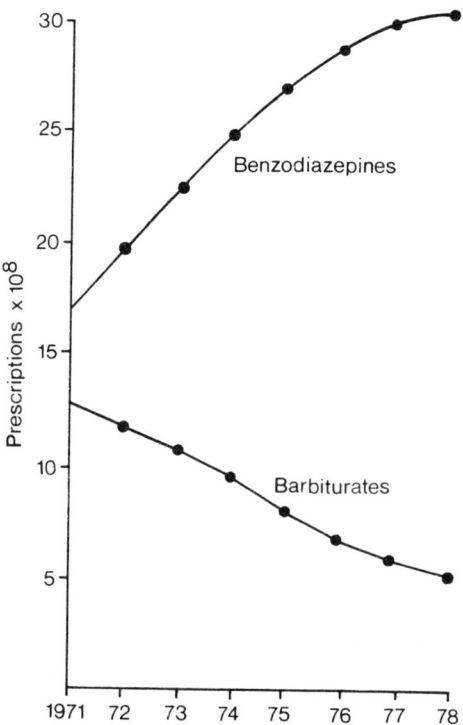

Figure 2.1 Prescriptions for tranquillisers in England and Wales, 1971–1978.

59% respectively, while the use of barbiturates decreased by a quarter [44]. In a review of six studies published in the ten-year period 1971–81, Marks [45] was able to show that the proportion of patients receiving multiple long-term repeat prescriptions rose from 27% in 1967 to 64% in 1977. This is particularly of concern as the duration of drug use may be the most important factor determining the risk of benzodiazepine dependence. He found that about half of repeat prescriptions for psychotropic drugs, particularly tranquillisers and sedatives, are provided on repeat prescription without the doctor seeing the patient. Furthermore, the more protracted the continuous treatment, the longer the interval between consulting the doctor. Overprescribing had reached such a height by the mid-1970s that in the UK during one year, 10% of adult males and 21% of adult females were prescribed at least one psychotropic drug and 4% of all GP prescriptions were for diazepam [46]. In 1979, prescribing of benzodiazepines reached an all time high of 30,871,000 prescriptions. Since then, it has been slowly falling but the extent to which overprescribing has taken place is perhaps best demonstrated by a survey in 1984 [47] which showed that 3% of adults in the UK had taken a benzodiazepine for a year or more.

Although the fall since 1979 has been an encouraging sign, this has been entirely due to a reduction in prescribing of benzodiazepine anxiolytics. The prescribing of benzodiazepine hypnotics has continued to increase since 1979 (although from 1982 it appears to have plateaued off). Moreover although there has been a marked decline in the prescribing of longer acting benzodiazepine preparations, there has been a concurrent rise in the prescribing of shorter acting benzodiazepine preparations. This is particularly worrying, for as the British National Formulary rightly points out: 'withdrawal phenomena are more common with the short-acting benzodiazepines'. This is because the steeper the fall in serum concentrations, the more severe will be the withdrawal. Shorter-acting benzodiazepines rose from a figure of 7% of all benzodiazepines prescribed in the UK in 1977 to nearly 53% in 1986.

Benzodiazepines and illicit drug users

Benzodiazepine misuse appears to be increasing among illicit drugtakers, particularly polydrug users [48]. As with barbiturate-taking [49], benzodiazepine misuse is frequently associated with the misuse of alcohol [48]. The black market availability of benzodiazepines is said to be particularly high in Scotland where methadone is only rarely prescribed by the drug clinics and where benzodiazepines are commonly used to help opioid withdrawal [50]. No studies have been done to estimate the prevalence of this form of drug misuse.

Mechanisms of action

Over the last few years, there have been some major advances in our understanding of the mechanism of action of benzodiazepines that have profound implications for general practitioners.

In 1977, Squires and Braestrup [51] in Copenhagen and Mohler and Okada [52] in Basle discovered that the mammalian brain possesses specific receptors for benzodiazepines by the use of radio-labelled diazepam. These receptors were later shown to be distributed throughout the brain although they are assumed to act primarily on subcortical structures such as the amygdala and hippocampus of the limbic system. Benzodiazepines have been shown to act indirectly through these receptors by enhancing the effect of gamma-amino-butyric acid (GABA), an inhibitory neurotransmitter. The existence of a naturally occurring benzodiazepine-like substance within the brain has been postulated.

Dependence on benzodiazepines

The demonstration of specific benzodiazepine receptors stimulated a great deal of other research. Although a steady stream, amounting to several hundred papers on benzodiazepine dependence had appeared in the literature since benzodiazepines were first introduced in 1960, these were all reports of high dose use. Later Covi and his colleagues in 1973 [53] and several American single case studies in the late 1970s indicated that benzodiazepine dependence could also occur after normal dosage. In 1981, Tyrer, Rutherford and Huggett [54] reported 40 patients with symptoms of dependence on therapeutic doses of benzodiazepines and later that year, Hallstrom *et al.* [55] published a paper suggesting that a distinct abstinence syndrome could occur on withdrawal from normal therapeutic doses. This indeed was later demonstrated and, moreover, the syndrome was shown to be clearly distinguishable from a simple re-emergence of pre-existing anxiety [56, 57, 58]. Key symptoms of the syndrome result from heightened sensory perception and include hyperacusis, photophobia, paraesthesiae, hyperosmia and hypersensitivity to touch and pain, gastrointestinal disturbances, headaches, muscle spasms, vertigo and sleep problems [47, 49, 50].

Implications for repeat prescribing

On the basis of the frequency of occurence of this withdrawal syndrome, it has been estimated that there are about 500,000 people dependent on therapeutic doses of benzodiazepines in the UK [59]. All of these people have been receiving repeat prescriptions of benzodiazepines from their GPs, some of them for many years. It has in fact been shown that withdrawal symptoms may follow a treatment as short as four to six weeks [60, 61]. Thus any monthly repeat prescription given for this class of drugs will put the patient at risk of developing dependence. It has also been claimed that benzodiazepines are no longer effective in the treatment of anxiety after one to four months of continuous treatment [62, 63]. To prescribe a drug that is ineffective and at the same time to expose the patient to a risk of becoming dependent on that drug, some would say, is negligent practice. In this context, it is interesting to read [64] that more than 1000 patients dependent on benzodiazepine tranquillisers have sought legal help to sue drug companies and doctors for negligence in supplying and prescribing these drugs. Eighty firms of solicitors across the country have formed an association to fight what will be the largest battle of its kind in British courts. This may be the tip of the iceberg as there are probably over three million long-term benzodiazepine users in this country [65]. Furthermore, with the introduction of the Consumer Protection Act 1987, which became law in March 1988, it is now easier to sue drug companies. This will undoubtedly lead to a further and even greater flood of litigation. Anyone making such a claim against the drug company is likely to be advised to also sue their GP.

Not only is long-term medication likely to be ineffective, and cause dependence but other harm can be engendered by what could be termed covert problem drug use as benzodiazepines are not often recognised as being the cause of the problem. There is little doubt that by overprescribing benzodiazepines, doctors have been responsible for many unnecessary road traffic, industrial and domestic accidents in people of all ages, and have reduced the quality of life of their elderly patients by causing memory impairment and an increased risk of falls. In 1981, there were 520,000 accidents at work from which 756 people died. In 1980, when prescribing of benzodiazepines was virtually at its peak, two million people were treated for home injuries in England and Wales and, of these, 6,222 died, 58% of them as a result of falls. It is not known to what degree benzodiazepines contributed to these figures, but the fact that they impair psychomotor performance makes it likely that they play a significant part. In addition, the drug may cumulate in the body and cause such adverse reactions as over-sedation, ataxia, dysarthria, motor incoordination, diplopia, muscle weakness, vertigo and mental confusion, poor memory and concentration, all of which may contribute to accidents.

Cumulation commonly occurs when there is metabolic degradation to N-desmethyldiazepam, which is pharmacologically active as a tranquilliser. It has a half-life of more than 100 hours and is a major metabolite of diazepam, clorazepate, medazepam, prazepam, ketazolam, and to some extent chlordiazepoxide. Similarly, clobazam has a long-acting metabolite N-desmethylclobazam. The long half-life allows cumulation of this metabolite to occur readily. Within a month of treatment, it reaches higher plasma and body concentrations than the parent compound [66]. Nitrazepam which has a moderately long half-life of its own (30 hours) also tends to cumulate.

The short-acting benzodiazepines lorazepam, oxazepam and temazepam which have half-lives of around 6–24 hours tend not to accumulate, although they may do so, particularly in the elderly. Triazolam has a half-life of less than four hours. However, short-acting benzodiazepines are not without their problems. Kales *et al.* [67] have shown that they will induce a rebound insomnia on withdrawal after single, nightly doses for two weeks. Tyrer and colleagues [68] have shown that the severity of withdrawal phenomena are greater in shorter-acting benzodiazepines, being related to the rate at which these drugs and their active metabolites are excreted and metabolised.

Benzodiazepines are widely prescribed for their anxiolytic, hypnotic, anticonvulsant and muscle-relaxant properties. The following are currently prescribable on the NHS limited list (although any benzodiazepine is prescribable on the NHS by parenteral or rectal administration).

As anxiolytic drugs: chlordiazepoxide, diazepam, lorazepam and oxazepam.

For their anticonvulsant properties: clobazam (the FP 10 should be endorsed 'S3B') and clonazepam (Rivotril). Intravenous diazepam is the treatment of choice for status epilepticus and works within 3 minutes (intramuscular administration of diazepam results in a slow and erratic absorption that yields lower peak plasma concentrations than after oral administration).

For their hypnotic effects: loprazolam, lormetazepam, nitrazepam, temazepam, triazolam.

As muscle relaxants: diazepam and many other benzodiazepines have muscle-relaxant properties.

Besides their main effect of potentiating the actions of gamma-amino-butyric acid (GABA), benzodiazepines have a subsidiary effect of depressing noradrenaline and 5-hydroxytryptamine activity in the septo-hippocampal system and possibly other limbic pathways. In addition, there is some evidence that an increase in endogenous opioid activity may occur.

Side effects of short-term administration

All benzodiazepines impair cognition and psychomotor function. The combination of disturbed judgement and delayed reaction times is likely to worsen driving skills and anyone taking benzodiazepines should be advised not to drive. This applies not only to those patients taking benzodiazepines during the day, but also to those who are taking benzodiazepine hypnotics with a long duration of action such as nitrazepam.

Memory may also be impaired. In one study all benzodiazepine hypnotics tested, with the exception of lormetazepam, significantly impaired short-term memory when subjects were tested the morning following ingestion. No other side effects were present on testing and those affected were completely unaware of the problem. Short-term memory is particularly needed for skills requiring higher cerebral functioning.

Long-term memory is also affected by many benzodiazepines, and this occurs anterogradely (i.e. from the time the drug is administered onwards), without any serious reduction in the level of consciousness. As a result, if late-night awakenings occur, which is common following the use of short-acting hypnotics, there can be difficulty in remembering whether the drug has been taken or not. Amnesia is not so common with temazepam, lormetazepam, oxazepam, or chlordiazepoxide, but may be regularly encountered following the use of diazepam, lorazepam, nitrazepam and triazolam.

Side effects from long-term administration

Possible organic brain damage
The ability of some subjects to perform complex tests of psychomotor function becomes permanently impaired following long-term benzodiazepine use and it has been suggested that this may reflect a lowering of intelligence. CT scans of the brains of 20 long-term users showed a reduction in brain size and appearance similar to, but less severe than, those seen in chronic alcoholism [69].

Tolerance
This group of drugs does not induce liver enzymes and metabolic tolerance does not occur. However, to a limited extent, as with all CNS depressant drugs, neuroadaptive tolerance to the sedative/hypnotic actions of benzodiazepines does occur, although not apparently to their anxiolytic activity.

Withdrawal phenomena
The specific benzodiazepine withdrawal syndrome has already been described. It appears within two to three days of stopping or reducing the dosage of a short-acting benzodiazepine and within seven days of stopping or reducing a long-acting one. It usually lasts about two weeks but can persist for two months or even longer. The syndrome is reported to occur in 15-45% of long-term benzodiazepine users even on tapered withdrawal, but it is important to note that almost 55-60% of such patients experience no clinically significant withdrawal symptoms when they stop taking benzodiazepines.

A rebound increase in pre-existing anxiety is commonly reported on benzodiazepine withdrawal and may be confused with the original symptoms for which the drug was first prescribed. Rebound anxiety occurring the morning after therapy with short-acting benzodiazepine hypnotics has also been reported.

Rebound increased REM sleep in the latter third of the night happens after only a few days' treatment with the short-acting benzodiazepine hypnotics, temazepam and triazolam. It is usually associated with disturbing anxiety-laden dreams and may be accompanied by frequent awakenings. Rebound insomnia may also follow the discontinuation of any benzodiazepine hypnotic, even after only a few days' use. This indicates the rapidity with which physical dependence and withdrawal effects may occur, and again this may be confused with the original symptoms for which the drug was first prescribed, reinforcing the patient's desire to continue treatment. Dependence on these drugs is thus readily established and overcome only with great difficulty.

Amphetamines

With the introduction of benzedrine in 1935, amphetamines were first brought into general medical use and soon gained widespread acceptance. By 1946, benzedrine was recommended for the treatment of 39 different disorders including migraine and impotence [70] and during World War II some 72 million amphetamine tablets were issued to British troops [71]. Hitler is said to have had five injections of methylamphetamine plus amphetamine tablets every day [71] and it has been suggested that as a consequence he may have been suffering from amphetamine psychosis. By the 1960s, the use of amphetamines was mainly confined to the treatment of obesity and depression. In spite of this in 1961, 2½% of all NHS prescriptions were for these drugs. In 1969, Dr Frank Wells and a number of other GPs and pharmacists in Ipswich were able to show that a voluntary total ban on amphetamine prescribing could be effective and was beneficial to patients. Prescriptions for CNS stimulants fell from five and a half million in 1966 to three million in 1971 and have been declining ever since.

As amphetamine prescribing declined, drugs that could be used in the treatment of obesity, that were safe and free from the problem of dependence, were sought by the drug companies. A number of alternatives were introduced, and most of them, being derived from amphetamines, acted by potentiating central catecholamine pathways. These amphetamine derivatives included diethylpropion (Apisate, Tenuate Dospan), mazindole (Teronac) and phentermine (Duromine, Ionamin), and subsequent experience has shown that they all have a potential to cause dependence, albeit less than the parent compound. They are now controlled under Class C (the least harmful of the controlled drugs) and various regulations apply to them including handwriting requirements for prescriptions, the signing of requisitions if purchased for stock, and regulations concerning the destruction of controlled drugs. Many GPs now consider it correct practice not to prescribe any appetite suppressants at all, but if a prescription is felt to be necessary, then fenfluramine (Ponderax), which is not a controlled drug and acts through serotonergic pathways, is probably less open to misuse, although rebound depression may follow its withdrawal [72], and hallucinations have been reported if high doses are taken [73].

Amphetamines themselves are Class B controlled drugs. There are now only two commercially available amphetamine preparations in medical use: Dexedrine (dexamphetamine) and Durophet (amphetamine and dexamphetamine). Ritalin (methylphenidate) was widely misused then discontinued in 1985 but it is still occasionally sold on the black market.

At present there are only two accepted indications for amphetamines in general medical practice. These are for the treatment of narcolepsy and, very occasionally, hyperactivity in childhood. Care should be taken in making the diagnosis of narcolepsy as great reliance is placed on the history given by the patient. In the past, it has been known for an intelligent drug user to give a clear history of narcolepsy and to elicit hospital letters giving a firm diagnosis of that condition, thus procuring a lifelong cheap supply of amphetamine. The GP, of course, always retains the right to question the accuracy of any diagnosis and should do so if he suspects such a case.

Prescribed amphetamines are becoming increasingly rare as a source for drugtakers. In contrast, illicitly manufactured amphetamines are becoming increasingly plentiful. The usual black market form is amphetamine sulphate, a white crystalline powder which can be readily manufactured by a simple process in home laboratories. Methylamphetamine (methedrine) use is still occasionally encountered because although licit supplies are unavailable in the UK, it can be readily manufactured from ephedrine in a clandestine home laboratory. The number of seizures of amphetamines in 1985 was about five times the number in 1980 and the rate of increase over that period was similar to the rate of increase for heroin [74]. This evidence suggests that in addition to our heroin epidemic there has also been an epidemic of amphetamine use. Amphetamines are not notifiable drugs and, partly as a result of their cheapness, amphetamine users do not develop problem drug use to the same degree as heroin users. Hence they are less motivated to seek help and are further discouraged from help-seeking by the lack of substitute prescribing. For these reasons, if an epidemic of amphetamine taking does occur it is likely to remain hidden. Although the extent of seizures is a reflection merely of availability, there is a well known association, that has already been described in this book, between availability and drugtaking, particularly if the drug is cheap to purchase on the black market. In harsh economic terms, the homeless drugtaker may find it cheaper to spend his last few pence on amphetamines than to eat or sleep. The expected cocaine explosion has failed to materialise as yet in the UK, although its use is increasing. This may be partly explained by the ready availability of cheap amphetamine. Amphetamine use in Britain is a cause of growing concern, particularly the increase in the incidence of amphetamine injecting in the light of HIV infection.

Mechanism of action

All CNS stimulants appear to have the same mechanism of action resulting in increased plasma levels of catecholamines and potentiating their effects. It is not surprising, therefore, that drugtakers commonly find it difficult or impossible to distinguish between them. Thus 'speed' or 'blues' are terms used by drugtakers to describe any amphetamine-like drug, although 'speed' originally referred to illicitly manufactured amphetamine sulphate and the term 'blues' was originally 'French blues', the street name for Drinamyl. Drinamyl (dexamphetamine plus amylobarbitone) was a highly successful blue-coloured combination drug manufactured by Smith, Kline, and French Laboratories Ltd. It was discontinued in 1978 because of its dependence potential, but was so successful that since that time manufacturers have tended to market the tablets of CNS stimulant drugs in a blue colour as this helps them to sell better.

There are some minor differences between the individual amphetamine drugs, particularly over duration of action and potency, but the similarities are more striking than the differences.

Amphetamines also have the same mechanism of action as cocaine with the exception that they do not block nerve conduction.

Tolerance to amphetamines is achieved to a remarkable degree. From a therapeutic dose of the order of five to ten mg, a regular user can rapidly increase the dose to several hundred milligrammes. This is a further difference to cocaine where tolerance occurs but only to a small degree.

The clinical effects of amphetamines

Amphetamines and cocaine have almost identical central excitatory and peripheral effects, except that amphetamines last considerably longer (several hours as opposed to less than one hour) and have no local anaesthetic action.

Often, the heavily dependent user will become distressed by the excitatory effects of the drug and will take barbiturates or benzodiazepines to 'come down'.

It has been accepted recent practice not to prescribe to relieve the symptoms of amphetamine withdrawal and perhaps as a result, many professionals underestimate the distress regular users experience when withdrawing from these drugs. They have as many emotional and psychological difficulties coming off amphetamines as heroin users have coming off opioids. By contrast, there is often a tendency to overestimate the problems of heroin withdrawal. With a view to AIDS prevention, there is now considered to be a case for short-term prescribing of dexamphetamine to some amphetamine injectors.

The psychic effects of amphetamines are also well-documented. These can be divided as follows:

Low dose amphetamine psychic effects
These may be observable in all amphetamine users. They have the appearance of being speeded up (hence the derivation of the term 'speed'), they are energetic and do not feel the need for either sleep or food while under the influence of the drug. Low doses of amphetamines do not disrupt thought patterns, so that individuals are able to think rationally, although they are prone to excessive mood swings, particularly when withdrawing from the drug.

Amphetamine psychosis
This has been recognised since 1938 when it was first described by Young and Scoville. It is a toxic effect of the drug and is commonly seen among drug users who are taking high doses of amphetamine. There seems to be no fixed dose above which an amphetamine psychosis will appear and variations occur according to the individual concerned. The psychotic state normally persists for several days after cessation of the drug.

Amphetamine psychosis may be hard to distinguish from acute paranoid schizophrenia. Auditory hallucinations and sometimes visual hallucinations may occur. Feelings of persecution are often present, although these are not usually intertwined in a complex system of irrational thought.

The classical description by Connell [75] has never been surpassed. More recently, it has been suggested that a common neurochemical pathway of stimulation of a catecholamine system or systems in the CNS is responsible for both amphetamine psychosis and schizophrenia [76, 77]. An amphetamine psychosis will wear off, usually within a few days of stopping the drug, and may be only distinguishable from acute schizophrenia by its temporary nature.

The amphetamine abstinence syndrome
This syndrome is characteristically divided into two phases. The immediate withdrawal phase is typified by extreme fatigue, followed by prolonged, but disturbed sleep. Upon waking, such individuals experience excessive hunger and eat voraciously. After two or three days, the second phase is entered; irritability, lassitude, and a moderate (occasionally severe) depression. This phase may last for weeks or sometimes months. Sometimes an apparently intractable state of depression and extreme lethargy is evident. It would seem that chronicity of amphetamine use may be related to the length of time during which this second phase persists. Patients who have used amphetamines every day for 15 years or more are at risk of becoming intractably and severely depressed on withdrawal. Such patients may

need a specialist referral for consideration as to whether a maintenance prescription for amphetamines would be appropriate.

Cocaine

Cocaine is derived from the pulped leaf of the South American coca plant, *Erythroxylum coca*. Historically the coca leaf has been chewed by South American Indians since about 2,500 BC, as an aid to arduous work, a practice which still continues today.

Cocaine was first extracted by the German chemist Friedrick Gaedcke in 1855, and by the 1880s it had become widely used in patent medicines and cola drinks for its stimulant properties. The rejuvenating effects of Mariani wine were even praised by Queen Victoria.

Cocaine was also the first local anaesthetic ever to be discovered and, following a suggestion by Sigmund Freud, it became regularly used in ophthalmic procedures. Freud also tried it as a cure for morphine dependence on his friend and fellow scientist, Ernst von Fleishl but von Fleishl responded by transferring his dependence onto cocaine. In spite of this Freud himself often took cocaine and made a number of studies of its effects. Later he became so disillusioned with the drug as more and more reports appeared linking it with dependance, that he eliminated all his studies of cocaine from his autobiography.

As time passed, concern throughout the western world mounted over the increased use of cocaine and its dependance potential. In 1906, the Pure Food and Drug Act was introduced prohibiting the use of cocaine in Coca-Cola in North America and caffeine was substituted. In Britain, legislation was brought in during the First World War to make cocaine a controlled drug. Under current UK legislation it is a Class A drug (the class reserved for the most dangerous drugs) and, as with heroin and Diconal, a special licence issued by the Home Office is required if any doctor wishes to prescribe it to treat anything other than physical illness.

Prevalence

Because of its expense, cocaine was once exclusively a drug for the 'jet set'. This is no longer the case. As the effects wear off very quickly in comparison with amphetamine, cocaine is still a relatively expensive stimulant, but its use is spreading in Britain among all social classes. Over recent years there has been a rising trend in offences involving cocaine and an increase in the quantity of cocaine seized. Considerably

80 Drug Misuse

more cocaine is now manufactured in South America than is needed for both American continents and Europe is said to be targeted for the surplus, although there is no conclusive evidence that this is happening as yet.

Cocaine formulation and routes of administration

In the United States and South America cocaine is used in a variety of different forms, but in Britain the most commonly found is cocaine hydrochloride, a white crystalline powder, often mixed with similar looking powders such as mannitol. The powder is usually arranged on a mirror or glass table in thin lines containing about 25 mg of cocaine and then inhaled into the nose through a straw or rolled paper. Cocaine may also be injected, either alone or with heroin, the combination being known as a 'speedball'. Regular cocaine takers use the heroin in the speedball to control the excitatory effects of cocaine. By contrast the chronic opioid taker will use the cocaine in a speedball to heighten the euphoric effect of heroin.

Cocaine can also be smoked, a practice particularly prevalent in America, but not as yet in Britain. The smoking form of cocaine is known as 'freebase', a name which derives from the process of 'freeing' the cocaine from the hydrochloride by mixing it with a volatile chemical like ether and then heating it up. Because of its relative water insolubility freebase cannot be sniffed, so tin foil or water pipes are used to smoke it. Freebase gives a more intense feeling because some of the impurities have been burned off, and more cocaine is absorbed but the production process is dangerous; one famous American comedian burned himself severely trying to produce freebase. Later, a much safer method of making cocaine base was discovered using ordinary household sodium bicarbonate, and underground chemists began producing cocaine base in small pellets or 'rocks' using the new technique. This is 'crack', the name deriving possibly from the cracking sound made by the pellets of cocaine as they are smoked. Crack is not pure cocaine but many users think that, because they are getting rid of some impurities, it is safer to take. In fact the reverse is true; because greater quantities of cocaine are absorbed by smoking, the dangerous toxic effects of the drug are more common. Whatever the street name or the processing methods, from a clinical standpoint there is no difference between smoking freebase or smoking crack. Some users think they can smoke cocaine hydrochloride in the same way that heroin is smoked on tin foil. But all that happens is the cocaine chars and any perceived 'high' is illusory.

Mechanism of action and comparison with other drugs

Cocaine acts both centrally and peripherally. Centrally, it blocks the uptake of the neurotransmitters dopamine and noradrenaline. It also increases dopamine receptor density. Peripherally, it acts by both increasing the level of circulating adrenaline and noradrenaline, potentiating both inhibitory and excitatory effects [78]. It also sensitises the tissues to the action of these catecholamines.

In addition, it increases myocardial oxygen demand. Amphetamines also work in this way but so too do the tricyclic antidepressants which do not produce euphoria. The euphoric actions of both cocaine and amphetamines can be blocked by pimozide and other dopamine antagonists [79]. Descriptions of the euphoria produced by cocaine are almost indistinguishable from those given by the amphetamine user. Furthermore, under experimental conditions, subjects familiar with cocaine cannot distinguish it from dexamphetamine when the drugs are given intravenously [80]. These pieces of circumstantial evidence suggest that cocaine and amphetamines have an identical site of action with regard to their euphoric effects, which are facilitated via the neurotransmitter dopamine.

Cocaine, however, differs from amphetamine both in its considerably shorter duration of action and its ability to block nerve conduction when brought into direct contact with nerve tissue. It is in fact the only local anaesthetic to cause vasoconstriction and mydriasis, and it is mainly its potential for misuse that has limited its clinical application in local anaesthesia. Cocaine continues to be used as a local anaesthetic in minor ENT surgery such as nasal cautery and at one time, it was used extensively in ophthalmological procedures, but this was stopped as it sometimes caused sloughing of the corneal epithelium.

The clinical effects of cocaine are considerably shorter-acting than those of the amphetamines. This is in line with cocaine's short plasma half-life of approximately one hour.

The clinical effects at low or moderate dose

(1) Euphoria

This is often said to be associated with feelings of great mental and physical power. This euphoric effect, which is the result of dopamine stimulation of the CNS, occurs within six seconds from freebasing, within 15 seconds from injecting, and within five minutes from sniffing cocaine.

Freebasing is also said to result in a more intense euphoria than other routes of administering the drug. The psychic effects of cocaine peak at 15–30 minutes and have mainly disappeared within an hour. Some heavy users have been known to inject cocaine intravenously every ten minutes leading to a cumulation of the drug in the body.

(2) Stimulation of the CNS
This is of short duration characterised by increased alertness, and is a feature of sympathetic stimulation of the nervous system. In addition, there is suppression of REM sleep, decreased hunger, mydriasis, an increased respiratory rate and increased muscular activity.

(3) Effects on the cardiovascular system
Small doses of cocaine may slow the heart as a result of central vagal stimulation but at moderate doses there is tachycardia and vasoconstriction, the combination leading to a rise in blood pressure [80]. Vasoconstriction and heat production from increased muscular activity together lead to a rise in body temperature, and cocaine is also thought to act directly on the temperature-regulating centre in the brain.

The clinical effects of high or toxic doses of cocaine

(1) Effects on the CNS
There are tremors and EEG changes of persistent low voltage fast waves, occasionally leading to tonic-clonic convulsions. There is also stimulation of lower motor centres and enhancement of cord reflexes. The vasomotor and vomiting centres are commonly stimulated causing emesis. Attacks of anxiety or panic occur and there is restless agitation, insomnia, anorexia, and digestive disorders. Prolonged sleeplessness leads to a confused state of exhaustion. Psychiatric complications are common with formication, manic-type euphoria, or sometimes depressive-like dysphoria. Paranoid psychoses mimicking acute paranoid schizophrenia are frequently seen. This central stimulation is quickly followed by depression of the central nervous system. Death is uncommon but if the medullary centres of the brain become depressed, death may result from respiratory failure.

(2) Effects on the CVS
A large intravenous dose or freebasing repeatedly over a short period of time may cause cardiac failure from a direct action on heart muscle. Less severe toxic effects include myocardial rhythm disturbances and

impotence. Anyone suffering from hypertension, cardiovascular disease or thyrotoxicosis is at special risk and should be strongly warned if found to be using cocaine.

A single dose of 1.2 grams may be fatal, but some people have an idiosyncratic reaction which renders them oversensitive to the effects of cocaine. In such cases, death from cardiovascular failure may occur quite suddenly after doses as low as 20 mg.

The effects of repeated cocaine use

(1) Ulceration or perforation of the nasal septum may occur when cocaine hydrochloride powder is sniffed repeatedly. This may be a result of intense vasoconstriction leading to avascular necrosis, but possibly the local anaesthetic action of cocaine may also play a causative role, in much the same way as a diabetic neuropathy will lead to trophic ulceration of the foot.
(2) Weight loss and emaciation may occur from persistent anorexia.
(3) Prolonged sleeplessness often leads to a state of mental confusion; there may also be chronic depression, fatigue, irritability and loss of libido or impotence.
(4) Tolerance to the convulsant and cardio-respiratory effects of cocaine has been reported [81] but tolerance to the other effects of the drug is often said not to occur. Indeed it is a widely held view that there may be an increased sensitivity of the CNS to repeated doses of cocaine [82]. However, with the increasing habit of freebasing it is now recognised that tolerance to the euphoric effects of the drug also occurs and many freebasers become anhedonic, i.e. incapable of enjoying pleasure.
(5) Withdrawal effects. Until quite recently it was said that there was no clear evidence of a cocaine withdrawal syndrome. This is now known to be incorrect; mild feelings of sleepiness, hunger and depression are commonly experienced as the effects of the drug wear off [83]. Abrupt cessation of chronic cocaine use leads to rebound increased REM sleep with excessive dreaming. The increasing habit of smoking 'crack' has highlighted many cases of severe post-use depression.
(6) Psychic dependence, as manifested by drug-seeking behaviour patterns has been recognised for over a century. If laboratory animals are given free access to cocaine under experimental conditions, they will continue to take it, in preference to food and water, to the point of death [84]. The pattern of dependence where the user neglects his/her responsibilities and focuses on the drug is most commonly encoun-

tered in heavy cocaine users and freebasers, although psychic dependence can occur when the drug is taken by any route. However, Andean Indian coca leaf chewers who only absorb small quantities of the drug, and who take it to reduce hunger and fatigue and to give them a sense of well-being while they are working, are said generally to have little problem in stopping the drug when they descend to low altitudes.

The fact that tolerance and withdrawal effects were not recognised until recently has led to the belief even in medical circles that cocaine use is without significant hazards or addiction potential. This erroneous belief is unfortunately still widely held and has helped to establish the drug in North America. If we are to avoid cocaine use in Britain on a similar scale, it is important that this belief is discarded and that there be as much education about cocaine as there is about heroin.

PSYCHEDELICS

The psychedelics comprise a group of drugs which include both synthetic and naturally occurring substances. They are taken primarily for their intense effects upon the mental processes of perception, thought and feelings. As hallucinations are an invariable accompaniment of their use they are sometimes referred to as hallucinogens. Many other drugs (e.g. CNS stimulants, anticholinergic drugs and antihistamines) will cause hallucinations in high doses, but because they are not taken primarily for this effect, they are not classified under this heading.

All these drugs are taken orally, although phencyclidine is also smoked or injected:

Synthetic drugs
- LSD
- mescaline
- hallucinogenic amphetamines
- phencyclidine and analogues

Naturally-occurring drugs
- magic mushrooms
- fly agaric
- mescaline
- morning glory seeds
- grated nutmeg and mace
- ergot

D-lysergic acid diethylamide (LSD)

Historical Background

Naturally occurring psychedelics have been taken for their effects for several hundred years. The Druids are thought to have eaten hallucinogenic mushrooms during ceremonial rituals. The Mexican habit of chewing discs sliced from the top of the mescal cactus, was described in the early sixteenth century. It is thought to have originated as an Aztec custom [85]. Ergotism, often called St Anthony's Fire because of the painful side effects of prolonged peripheral vasoconstriction causing gangrene in the fingers, toes and ears, occurred in epidemics in the Middle Ages when rye bread contaminated by fungus was eaten.

Synthetic psychedelics were first introduced after Albert Hofmann discovered LSD in 1938. He was employed by Sandoz to prepare analogues of ergot in the hope of deriving a new stimulant drug. LSD was the 25th such analogue (hence LSD 25). Preliminary tests on animals were disappointing and further work was shelved until 1943 when Hofmann had 'a feeling that it would be worthwhile to carry out more profound studies'. During the preparation of a fresh quantity, Hofmann unwittingly ingested a minute amount and precariously cycled home under its influence. Later he described his experience: 'At home I lay down and sank into a not unpleasant intoxicated-like condition, characterised by an extremely stimulated imagination. In a dream-like state, with eyes closed, I perceived an uninterrupted stream of fantastic pictures, extraordinary shapes with intense kaleidoscopic play of colours. After some two hours the condition faded away.'[86]

LSD was later marketed by Sandoz and was widely used by psychiatrists for both research and treatment in the 1950s and early 1960s, particularly for the treatment of drug and alcohol dependence.

It was believed to have the ability to release a stream of repressed recollections and responses stored in the subconscious mind and was particularly valued by psychotherapists. However, an alarming increase in the non-medical use of LSD by young people led to it becoming legally controlled in 1966, and shortly after this, therapeutic prescribing of LSD virtually ceased. Having been heralded as a therapeutic panacea, it had increasingly fallen from favour.

During the 1950s and early 1960s, the US military and intelligence services had been attracted to the possible use of LSD as a brainwashing or truth drug, and had arranged for a number of University departments to conduct tests on student volunteers. Two Harvard psychologists, Timothy Leary and Richard Alpert, became interested when they heard students talking of their experiences. Leary and Alpert conducted their own experiments on the value of psychedelic experiences. They conceived of LSD as a 'chemical key' that would open up the mind to new experiences of self-awareness and enlightenment which (so they believed), if taken by sufficient numbers of people would join them together in a 'Brotherhood of Love', and benefit mankind as a whole. Leary became a public crusader urging people to 'turn on, tune in, and drop out'. The authorities reacted by sacking him but the idea of LSD as a means to self-improvement caught on among students, intellectuals, artists, and musicians. Eventually it spread to include a wider group who wanted to take it as a fun drug rather than to improve their aesthetic appreciation or expand their mind.

Sandoz withdrew the drug from the market in 1966 as public concern mounted about its misuse. The media overreacted and told horror stories of brain damage, deformed babies, murder and suicide as a result of LSD use.

Although this was an overreaction, LSD, psilocin and psilocybin are all Class A controlled drugs. They are controlled as much for their potential to cause widespread social harm as for their individual effects.

LSD can be relatively easily synthesised in a home laboratory. It is the most powerful of all the psychedelic drugs, the usual dose varying from 100-150 micrograms. It is usually distributed as microdots on paper carrying distinct designs such as Toadstool, Red Heart, E.T., Palm Trees, and Pink Panther. Although widely used on a one-off, sporadic, or occasional basis, regular use of LSD appears to be substantially less than most other illicit drugs such as cannabis, amphetamines or heroin.

Mechanism of action

The shape of the LSD molecule has a resemblance to both 5-hydroxytryptamine (serotonin) and the sympathomimetic amines, adrenaline and noradrenaline. It is likely that this molecular similarity helps to explain the biological effects of the drug [87]. Although LSD affects dopaminergic activity, it is likely that its psychic effects are mediated mainly via serotonergic pathways [88, 89].

Clinical effects

About 35-45 minutes after ingestion, sympathomimetic drug effects appear: the pupils dilate, the blood pressure is slightly raised, and there is a tachycardia. There may be tremors, piloerection (gooseflesh), weakness, nausea and a raised body temperature.

Psychic effects

Vivid visual hallucinations and pseudo-hallucinations occur. Time seems to be slowed down. There may be synaesthesia – one sensation merging into another. Thus, those under the influence of the drug may speak of tasting colour or touching sound. Colours and forms alter. The body image becomes distorted and ordinary sounds increase in intensity. Although the half life of LSD is only three hours, psychic effects generally last from 6–18 hours and occasionally up to 48 hours.

Adverse effects

(a) The 'bad trip'
Mood changes are common while under the influence of the drug and a distressing dysphoria may arise associated with anxiety or panic. Parts of the body may seem to become detached and the ego fragmented. Some bad trips have been recorded as leading to attempted suicide, although this is an unlikely consequence. The suicide risk from LSD use has probably been exaggerated in the past. Rather than death by suicide, accidental fatalities while under the influence of the drug are much more likely, for example by falling from a window or walking in front of a car or train.

(b) Postulated genetic and neoplastic effects from chromosomal damage
The finding of LSD-induced chromosomal damage led to a speculation that LSD is a carcinogenic agent and causes birth defects. Although there have been reports of leukaemia associated with LSD use, it has not been clearly established that LSD causes leukaemia. Similarly there is no clear evidence that LSD users have an increased incidence of congenital birth defects. Many other drugs, including aspirin and caffeine, have now been shown to cause chromosomal damage and this finding is probably of very little clinical significance. A teratogenic or carcinogenic consequence of LSD use is therefore unlikely.

(c) Psychosis
Repeated use of LSD can lead to a prolonged psychosis which resembles schizophrenia [90, 91]. Although this lasts for several weeks

or months, it will eventually clear completely and permanently. It has been suggested on rather flimsy evidence that those who develop temporary schizophreniform illness with LSD have an inherent predisposition to schizophrenia.

Frequent LSD use has been claimed to lead to a condition where the capability for abstract thought is lacking [92]. This could be a mild drug-induced schizophreniform effect.

(d) Flashbacks

These were originally described in the mid 1950s by Cooper [93]. They are the sudden recurrence of psychic effects previously experienced while under the influence of LSD. For example, a particular hallucination may recur months or even years after complete cessation of LSD use.

(e) Violence

This has occasionally been reported in association with LSD use but is unusual. LSD was implicated in the ritualistic killing of Sharon Tate and others by Charles Manson's followers in 1969.

(f) Tolerance

Tolerance occurs rapidly but no *withdrawal syndrome* has been described.

Mescaline

A weak psychedelic drug, which was brought to prominence in the UK by the novelist Aldous Huxley who wrote about his experiences when taking the drug [94]. It is rarely seen in this country.

Hallucinogenic amphetamines

These are all amphetamine analogues of mescaline. They are clandestinely produced in home laboratories in the United States and the common ones are known by the following abbreviations: MDA, MDMA, TMA, PMA, DOB, DMA, DOM, (also known as STP) and DMT. Although common in the States, MDMA (3,4, methylenedioxymeth-amphetamine, which also goes under the name of 'Xstasy') and STP are about the only ones ever seen in this country, and surface only very occasionally. All the drugs in this group are controlled in the UK by generic legislation introduced in 1977.

Phencyclidine and its derivatives

Phencyclidine (Angel Dust, PCP) and three of its derivatives are explicitly controlled in the UK. It was first introduced as a general anaesthetic but quickly fell from favour because of post-operative delirium. It is widely misused in the United States but is rarely seen in this country. At low doses, it gives a feeling of weightlessness, euphoria and intoxication. At higher doses, visual hallucinations and synaesthesia occur. Unlike other psychedelic drugs it is sometimes smoked or injected. Although a single dose of phencyclidine can lead to a psychosis persisting for up to two weeks, the harm from this drug has been generally overestimated. An abstinence syndrome, similar to the amphetamine abstinence syndrome, is recognised in regular users [95].

Magic mushrooms

Psilocybe semilanceata, also known as Liberty Cap, grows wild in the UK. The active principal is psilocybin which has about one-hundredth the potency of LSD. About 20–30 mushrooms are needed to produce an effective dose. Possession of the mushrooms is not a legal offence but in 1981 a Court of Appeal ruling in the case of R. *v.* Robert Stevens upheld a charge of possession when the plants had been shown to have been dried and crushed. Intoxication is not especially dangerous unless other similar mushrooms have been ingested by mistake.

Fly agaric

Amanita muscaria or Fly Agaric is the red-capped, white-flecked mushroom of fairy tales. Sometimes doctors are consulted because of mushroom poisoning with *Amanita muscaria*. Symptoms commence from 30 minutes to two hours after ingestion. They include salivation, sweating, lacrimation, blurred vision, abdominal cramps, watery diarrhoea, constriction of the pupils, and hypotension. Death can sometimes occur but is rare. In any suspected case the National Poisons Information Service (NPIS) may be contacted and the patient transported to hospital. The telephone number of the NPIS is 01-635 9193. It runs a 24-hour service.

Grated nutmeg and mace (part of the outer covering of nutmeg)

Both of these spices contain the psychotomimetic agent myristicin. After ingestion and a latent period of several hours, atropine-like effects become prominent: dry mouth, tachycardia, facial flushing, excitement, hallucinations, and depersonalisation. Although misuse is recorded, it is rarely seen in the UK.

Morning glory seeds and ergot (the active principal in rye fungus)

Both contain naturally occurring alkaloids similar to LSD.

MISCELLANEOUS DRUGS

Drug misuse may also occur with drugs that do not belong to any of the groups already described. Some of the drugs are rarely encountered, others are more common. Sometimes substances, not normally thought of as drugs, are used to obtain euphoria. In Britain, unusual ways of obtaining euphoria include the chewing of Khat twigs (a CNS stimulant) [96, 97], snorting Pernod [98], and injecting peanut butter. More commonly, drug misuse occurs with both prescribed drugs and over the counter (OTC) preparations such as cyclizine, pemoline, and caffeine.

Misuse of prescribed drugs may particularly occur with chlormethiazole (Heminevrin) [99], salbutamol (Ventolin) inhalers, anticholinergic drugs especially benzhexol (Artane) [100], and anticonvulsants such as phenytoin. Phenytoin has in the past been frequently prescribed to barbiturate takers in the hope of preventing withdrawal convulsions. The usual result is that phenytoin itself becomes misused increasing the risk of seizures [101].

Sometimes OTC combination preparations are misused such as Phensedyl (promethazine, codeine and ephedrine), Actifed (triprolidine and pseudoephedrine) or Gee's Linctus (camphorated opium tincture, squill oxymel and tolu syrup). Severely disturbed drugtakers may be encountered who take drugs by the handful not caring what they are. In this situation it is the availability of the drug rather than its dependence potential that determines whether it is misused. Thus paracetamol is commonly misused by such people. Regular drug users will, as a general rule, look for substitutes if they are unable to obtain the drug of their choice. These substitutes are not always from the same class of drugs. This is particularly found with polydrug misusers

– drug misusers taking several different drugs at the same time. Polydrug misusers will often increase the usual amount taken of one class of drugs (e.g. amphetamines) if another class (e.g. opioids) is in short supply.

Some of the more commonly misused of the miscellaneous drugs are described below.

Chlormethiazole

Since it was introduced in the late 1950s, chlormethiazole (Heminevrin) has been used widely in the treatment of alcohol withdrawal because of its potent anticonvulsant and associated anxiolytic and hypnotic properties. In 1981, it was the most popular drug for alcohol withdrawal in Britain [102]. Chlormethiazole has, however, been shown to cause dependence in its own right [99] and in combination with alcohol its bioavailability becomes increased with a potentially fatal outcome [103, 104]. Cross-tolerance with alcohol also occurs and transfer of dependence may be rapid [105]. In spite of this a recent survey suggested that half of all alcoholics requiring detoxification in Britain are managed at home by general practitioners who favour chlormethiazole and are prepared to continue its prescription for long periods [106].

In a rapidly reducing regimen over 6 days, chlormethiazole has been shown to be highly effective [107], and there is no place for a prescription over a longer period. In addition, wherever possible the use of chlormethiazole in this context should be confined to inpatient treatment only, but if prescribed in general practice the drug should be dispensed on a daily basis.

For those who have been taking the drug for long periods, abrupt withdrawal commonly leads to an abstinence syndrome consisting of restlessness, insomnia, tremors, and grand mal epileptic fits. Abrupt withdrawal of large doses (five grams daily or more) may precipitate an organic psychosis characterised by disordered thought patterns, visual and auditory hallucinations and sometimes paranoid features [108, 109, 110]. This has also been described in the case of an elderly man who had been taking two grams of chlormethiazole for two years (110). When the psychosis occurs it develops 24–48 hours after stopping the drug and may last for 8–20 days.

Benzodiazepines [111] and beta blockers [112] have also been shown to be effective and safe alternatives to chlormethiazole and should be preferred as drug treatment of alcohol withdrawal if this is considered necessary.

Cyclizine

For many years it was thought to be the dipipanone content of the drug which led drugtakers to seek out Diconal (dipipanone and cyclizine). By the early 1980s, misuse of Diconal had become such a problem that legislation was introduced to stop doctors prescribing it in the treatment of dependence unless they had a special licence to do so. Shortly after this, the ROMA rehabilitation project reported to the Home Office that several of its residents had been misusing Marzine (cyclizine) tablets and since then there have been several other reports of cyclizine misuse.

In retrospect it may well have been that cyclizine increased the dependence potential of dipipanone for there is anecdotal evidence that when cyclizine is misused now, it is commonly done in conjunction with another opiate. In the light of this, it is interesting to note that methaqualone, when on its own, is a relatively harmless drug, yet when it was combined with an antihistamine, diphenhydramine, and marketed as Mandrax, it became highly sought-after by drugtakers.

When it was realised that cyclizine on its own had become a drug of misuse, the Pharmaceutical Society of Great Britain advised that products containing cyclizine, such as Marzine or Valoid, should be sold personally by pharmacists. This seemed to have the desired effect of reducing its availability, although there is no doubt that misuse has subsequently occurred. The Wellcome Foundation has now reformulated its Marzine preparation. The new product, Marzine R.F., contains cinnarizine 15 mg per tablet instead of cyclizine, and although cinnarizine does have some centrally acting properties, it is hoped that this will help to solve the problem.

Pemoline

Pemoline was originally controlled under the Drugs (Prevention of Misuse) Act 1964 and for a short period was included in Part III Class C of Schedule 2 to the Misuse of Drugs Act 1971. It was deleted from this Act by a modification order in 1973 on the grounds of its low potential for misuse.

Very large amounts of licitly produced tablets containing pemoline are produced by UK companies for export, principally to Nigeria. During 1979 and 1980, illicit amounts totalling 227,500 tablets were seized by police forces. Since then there have been sporadic seizures of smaller quantities.

Pemoline is a weak CNS stimulant. With very high consumption, psychoses have been described but such complications are rare. The extent of pemoline misuse in the UK is difficult to quantify because it is not detectable by routine urine screening and because the tablets are generally sold on the black market as 'blues' or 'speed' so that most people taking them think that they are amphetamines. There is to date no evidence that pemoline misuse constitutes a social problem.

Caffeine

As well as being the active constituent of tea and coffee, caffeine is also found in coca, chocolate, cola drinks, and compound analgesic preparations. At the time of writing there are 89 over-the-counter analgesic preparations of which 32 contain caffeine.

Although tea drinking is said to date back to the 27th century BC, legend has it that coffee was discovered by the prophet Mohammed, and tea by Dharma, the Buddhist son of an Indian monarch. Tea came to England around 1660 AD and achieved great popularity. Coffee followed and from 1680–1730, London became filled with coffee houses. These became famous as literary centres and were frequented by such figures as Sheridan, Dryden, Swift, and Hogarth. But in addition they were 'places of robust political intercourse – places to campaign, recruit and speechify'. The authorities felt threatened and eventually closed these establishments 'because in them harm has been done to the King's majesty and to the realm by spreading of malicious and shameful reports'.

Some 120,000 tonnes of caffeine are consumed each year worldwide – equivalent to about half a cup of instant coffee a day for everyone on the planet. We British consume twice that per capita usually as either coffee or tea. Problems associated with the use of caffeine are not easy to identify because consumption is so widespread.

Actions

The ingestion of 250 mg caffeine (the equivalent of four cups of instant coffee or three cups of percolated coffee) has been shown to increase the circulating concentrations of, and potentiate the effects of, adrenaline and noradrenaline. Its actions are therefore very similar to a mild amphetamine. There are, however, effects that are specific to caffeine and the other xanthines (such as theophylline). There is a short-lived dilatation of systemic blood vessels which together with the increased cardiac output (a sympathomimetic effect) will cause a temporary increase in organ perfusion. The exception to this is the cerebral vasculature as caffeine promotes a decrease in cerebral blood flow caused by vasoconstriction. It is this vasoconstriction that is thought to be reponsible for the known therapeutic effect of caffeine in the relief of headache. All xanthines have the effect of causing relaxation of smooth muscle, hence theophylline's use in the treatment of bronchial asthma.

Caffeine acts as a diuretic in two ways: by increasing renal blood flow and hence glomerular filtration rate, and by inhibiting the tubular reabsorption of sodium. Caffeine also increases the secretion of acid and pepsin from the stomach and should be avoided in all who have a predisposition to peptic ulceration (decaffeinated coffee stimulates gastric acid secretion too). Large doses of the drug can cause vomiting and convulsions but fatal poisoning with caffeine is rare. One retrospective study shows that large doses of caffeine (600 mg or more/day) increase the risk of first trimester abortion [113]. There is conflicting evidence as to whether coffee drinking increases the risk of myocardial infarction but on balance this evidence does not support a significant independent relationship [114].

Tolerance, withdrawal effects and dependence

Tolerance readily occurs and withdrawal effects have been demonstrated. Regular caffeine users taking more than 400 mg per day (more than six cups of tea or instant coffee per day) have been shown to exhibit decreased alertness and contentedness but increased sleepiness, irritability, nervousness, and headache. The caffeine withdrawal syndrome starts 12–16 hours after the last caffeine ingestion.

Drugseeking behaviour has been demonstrated by adjusting the caffeine content of coffee. An increase in caffeine content results in a decrease of coffee consumption, whereas a decrease in caffeine content results in an increase in consumption. These effects occur even when the adjustment of caffeine content are only small (one-third of a cup of instant coffee) [115]. Dependence on a large scale clearly occurs even with what most people would see as moderate tea or coffee drinking. In spite of this there is little or no apparent social or individual harm in the majority of cases. Indeed, just as with coca leaf chewing by Andean Indians, caffeine consumption is generally viewed as an aid to work by increasing concentration and speed of working. In a few cases, extreme forms of caffeine dependence are encountered, for example where an individual will get through several pounds of coffee in one week, or consume several litres of cola drinks per day. 'Colaholism' is more common in the United States than in this country but is occasionally seen here.

Designer drugs

Chemically simple drugs of misuse, particularly amphetamine and the hallucinogenic analogues of the amphetamine series, have been manufactured in home laboratories since the 1960s. The synthetic hallucinogens have been manufactured mainly in the USA and have only rarely been seen in this country. They seem to have been adequately controlled in the United Kingdom by generic legislation introduced in 1977.

Developments over the past 20 years have made it possible for virtually any organic compound to be synthesised in a laboratory and any properly trained organic chemist can, with relative ease, produce analogues of drugs of dependence considerably more potent than existing drugs.

In 1979, in California, the first of a new breed of illicitly manufactured synthetic analogues appeared. Alpha-methyl fentanyl was manufactured from a clandestine home laboratory and like fentanyl was about 35 times more potent than heroin. It was diluted with lactose and packaged in the same way as heroin and when a dealer unveiled it to local heroin users, he called it China White (the street name for the finest South East Asian heroin).

Following this, a number of analogues of both fentanyl and pethidine appeared and received considerable media coverage. Journalists coined the name 'designer drugs' for them and this term seems to have gone into general use, although the majority of these analogues have not been designed from scratch.

Legitimate manufacturing chemists synthesise a vast number of analogues of known drugs in the hope of discovering new and useful drugs. Most of these synthetic analogues, for one reason or another, do not get to be manufactured, but the method of synthesis is published in a journal known as *Chemical Abstracts* and available for anyone to read. All an underground chemist has to do is therefore purchase the ingredients and read the instructions for manufacture. An exception to this was para-fluoro fentanyl, which appeared in California in 1981 and was a previously unknown fentanyl analogue. Clearly the manufacturer was a talented chemist.

Many designer drugs have extremely high potency. 3-methyl

fentanyl, for example, is about 1,000 times more potent than heroin and has caused a considerable number of accidental deaths from overdosage in American drug users. In all, more than 100 deaths from fentanyl analogues have been recorded in the United States.

Another problem is that clandestine laboratories are not subject to the same quality control as those which manufacture drugs legally. A synthetic analogue of meperidine (the American name for pethidine) can be produced by converting an ethyl carboxylate ester ($-COOC_2H_5$) to the propionate ester of an alcohol ($-OCOC_2H_5$). The result is a drug known as MPPP 1-methyl-4-phenyl-4-propionoxy-piperidine). If too much heat or acid is used in the process, small amounts of an impurity MPTP (1-methyl-4-phenyl-1,2,5,6-tetrahydropyridine) are produced. This impurity has the ability to induce an irreversible form of Parkinson's disease and at least seven people in the USA are known to have developed this condition. This discovery, although disastrous to the individual user, has been beneficial for medical research into Parkinson's disease.

Currently designer drugs fall into five different classes:

Analogues of fentanyl

Fentanyl (marketed as Sublimaze and Innovar) is a short-acting, highly potent opioid which is used as an anaesthetic during surgery. So far, 18 fentanyl analogues have been identified as emanating from clandestine laboratories in the USA.

Analogues of pethidine

MPPP is about five to ten times more potent as an analgesic than pethidine. Another pethidine analogue, PEPAP (1-phenylethyl-4-phenyl-4-acetyloxy-piperidine) has recently surfaced in the United States. This drug has also been found to contain a by-product that is chemically related to the neurotoxin, MPTP.

Analogues of amphetamine

These are derived from ring methoxylated derivatives of amphetamine (MDA, DMA, PMA, TMA, MMDA), methamphetamine (MDMA), and phenethylamine (mescaline, BDMPEA). Generally speaking they all tend to produce mescaline-like hallucinogenic effects.

At low doses there is an increased motor activity, heightened level of sensory perceptions, analgesia and varying levels of intoxication. There may be either euphoria or fright, sensory distortions/hallucinations, nausea, vomiting, jaw clenching, flushing, elevated blood pressure, mydriasis and ataxia. With increasing doses muscular rigidity, tremors and stereotypic behaviour may predominate followed eventually by convulsions and death.

Two of the series, MDA (3,4-methylenedioxyamphetamine) and MDMA (3,4-methylenedioxymethamphetamine) which is also known as 'Xstasy' have been widely available in the United States. A single high dose of MDA can be shown to produce brain damage in rats and it is likely that MDMA may produce similar effects.

Analogues of phencyclidine and methaqualone

In the 1970s, three phencyclidine (PCP) analogues, together with the methaqualone analogue, mecloqualone, were all controlled explicitly in the USA and in the UK. There remain at least 32 other phencyclidine derivatives at present not controlled.

Profits from designer drugs are potentially huge. In the USA, a 2,000 dollar investment in glassware and chemicals will yield a kilogram of 3-methyl fentanyl, worth about one billion dollars on the street. Furthermore, organised gangs profiteering from the illicit drug market, do not have to face the risk of illegal importation if they arrange for their drugs to be manufactured from a home laboratory.

Although to date no fentanyl or pethidine analogues have appeared in the UK, there is no doubt among experts that it is only a matter of time before they do, and that, once established, the manufacture of these drugs will rapidly increase. Following advice from the Advisory Council on the Misuse of Drugs, the government introduced legislation in 1986 to control certain generic forms of fentanyl and pethidine which covers all known and expected analogues of these two drugs.

Alcohol and its relationship to drug misuse

Many readers of this book will have been struck by the similarities between problem drinking and drug misuse. Just as those drugs described are capable of inducing dependence and the neuronal changes that lead to tolerance and withdrawal effects, so too is alcohol. Both alcohol and drugs of misuse are taken primarily for their psychic effects, but sometimes also to alleviate the discomfort of an abstinence syndrome. Looking in greater detail at some of the similarities, the excessive use of alcohol by binge drinking can lead to physical harm from road 'traffic' [116] and other accidents [117], hypertension [118] and cardiac arrhythmias [119]. These consequences have also been found as a result of drug misuse. Driving skills have been shown to be impaired by nearly 200 psychoactive substances [120] and of these just over 100 are especially hazardous [121]. Of particular note because of their widespread use and the long half-life of their active metabolites are cannabis and diazepam. Additionally, cannabis use is almost certainly a frequent unrecognised cause of industrial accidents. Some industries are now beginning to take this problem seriously as shown by a recent study of offshore oil and gas rig workers [28]. Hypertension and cardiac arrhythmias are a well recognised feature of amphetamine and cocaine use [122].

Regular heavy drinking may cause malnutrition [123], cerebral atrophy [124], loss of libido and reduced sexual activity [125]. Similarly, malnutrition is a frequent accompaniment of heavy drug use, particularly of CNS stimulant drugs [126]. Cerebral atrophy has been demonstrated by CT scan in association with long-term benzodiazepine use [69] and chronic glue sniffing [10]. The effects of drug misuse on sexual function are complex. The same drug can act as a sexual enhancer in one situation and be inhibitory in another [127, 128] for different individuals or for the same individual at different times. Generally speaking, however, high dose or long-term drug misuse has a negative effect on sexual activity. Heroin in particular reduces libido, prevents orgasm, and causes impotence [129].

Women who drink may develop menstrual irregularities or amenorrhoea [125]. Conception is unlikely in very heavy drinking women [125], but when it does occur there is an increased risk of fetal abnormalities, including the fetal alcohol syndrome [130], spontaneous abortion, stillbirth, and intra-uterine growth retardation [131]. Opioids also cause menstrual irregularities and prolonged amenorrhoea [132] thus reducing fertility. Furthermore, many drugs, like alcohol, are capable of affecting pregnancy adversely. Fetal malformations are a recognised associant with barbiturate [133], amphetamine [134] and benzodiazepine [135] use; spontaneous abortions are increased by cocaine [136], the stillbirth rate is raised by heroin use [137]; and intra-uterine growth retardation is a feature of maternal opioid use, having been demonstrated in 20-47% of cases.

On the psycho-social side, there are also many similarities between alcohol and drugs. Alcohol causes an impairment of psychomotor performance, cognition, and memory. So, too, do benzodiazepines and barbiturates and these drugs, like alcohol, are central nervous system depressants. Benzodiazepine and barbiturate [138] intoxication will cause ataxia, dysarthria, nystagmus, affective lability, and truculent behaviour; characterising a syndrome that is essentially similar to that found with alcohol intoxication. Indeed, it is not uncommon for benzodiazepine and barbiturate users to be accused of being drunk. Cognition, memory, and psychomotor disturbance are seen to a lesser degree with cannabis use [139], but these 'hidden' problems are no less important when it comes to driving or operating machinery, as space-time coordination is particularly affected. The adverse effects of drugs on driving skills have tended to be overlooked since the introduction of the breathalyser as an immediate roadside test for alcohol, as fewer blood or urine samples are now obtained to test for drugs.

There are many other close parallels between drugs and alcohol. Both drinkers [140] and drugtakers [141] tend to be low in self-esteem and depressive symptomatology is ubiquitous among substance misusers. True depression among drinkers is also more common than in the general population, although, not unexpectedly, this is considerably less than the numbers who complain that they are depressed. In one overview of the literature 70-98% of 'alcoholics' had symptoms of depression but only 3-10% were regarded as being clinically depressed [142]. It may well have been, however, that there was a tendency for interviewers to overcompensate for withdrawal dysphoria and the difficult social circumstances of many of those interviewed. Other substance use is also associated with depression. It is seen as a withdrawal effect following high dose amphetamine or cocaine use (particularly after freebasing). It is also seen in association with heroin use and one study reported that 23% of deaths from heroin use were by suicide [143]. There is also a high rate of attempted and successful suicide among heavy drinkers [144] and feelings of conflict and guilt are as common when there is a recognition of dependency on the part of the drug user as they are in the drinker.

A 'general depressant withdrawal syndrome', identical to the alcohol withdrawal syndrome, and featuring anxiety, tremors, and sometimes phobias and delirium tremens has been described resulting from such drugs as barbiturates, benzodiazepines, glutethimide, meprobamate, and methaqualone [138].

Crime [145], violence [146], unemployment [147], financial stresses, family and marital disharmony [148], and child neglect and abuse [149] are all known to be associated with heavy drinking. Similarly there is a strong link between drug use and crime. About 30% of persons arrested for housebreaking offences in Edinburgh have been found to be either 'regular drug users', or had links with drug use [150].

Violence also occurs in drugtakers who take CNS depressants and, as with alcohol, this is traditionally explained by the disinhibition of aggressive impulses. Feelings of self-hatred are often projected onto others by drugtakers in a manner similar to that seen with drinkers, but in some drug-induced psychoses, for example paranoid delusions from amphetamine use, may have a role in precipitating violence. Family disruption also occurs in association with drug misuse and children are often the innocent victims. Drug misuse was recorded as a significant stress factor in the families of 4% of the 6,562 children placed on the NSPCC child abuse registers between 1977 and 1982 [152].

Both dependent drinking and dependent drugtaking are relapsing disorders, and longitudinal studies bear many similarities. Both drinking and drug use are influenced by socio-cultural factors and are increased by increased availability. As has been shown, the similarities between alcohol and drug misuse are so great that it is not surprising that many workers in the field consider alcohol to be just another drug.

What, then, are the diffferences? The main difference in this country is that alcohol consumption is legal, whereas most drug misuse is against the law. Not all drug misuse, however, is illegal - for instance, drinking three bottles of codeine linctus, which can be bought over the counter, gives the body as much opiate as $\frac{1}{4}$ gram of street heroin and is frequently resorted to by heroin users if they are unable to obtain their normal supply. Other differences are sometimes put forward. Some say that drinking alcohol is socially acceptable whereas illicit drug use is not. Yet with an estimated 5.5–6.9 million regular users in the UK in 1979 (11–14% of the adult population) [152], cannabis use can hardly be said to be socially unaccepted.

Other socio-cultural and age differences between problem drinkers and drugtakers that were apparent in the 1960s and 1970s are no longer so marked. Thus, whereas 'younger clients were significantly more likely to be drug addicts, and older clients were more likely to be alcoholics' [153], drugtakers who started in the 1960s are now getting older and it is now much more common to see young problem drinkers [154]. Some cultural barriers that were originally present against heroin use but not drinking have now broken down [155] and as drugtaking has increased, so the differences in lifestyle and sophistication between drugtakers and drinkers, that was so noticeable in the 1960s and 1970s, is now disappearing.

Nevertheless there are still some differences apparent between drinkers and drugtakers but these are really no greater than they are between the users of individual drugs. For example, because of the high cost of some drugs such as heroin or cocaine, dependent users often have a history of criminal involvement or prostitution in order to maintain their drug supply. Problem drinkers do not usually resort to this but then neither do regular amphetamine users or cannabis smokers. Cocaine users, in spite of dropping down the social scale in recent years, still tend to be of a higher social class than heroin users or drinkers. Takers of LSD tend to be more interested in their own inner vision than many takers of other drugs or drinkers. To what extent these differences can be attributed to the attraction of an individual to a particular substance because of its effects, and to what extent they are directly or indirectly attributable to the drug itself is not always easy to ascertain. However, it is clear that many drinkers turn to drugtaking just as many reformed drugtakers become problem drinkers. The latter problem is so common that drugtakers should be specifically warned against it.

Another indication of the close relationship between drinking and drugtaking is the fact that many drugtakers use alcohol as just another drug. With an increasing trend towards multiple drug use this is now a frequent occurrence with alcohol playing a leading role in the mixture of drugs abused [156]. Occasionally this use of alcohol is emphasised by a change in its route of administration. It is not unknown for alcohol to be injected, and 'snorting' Pernod has been reported [98]. The trend towards multidrug use is of concern as the combination of two mind-altering substances produces not only successively greater impairments, but also tends to increase unpredictability in the user [157].

The similarities between alcohol and drug misuse have prompted initiatives on combined treatment and a number of treatment centres both in the UK and abroad now have several years experience with this approach. Glatt was an early pioneer of combined treatment in his units at St. Bernard's and Warlingham Park and commented that both 'alcoholism and drug dependence' are problems of multifactorial causation requiring an integrated multi- and inter-disciplinary approach; for example, as regards treatment by the employment of psychological, social, and pharmacological techniques'.

Combined treatment regimes have had a varying degree of success. There have been some remarkable achievements, but also some notable failures. More often than not the failures have been due to a failure of the staff rather than the patients to relate to both groups. The ones set up from the beginning as combined treatment units have generally fared better than those that have been asked to adapt by taking on an extra client group.

Originally it was thought that only professional [158] and therapeutic [159] drug dependents could be readily treated together with problem drinkers. Then some early studies showed that joint treatment could be successful if the 'unique needs of each group' were catered for [160, 161]. More recent work has shown that the treatment of all types of drug user is effective when alcohol and drug dependent patients are admitted to the same treatment programme. In a study of 689 patients in a multimodel 60 day programme in 1980, Aumark found no significant difference between patients from segregated and integrated programmes [162]. La Porte *et al.* also evaluated combined treatment [163] and commented that despite the fact that the two populations differed notably in terms of age and intelligence, the main finding was that the vast majority in both groups felt comfortable with each other and were of the opinion that combined treatment was helpful. Since that time the epidemic of drug misuse in the UK has tended to iron out these differences so that a combined approach now should be technically easier as well as being more cost-effective.

It is interesting to note that some of the most successful self-help groups for people with alcohol and drug problems are run on almost identical lines. Alcoholics Anonymous, Al-Anon, and Al-Ateen and their sister groups in the drugs field, Narcotics Anonymous and Families Anonymous, all have the same basic format with the same 12 steps.

There is scope for further initiatives in the community and voluntary sectors on combined treatment, and training could also be done more effectively if resources and expertise for substance misuse were combined. The relationship between alcohol and drug problems is now more clearly seen and perhaps practical advantage will accrue from this in the future.

Chapter 3

Medical Conditions Arising from Drug Misuse

Overdoses

Many drugtakers purposefully overdose when they see no other solution to their problem. Alternatively, overdoses, some of them successful, may be a cry for help and some are completely unintentional. Unintentional overdoses are a particular feature of barbiturate misuse because of the dangerously low margin of safety of these drugs. They also may be a feature of polydrug use if there is summation of drug effects, especially if alcohol is taken in combination with other CNS depressants.

Opioid overdoses can be rapidly reversed by an intramuscular or intravenous injection of 0.4–2 mg of naloxone (Narcan) initially, with increments every 2–3 minutes to a maximum of 10 mg if given intravenously. The effect is usually dramatic although short-lived; the moribund patient regains consciousness and usually sits up and starts talking. A heavily dependent opioid user may, however, be thrown into severe opioid withdrawals. As the effect wears off after only 15–20 minutes, it is as well to reserve its use until as late as possible. Thus the unconscious patient is best treated by maintaining a good airway with the patient lying on his side in the recovery position, whilst monitoring the circulation and respiration. Naloxone should be given just before the ambulance arrives or earlier if the respiration becomes shallow and the lips cyanosed.

Naloxone is also claimed to be of marginal benefit in stimulating the respiratory centre when barbiturate overdose causes respiratory failure, although it has no effect in antagonising other actions of barbiturates. Every GP should carry at least 2 × 1ml (0.4 mg) ampoules of naloxone in his or her emergency bag as its use may be life-saving.

Hypothermia

Significant hypothermia – where the rectal temperature is below

36° C – is a particular feature of both alcohol and barbiturate poisoning and may require specific treatment.

Pyrexia

A mild pyrexia, commonly 37.5° C, may be seen in any person going through acute drug withdrawals. Any drug user with a temperature of 38° C or more is likely to be suffering from an intercurrent infection and the clinician must be alert to the possibility of septicaemia in the intravenous drugtaker as this can be life-threatening. If septicaemia is suspected, at least two blood samples should be taken in special culture medium at different times, preferably at the height of a fever. This may be best done in a hospital setting where the patient can be closely monitored. Intravenous drugtakers who have congenital heart defects are at high risk of developing subacute bacterial endocarditis (SBE). They should be particularly warned not to inject. AIDS is becoming an increasingly likely cause of pyrexia from opportunistic infections and may well soon be the most likely cause of an unexplained pyrexia in a drugtaker. It must not be forgotten that cocaine and, to a lesser extent, amphetamines may cause a pyrexia as a direct drug effect.

Respiratory complications

All CNS depressant drugs, including the opioids, have a direct depressant action on the respiratory centre in overdosage which may be life-threatening. Respiratory rate reduces and this is frequently accompanied by hypoventilation. Shallow respiration together with cyanosis denote respiratory failure and attention should be directed towards life support and immediate access to intensive care. As stated above, in the case of opioid overdosage, an injection of as little as 0.4 mg naloxone (Narcan), preferably intravenously, can be life-saving.

Acute pulmonary oedema may also occur in association with an overdose of opioid drugs. It is non-cardiac in origin and its cause is not fully understood. It may be an allergic phenomenon.

All CNS-depressant drugs will also depress the cough reflex allowing secretions to develop and collect in the bronchial tree; bronchitis and pneumonia are therefore often seen in drug users. Chronic inhalation of toluene may directly affect the alveolus and cause a reduced diffusion capacity.

Cardiovascular complications

Sympathomimetic effects, tachycardia, vasoconstriction and a raised blood pressure are commonly observable in users of CNS stimulant drugs, particularly cocaine and amphetamines. This is because these drugs act peripherally by increasing the levels of circulating adrenaline and noradrenaline. Small doses of cocaine will, however, slow the heart rate by vagal nerve stimulation. Very large doses (e.g. 1 gram or more) of cocaine, either from intravenous administration or frequent freebasing, are toxic to the myocardium and may precipitate cardiac failure.

Tachycardia, vasoconstriction and a rise in blood pressure are also observable in those withdrawing from CNS depressant drugs, particularly barbiturates and alcohol.

Some volatile substances, particularly halons and, to a lesser extent, toluene, butane, propane, n-hexane, petrol and trichloroethylene appear to sensitise the myocardium to the effects of circulating catecholamines. An increase in the level of endogenous catecholamines as may occur in 'fright and flight' reactions may precipitate a cardiac dysrhythmia which can on occasion be fatal. In 1970, Bass reported a number of deaths from aerosol inhalation in boys who had run away when they had been approached [1]. Halons also depress myocardial contractility and hence lower cardiac output. Toluene use may, in addition, lead to reversible right heart failure.

CNS effects

The state of cerebral excitation caused by the use of CNS stimulants may cause some drugtakers to have grand mal convulsions. This is especially so following the use of high doses of cocaine. Toluene sniffing may also cause convulsions in some people. Also as the withdrawal effects of any drug of dependence are almost invariably the opposite of its clinical effect, the withdrawal of CNS depressant drugs will lead to a state of cerebral excitation. The withdrawal of barbiturates in particular may provoke, in dependent subjects, grand mal convulsions and a period of insomnia lasting for about five weeks. The convulsions occur in people who are not inherently epileptic. The withdrawal of other CNS depressant drugs, including alcohol and benzodiazepines (but not including opioids) may also induce epileptic seizures.

Convulsions may cause physical damage, not only to the brain, but also by injuring other parts of the body. Fatal inhalation of vomit has also been known to occur during a fit. Barbiturate users should therefore be protected by detoxification, preferably in a hospital or other specialised unit.

Difficulties arise when the drugtaker claims to be an epileptic as the anticonvulsants prescribed are almost invariably abused and the drugtaker may lie in order to obtain anticonvulsant drugs. A history of epilepsy from childhood should be viewed with suspicion until confirmed by another source. A history of later onset epilepsy, starting, say, at about the age of 17, should in this patient group be assumed to be withdrawal convulsions until proved otherwise.

When investigating epileptiform convulsions an EEG should not be done while the drug user is taking barbiturates or other CNS depressant drugs including anticonvulsants. It must be remembered that the diagnosis of epilepsy is not made on the EEG result alone but may sometimes be made on the history alone with a negative EEG. Thus it is sometimes possible for other doctors to have made a diagnosis of epilepsy on the basis of a false history.

Cerebellar signs, including nystagmus and ataxia, are a feature of the excessive use of glutethimide (Doriden), phenytoin (Epanutin) and both acute and chronic toluene inhalation. Glutethimide is stored in the body fat and released in small packets so that clinical signs may be intermittent. Phenytoin is sometimes prescribed to barbiturate and other CNS depressant users in the erroneous belief that this will prevent withdrawal convulsions. Almost invariably the phenytoin itself is misused, not only increasing the risk of convulsions, but also causing disorientation and ataxia.

Most drugtakers appear to have difficulty taking anything as prescribed and some drugs, notably barbiturates and benzodiazepines, interfere with the memory processes and compound this difficulty. High dose barbiturate misusers are generally so chaotic that an unsupervised prescription is usually best abandoned except in dire circumstances. A difficulty arises when the drugtaker is truly epileptic.

As has already been mentioned, chronic glue sniffing [2] and chronic benzodiazepine taking [3] can be shown to be associated with cerebral atrophy by CT scanning.

A peripheral neuropathy is seen as a toxic effect of the inhalation of the aliphatic hydrocarbons butane, propane and particularly n-hexane which predominantly effects sensory nerves. It is occasionally seen in association with other volatile substance abuse (e.g. toluene) besides being a well-known effect of chronic alcohol use.

Optic neuropathy has been described in association with toluene and trichloroethylene inhalation, and toluene abuse has also been recorded as causing sensorineural deafness.

An encephalopathy due to lead poisoning from petrol sniffing may also occur.

Genito-urinary and sexual effects

Female opioid users frequently suffer from menstrual irregularities, most commonly amenorrhoea. Although the data is to some extent conflicting, this appears to occur indirectly through the inhibition of both luteinising hormone (LH) and follicle stimulating hormone (FSH) and hence the suppression of ovulation. Thus opioids abolish cyclical changes in FSH and the midcycle peaks of serum gonadotrophins, and the rise in serum progesterone in the latter half of the cycle fails to occur [4]. Morphine increases the serum prolactin level [5] whereas opioid antagonists [6] and opioid withdrawal [7] decrease serum prolactin. Methadone users seem to experience a lower incidence of amenorrhoea and anovulation than heroin users [8]. This may not be a straightforward drug effect as methadone users tend to have a better nutritional status and overall medical care [9].

Men who are using opioids have decreased serum testosterone levels and this can be reversed by naloxone [10]. In addition, one study showed that sperm mobility is considerably lower among heroin and methadone users than controls [11]. Sperm counts were not initially different between these opioid users and controls but after three days or more sexual abstinence, sperm counts were significantly higher in methadone users and methadone appears to reduce male fertility more than heroin both in studies on animals and man [11].

Both men and women who take opioid drugs suffer loss of libido. In a study of 500 heroin users Smith *et al.* [12] showed that low doses delay ejaculation and also increase the ability to sustain an erection. Higher doses, however, are associated with impotence, decreased libido and ejaculatory failure. These results support not only the fact that a few people claim that opiates are aphrodisiacs but also the finding of Gay and others that in general men and women regard heroin as a drug that decreases sexual pleasure [13].

Looking at drug use in general, not only can high and low doses of a drug influence the sexual response in different ways, but also the same drug can act as a sexual enhancer in one situation and a sexual inhibitor in another [14], both for different individuals or the same individual at different times. This is not surprising since the sexual experience is a complex interaction between physiological, psychological and sociological variables. The situation is further complicated because different researchers measure the sexual response using different parameters. Thus physiologists might judge that cannabis is a sexual inhibitor because it reduces the level of circulating testosterone in men, whereas a psychologist measuring the perceived height of sexual experience might deem it a sexual enhancer, as it tends to distort time sense, heighten sensory awareness, increase vividness of fantasy and reduce sexual anxiety [15,16,17,18].

Amphetamines, when given by intravenous injection, may be associated with erection [19] and produce an 'orgasm-like' effect [18]. However, they are not popular as sexual enhancers. High doses produce a diffuse loss of coordination and restlessness which interfere with sexual response. Chronic amphetamine users report a host of difficulties including loss of libido.

Cocaine is reported to increase libido and enhance sexual performance, somtimes producing multiple orgasms. Its local anaesthetic properties are also sometimes used to effect prolonged thrusting by some drugtakers by rubbing it on the head of the penis or clitoris [13], a practice that exposes them to the risk of genital injuries [13]. As with amphetamines, heavy or prolonged use is associated with lack of coordination and loss of libido.

Barbiturates and benzodiazepines have a similar effect on the sexual response as alcohol. In general, low doses disinhibit sexual behaviour and excitement and reduce associated anxiety. Higher doses reduce libido [18].

Users of amyl nitrite report that it prolongs orgasm and delays ejaculation [18]. Nitrites are particularly popular among homosexual men due to their property of relaxing the anal sphincter.

Hallucinogenic drugs redirect the mind inwardly, and this may work against the interactive elements of sexual intercourse [18]. Users of LSD report that it markedly alters the perceived quality of sexual experience, describing more 'complex' experiences and a deeper orgasm [16].

Many drug users do not have a regular sexual partner and others become involved in prostitution so venereal disease is common. The incidence of sexually transmitted disease appears to be declining following media publicity of the spread of HIV infection. It seems in general that people are changing their sexual habits. However it appears that the drug using population is more resistant to such changes than other groups. Women drugtakers are also at high risk of developing wart virus infection and are thus a high risk group for developing cancer of the cervix. Annual cervical smears are advisable.

Psychological effects of drug misuse

To avoid duplication, disturbances of affect have been included in the later section on psychiatric morbidity and drug use. This section comprises disturbances of perception, impairment of cognition and psychomotor function, and disturbances of memory; features which, it is interesting to note, rarely if ever result from opioid drugtaking, but which are commonly found in association with the misuse of other drugs.

Disturbances of perception

Visual disturbances are particularly found with the use of psychedelic drugs such as LSD. Colours become more vivid, outlines emphasised and objects appear to be magnified or reduced in size. Space is often distorted, with the room in which the person is situated changing its dimensions in an extreme way. After-images, with trailing colours on closing the eyes, are intensified and prolonged. Vivid visual hallucinations and pseudohallucinations (when the person experiencing them is aware that they are unreal) are almost an invariable accompaniment of psychedelic drug use.

Visual hallucinations can also result from other drug use but less frequently, and then usually only when high doses have been used. They are found as a toxic effect of high doses of cannabis, amphetamines and cocaine, and as a withdrawal effect from high doses of CNS depressant drugs such as chlormethiazole, benzodiazepine and barbiturates. Pseudohallucinations are a common result of volatile substance abuse. Benzodiazepine withdrawal commonly leads to intensification of perception; thus some patients experience photophobia. Auditory perception may also be intensified (hyperacusis) in benzodiazepine withdrawal, by the use of psychedelic drugs and, to a lesser extent, cannabis. Auditory hallucinations are a frequent effect of high doses of CNS stimulant drugs, particularly amphetamines and freebase cocaine. They are also found sporadically with other drug use, notably in association with the inhalation of volatile substances and accompanying withdrawal from chlormethiazole.

The intensification of other perceptions such as smell (hyperosmia), taste, and hypersensitivity to touch and pain may also be found with benzodiazepine withdrawal and cannabis or psychedelic drug use. Formication (the sensation of insects crawling over the body) is an occasional complaint of the high dose amphetamine or cocaine user or of someone withdrawing badly from barbiturates or other CNS depressant drugs. It commonly accompanies delirium tremens.

Impairment of cognition and psychomotor function

This is important as some drugtaking impairs the effective management of such complex tasks as driving or the operating of complex machinery. Many people do not realise that the use of such drugs as cannabis and benzodiazepines will impair their performance even at low doses. There is no doubt that this results in numerous unnecessary accidents at work and many fatal road accidents. It is of particular significance because some of these drugs, notably cannabis and diazepam, have active metabolites with very long half-lives. Cannabis, for instance, being stored in the body fat and slowly released can be detected in the urine for two weeks or more after a single 'joint' has been smoked. N-desmethyldiazepam, an active metabolite of diazepam, has a half-life of over 100 hours. Impairment of psychomotor function can be readily demonstrated with therapeutic doses of diazepam and in those people who are taking this drug regularly every day the situation is worsened because its active metabolite accumulates.

Time appears to be slowed to the user of cannabis and psychedelic drugs, and space-time coordination, so important for driving, is impaired. Disturbed judgement and delayed reaction times are a common feature of the use of all CNS depressant drugs. It is well known that alcohol impairs driving skills but before the advent of breath-testing, people were commonly charged with driving 'while under the influence of drink *or* drugs'. Since the introduction of the breathalyser, drugs appear in general to have been forgotten as a cause of road accidents.

Disturbances of memory

Short-term memory is also essential for the safe and effective operation of complex machinery in industry and for safe driving, as well as for ordinary day-to-day and higher intellectual functioning. Work performance will generally be impaired by the loss of short-term memory, but not usually to a level that is recognised by the employer or the employee. Just as with the impairment of psychomotor function and cognition there is no doubt that these effects go mainly unrecognised. Such covert problem drug use is undoubtedly common both inside and outside a working environment. Cannabis use interferes with short-term memory and benzodiazepines and barbiturates impair both long and short-term memory.

Psychiatric morbidity and drug use

It is sometimes claimed that those with underlying psychiatric disorders turn to illicit drug use because they are unable to cope with day-to-day life and drugs provide temporary relief. However, the prevalence of primary affective disorder in opioid users is comparable to that found in the general population (6%) whereas the prevalence of secondary disorder is generally reported to be in the region of 20-30%. Thus there is little doubt that drug misuse is a major cause of psychiatric illness and this is confirmed by the work of Hall *et al.* [20] who found that 58% of patients admitted to a psychiatric unit give a history of drug misuse. However, it is not always clear cut from direct questioning as to whether psychiatric illness has preceded drug misuse or whether it has been precipitated by taking drugs. Many people disguise the fact that they are taking drugs and in areas of high prevalence this may be of considerable significance. In the author's own practice in inner London, 231 routine attenders aged 30-34 years were randomly screened for substance misuse by questionnaire examination and urine testing. About a third were found to be currently misusing drugs and three-quarters of these had concealed their drug misuse when asked by direct questioning [21]. In view of these findings, any young person who presents with psychiatric disorder should not only be asked about their drugtaking habits but a urine sample should also be obtained for analysis for drugs.

It is very easy for a patient to be labelled with a psychiatric illness when in fact the psychosis is due to drugtaking and this wrong diagnosis may have profound long-term consequences for the patient concerned. This is particularly so with *schizophrenia*. High dose amphetamine or cocaine use can lead to a psychosis which is indistinguishable from acute paranoid schizophrenia except by its temporary nature. It lasts for several days. It has been suggested [22, 23] that amphetamine psychosis and schizophrenia are both caused by stimulation of CNS pathways mediated by catecholamine neurotransmitters. Cannabis psychosis also resembles schizophrenia but is shorter lived. Nevertheless, the regular daily smoker of cannabis may appear to be suffering from chronic schizophrenia and be treated as such.

Other drug use may also at times mimic schizophrenia. Repeated use of psychedelic drugs for example, can lead to a prolonged psychosis lasting several weeks or months. This resembles schizophrenia but eventually clears [24, 25].

Depression was commonly treated by amphetamines until the 1950s and early 1960s and indeed amphetamines are still occasionally prescribed for this purpose by some doctors [26]. Amphetamines fell into disrepute when it was realised that dependence on these drugs was adding to patients' problems - problems compounded by the fact that withdrawal from prolonged amphetamine use may lead to severe depression and in instances where these drugs have been used for several years, the depression may be intractable.

Until recently it was thought that cocaine use was not associated with physical withdrawal symptoms and as a result it became a widely held view, even in professional medical circles, that cocaine was a non-addictive drug. An abstinence syndrome was eventually recognised in 1976 [27] and this has become more pronounced with the increasing use of freebasing or smoking crack. Depression is a feature of this abstinence syndrome and regular freebasers or crack smokers may become anhedonic - completely incapable of enjoying any pleasure.

There is an interesting relationship between tricyclic anti-depressants and CNS stimulant drugs. Amphetamines, cocaine and tricyclics all block the uptake in the brain of the neurotransmitters noradrenaline and dopamine, and beta-adrenergic and dopaminergic receptor changes also occur following the use of these drugs. Animal research on neurotransmitter and receptor changes following chronic cocaine administration suggests that long-term effects may be reversible by treatment with tricyclic antidepressants and subsequent human research has shown tricyclics to be helpful in the treatment of cocaine dependence. One study showed that treatment with desipramine was associated with prolonged (more than twelve weeks) abstinence in eleven of twelve subjects who had been chronically dependent on cocaine [28]. Decreases in craving followed a time course consistent with desipramine's time course for neuroreceptor changes and it is interesting to note that most of the subjects did not meet the criteria needed to diagnose depression.

Depression is more readily demonstrable in those who are using opioid drugs. Dackis and Marks [29] showed the prevalence of major depression to be 17% in opiate users, a figure which rose to 32% three weeks post-withdrawal.

Some studies [30, 31] have suggested that family doctors appear to prescribe tricyclic anti-depressants and benzodiazepines as almost interchangeable drugs in the treatment of depression. However, a search of the literature [32] has failed to support claims that benzodiazepines have any true antidepressant effect. Claims that benzodiazepines cause depression are mainly anecdotal and there is no substantial proof that this is so. Depressive reactions have, however, been described in association with benzodiazepine withdrawal [33], occurring most frequently two to four weeks after withdrawal, in contrast to most other withdrawal symptoms which occurred mainly within the first two post-withdrawal weeks.

LSD, causing distortions of perception, may in vulnerable people be associated with severe disturbances of affect. Depression in association with LSD use is said to be noteworthy for its severity [34]. Similarly extreme forms of anxiety and panic are sometimes encountered in the user of hallucinogenic drugs.

Anxiety is a well recognised withdrawal effect of central nervous system depressants such as chlormethiazole, benzodiazepines and barbiturates. This withdrawal effect is frequently mistaken for the original condition for which these drugs were prescribed or taken, thus setting up a vicious circle of drugtaking, prolonging drug use and increasing the severity of dependence. High doses of cocaine or amphetamines will also cause anxiety, panic attacks and a state of restless agitation. There is anecdotal evidence that cannabis is frequently used for its anxiolytic properties.

Hypomania may be encountered with high doses of CNS stimulant drugs such as are found with repeated freebase or crack smoking. Pemoline-induced mania has also been described. A significantly high occurrence of hypomanic symptoms are associated with cannabis psychoses. However, cannabis use in manic patients appears to modify the symptomatology towards that of a schizophreniform illness [35].

Delirium which is a non-specific response to some intra or extra cerebral toxin, infection, metabolic or other system disturbance may be the result of high dose illicit drug use. The condition is usually reversible but the patient is best treated in a hospital setting.

Flashbacks are a well recognised complication of LSD and other drugs of the psychedelic group. They sometimes occur many years after the drug was last taken and are most commonly disturbances of perception, geometric pseudohallucinations, flashes or intensified colours and trailing phenomena (positive after-images) [36]. Flashbacks have been described as resulting from cannabis use *per se*. However, it is now generally accepted that, in almost every case, cannabis acts as a precipitant of a psychedelic flashback.

Thus, psychosis is a common consequence of illicit drugtaking – a finding which is not surprising in view of the fact that these drugs are taken primarily for their mind-altering properties. Drug dependence on its own is no longer sectionable under the Mental Health Act (1983) although of course a psychosis resultant from drugtaking is encompassed by the Act.

Medical hazards of injecting

Abscesses

Injection abscesses may be sterile or infected. Sterile (cold) abscesses are the result of injecting ground-up tablets such as Diconal, DF118 and methadone where the vein has been missed. Talc, the filler used in these tablets, is highly irritant to the tissues. Sterile abscess formation will occur when it is injected outside a vein.

Diconal causes particularly bad tissue reactions when injected in this way, sometimes with gross oedema of an entire limb or part of a limb e.g. 'boxing glove' hand, and this may last for several months. Barbiturate powder itself, rather than the filler, is also highly irritant to tissues. When a vein is missed, the skin above the injection site will slough off – a 'barb burn' – leaving an ulcer.

Infected (hot) abscesses result from using unsterile techniques, such as tap water to dissolve the drug, or using dirty needles or syringes. Most infected abscesses unless they are very large are best treated by antibiotics rather than lancing, as some drug users may be carriers of, or may be incubating, hepatitis or HIV.

Sterile abscesses are best left to resolve on their own. All ulcers should be cleaned and dressed, making sure that the nurse who does this wears gloves for his/her own protection.

Thrombophlebitis

The irritant effect of talc or barbiturates will also often cause a thrombophlebitis when injected into a vein. Commonly, the seasoned drug user will have used up all the superficial veins in his arms and legs. When this happens other veins may be used, such as the femoral or the jugular vein. The dorsal vein of the penis is not unknown to be used in this respect.

Gangrene

This may occur when a drugtaker injects, for example, barbiturates by mistake into an artery, as this commonly goes into spasm, cutting off the blood supply to the tissues distal to it. This happens most frequently with the femoral artery as a result of its proximity to the femoral vein. Many drug users have had a leg amputated as a consequence of this. All drug users who admit injecting into the femoral vein should be warned of this complication. Similarly, some drug users have had to have fingers amputated.

There are now several known cases where Diconal, after intravenous injection and subsequent circulation round the body, causes isolated arterial spasm and gangrene. The mesenteric artery seems to be particularly prone to this and the optic artery has also been noted to do this in one instance.

Septicaemia

This complication may occur in drug users who inject using unsterile techniques. Septicaemia is a serious illness and should be considered in any drug user who is pyrexial. Those who have a cardiac lesion are of course at special risk of developing subacute bacterial endocarditis.

Hepatitis

Hepatitis in a drugtaker is normally viral in origin, although sometimes a chemical cause may be found.

Drugs or toxins that may cause hepatitis either in overdose or as an idiosyncratic effect include an excess of alcohol, paracetamol overdose (which causes 40% of all cases of severe liver damage) and methyldopa, rifampin, para-aminosalicylic acid, and isoniazid.

Viral Hepatitis

Hepatitis A, B and non-A, non-B have all been shown to be more common in drug users, although there is conflicting evidence about hepatitis A. Several studies, including those from New York [37] and Melbourne [38] showed no increased incidence of hepatitis A but two Swedish studies, one from Gothenburg [39] and the other from Malmo [40] have demonstrated an increased prevalence among drug users.

Hepatitis A

This is spread by the faeco-oral route when there are poor standards of hygiene. The virus has an incubation period of 2-6 weeks. Although it is an unpleasant illness, there is almost invariably full recovery.

There is no carrier state, chronic active hepatitis A does not occur, and acute fulminating hepatitis A is rare. Nausea, anorexia, and jaundice are the usual clinical features. Very high SGOT levels in excess of 1,000 U/l are sometimes seen in the early stages of the illness. Those who contract hepatitis A or any form of viral hepatitis, should be advised to abstain from all alcohol during the course of the illness and for 3 months following recovery. Dietary restriction of fat need only be recommended if fatty foods cause the hepatitis sufferer to feel worse. Those who have been found to have hepatitis A should be advised to be scrupulous about their personal hygiene and to avoid preparing food for consumption by others, particularly if it is uncooked.

Hepatitis B

Prevalence of anti-HBs, a marker of previous infection has been shown to be less than 5% in the general population [41] but as high as 50% in homosexual men and prostitutes [41, 42], and in one study of drug users 88% had serological evidence of previous hepatitis B infection [43]. In this last study only 40% gave a history of hepatitis.

Drugtakers who are injecting with shared needles or syringes or who are involved in male prostitution are at a very high risk of contracting an infection with the hepatitis B virus (HBV). However, heterosexual contact, needlestick injuries, splashes of infectious fluids into the eye or onto mucous membranes may also transmit the virus. These, of course, are the same routes of spread as for human immunodeficiency virus (HIV) although HBV is much more infectious than HIV. HBV is a DNA virus which is unique to man in that it is partly single-stranded. In the viral core it also carries DNA polymerase, which when in an intracellular location is able to complete the DNA to make it fully double-stranded.

In the acute stage of HBV infection, the virus enters the liver cell and utilises intracellular mechanisms for its own replication. It exists free in the nucleus of infected cells but may become integrated with the cell DNA. Hepatocellular carcinoma cells have been shown to contain hepatitis B viral DNA integrated in this way. Carriers of hepatitis B and those with chronic active hepatitis B may also sometimes have integrated DNA. It is thought that such patients are likely to subsequently develop hepatocellular carcinoma.

Analysis of data held at the public health laboratories communicable disease surveillance centre, shows that there was a national epidemic of hepatitis B in the years 1984 and 1985 (see Fig. 3.1). This was reflected locally in many places. Analysis of surveillance forms in Glasgow from 1980–1983 showed an earlier rise in 1982 and 1983 which was due almost entirely to an increase in the number of drugtakers who had developed the illness as opposed to other groups (mainly male homosexuals) in which the incidence of hepatitis B remained almost static [8].

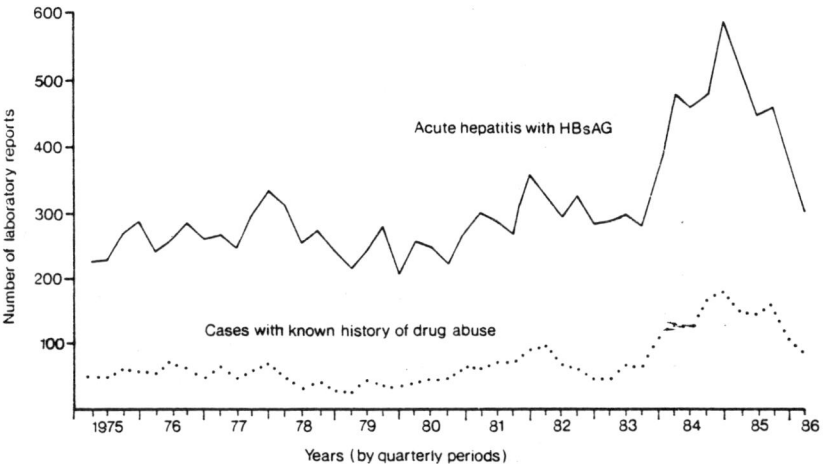

Figure 3.1 Acute hepatitis B: Laboratory reports, England and Wales 1975–1986. (Source: Communicable Disease Surveillance Centre.)

HBV is never spread by ordinary social contact. Infection is usually from contaminated syringes and needles or from male homosexual intercourse. Heterosexual intercourse is a less likely but still possible means of passing on the infection and, in theory, poor techniques of sterilising medical, dental, tattooing and acupuncture equipment may contribute to the spread of the virus. Anyone who has, or is at risk of having, hepatitis B should be advised never to share toothbrushes or razors.

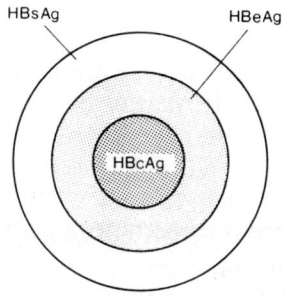

Figure 3.2 Make-up of hepatitis B virus.

The incubation period for this virus is 3–5 months. About two-thirds or more of the infections are anicteric, so a negative history does not exclude previous infection. The hepatitis B virus is made up as shown in Fig. 3.2.

Hepatitis markers

Using radioisotope immunoassay techniques, various hepatitis B markers can be detected in the serum of infected patients. The following are useful in diagnosing and staging the disease:

Table 3.1 Interpretation of results of serological tests for hepatitis B.

HBsAg	HBeAg	Anti-HBe	Anti-HBc IgM	Anti-HBc IgC	Anti-HBs	Interpretation
+	+	−	−	−	−	incubation period
+	+	−	+	+	−	acute hepatitis B or persistent carrier state
+	+	−	−	+	−	persistent carrier state
+	−	+	+/−	+	−	persistent carrier state
−	−	+	+/−	+	+	convalescence
−	−	−	−	+	+	recovery
−	−	−	+	−	−	infection with hepatitis B virus without detectable HBsAg
−	−	−	−	+	−	recovery with loss of detectable anti-HBs
−	−	−	−	−	+	immunisation without infection; repeated exposure to antigen without infection or recovery from infection with loss of detectable anti-HBc

HBsAg: surface antigen (Australia antigen).
HBeAg: e antigen. A crude marker of viral replication. However it is clinically useful as its presence in serum reflects infectivity. Carriers with this marker are at high risk of transmitting HBV.
HBcAg: core antigen. It is in fact HBV DNA. Although a much better marker of viral replication than HBeAg, it is not clinically useful as it is not detectable in serum.
anti-HBs: immunoglobulin antibodies to surface antigen denotes immunity to hepatitis B.

anti-HBe: antibodies to e antigen. The presence of this marker shows that viral replication has stopped.

anti-HBc IgM: macroglobulin antibodies to core antigen. This denotes an acute infection with hepatitis B virus.

anti-HBc IgG: immunoglobulin antibodies to core antigen. This marker is present in both acute hepatitis B infection and the carrier state.

Surface antigen (HBsAg) may be present in three different forms; as the outside coating of the complete virus (Dane particle), as particles which are subunits of this coating, or as filamentous aggregates of these particles. HBsAg may be detectable as early as 1–2 months prior to the onset of jaundice in acute HBV infection. If HBsAg is present for more than 6 months then the patient is either a carrier of hepatitis B or has chronic hepatitis B. Abnormal liver function test point to the latter, but liver biopsy is required to confirm the diagnosis.

Acute hepatitis B is maximally infective just before the onset of jaundice and this stage is sometimes accompanied by an urticarial rash, malaise, and arthralgia. HBsAg, HBeAg, anti-HBc IgM and anti-HBc IgG are all present at this time and when jaundice appears. HBeAg normally disappears within 3 months of symptoms and is replaced by anti-HBe. HBsAg normally disappears 3–5 months from the onset of jaundice and is replaced by anti-HBs. This denotes full recovery from the acute infection and immunity to further encounters with the virus.

Most people with acute hepatitis B have a relatively mild illness. However, about one in a thousand cases develop a *acute fulminant hepatitis B*. In this condition the patient progresses rapidly to liver failure and if this is not spotted before hepatic coma develops, death is said to occur in 80% of cases. A positive HBsAg, transaminase levels of more than 1,000 U/l, and a deteriorating clinical condition should alert the doctor to this possibility. Clinical signs of impending hepatic failure are deep

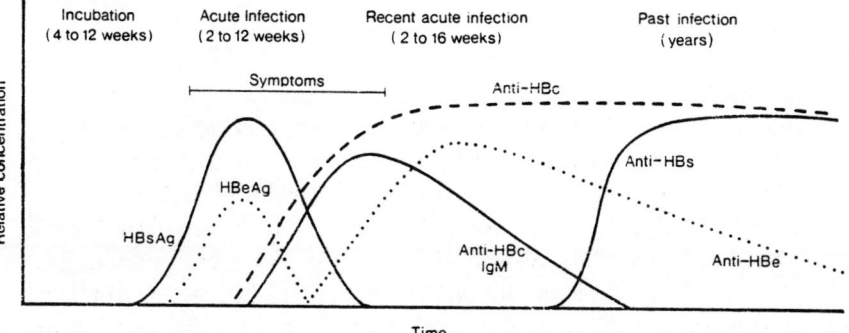

Figure 3.3 Profile of serological markers in typical acute hepatitis B infection.

jaundice, hepatic fetor, bleeding tendency (from prolonged prothrombin time), restlessness, dehydration, and impairment of consciousness.

Carriers of hepatitis B

In 5% of infected individuals, usually those with anicteric infections, HBsAg does not disappear from the serum. Diagnosis of the carrier state may be made when HBsAg has been present for more than six months. Some carriers also have persistent HBeAg markers and these patients are highly infectious. These so-called supercarriers sometimes occur in the absence of HBeAg if anti-HBe is also not detectable. Supercarriers do not remain highly infectious indefinitely. After a period varying from five to twenty years, the HBeAg disappears and is replaced by anti-HBe. The patient is then said to have low infectivity.

Chronic active hepatitis B

In this condition there is a chronic low grade hepatitis, progressing after a number of years to liver failure and death in 25–50% of cases. It is usually, but not always, accompanied by abnormal liver function tests and there may be a history of recurrent attacks of jaundice. The diagnosis is confirmed by liver biopsy. Normally about one-third of all carriers have chronic active hepatitis B.

There is a close link between chronic active hepatitis B and delta agent [44] infection which is sometimes also known as hepatitis D. The delta agent is an incomplete RNA virus which will replicate only in the presence of HBV. The RNA core is contained within a shell of delta antigen and the virus is completed by a covering of HBsAg. There is now no doubt that the presence of the delta agent considerably worsens the prognosis of hepatitis B. In the acute stage fulminant hepatitis is more likely. Twice the number of carriers will develop chronic active hepatitis in the presence of delta virus and 20% of these will progress to cirrhosis.

Unlike the clinically similar autoimmune chronic active hepatitis, treatment with corticosteroids alone, with few exceptions, is of no benefit. It probably serves only to potentiate viral replication delaying the loss of HBeAg from the serum, and is associated with clinical deterioration.

In combination with some viricidal drugs, however, such as vidarabine monophosphate, corticosteroids, if used as a pre-treatment, both increase the rate of seroconversion to anti-HBe, notifying inhibition of viral replication, and reduce side effects.

Treatment with interferons is theoretically very attractive because, not only do they have direct antiviral activity themselves, but they also enhance the body's own natural defence mechanisms against viruses. A hepatitis-like illness occurs three months after treatment and is followed by seroconversion from HBeAg to anti-HBe. A high proportion of cases seroconvert in this way, interferons seem to be currently the best treatment available for chronic active hepatitis B.

There are now a number of specialist centres in the UK involved in the treatment of this condition. If possible referral should be made at an early stage in the hope of treating the condition before substantial integration of viral DNA sequences occurs within the nucleus of the liver cell, with a view to reducing the future incidence of hepatocellular carcinoma.

Immunisation against hepatitis B

Passive immunisation
Intramuscular hyperimmune gamma globulin will provide some protection if given within 48 hours of possible infection. Carers who may have been accidentally pricked by a contaminated needle or bitten by a carrier should be considered for this.

Active immunisation
Active immunisation against hepatitis B has been available in Britain since 1982 and gives good antibody levels in 90% of cases. It is a course of 3 injections and should not be given to those who are pregnant or who are trying to conceive. Two weeks following the course of injections, patients receiving them should be tested for anti-HBs to confirm that they are immune. This vaccine is at present quite expensive but cheaper vaccines, derived from yeasts and synthetic polypeptides, will be produced in the near future. Highly purified surface antigen is used to stimulate antibody production (anti-HBs). Immunity to hepatitis B produced in this way will also prevent the completion of the delta agent by surface antigen, thus confirming a double immunity. Before they are offered active immunisation, patients at risk should always be tested for antibodies to surface antigen (anti-HBs) to ensure that they are not already immune.

In October 1982 the Joint Committee on Vaccination and Immunisation issued a summary of recommendations as to who should be vaccinated. Given the high cost of the vaccine, it was felt that its use should be restricted to health care personnel, patients in residential institutions for the mentally handicapped, renal dialysis patients, and spouses or other sexual contacts of HBV carriers who are anti-HBe negative.

At the time of writing new guidelines on the recipients of hepatitis B vaccine are about to be issued. It is hoped that these will include male homosexuals and intravenous drug users who have the greatest risk of contracting the disease.

Combined passive : active immunisation at birth
All infants born to HB carrier mothers (HBsAg positive), whatever the 'e' antigen/antibody status, should be given combined passive:active immunisation as soon as possible after birth. The doses given should be:

(a) hepatitis B vaccine 0.5 ml intramuscularly (active immunisation);
(b) hepatitis B immunoglobulin 2.0 ml intramuscularly (passive immunisation). Active immunisation only should be repeated at one month and six months of age.

Non-A, non-B hepatitis

At least two viruses are classified under this heading. It is diagnosed by exclusion when tests for both hepatitis A and hepatitis B are negative, and it may be as prevalent among drug users as is hepatitis B. The route of spread is similar to HBV infection, the main modes of transmission being via dirty needles and there is as yet no evidence that it is spread by either homosexual and heterosexual contact. As there is no screening test for this form of hepatitis, it may sometimes be transmitted by blood transfusion and accounts for 90% of all cases of post-transfusion hepatitis.

Chronic active hepatitis non-A non-B also occurs and is said to be more common than hepatitis B. There is considerable evidence that the infection may be followed in many patients by prolonged viraemia and the development of a persistent carrier state. Chronic liver damage may occur in as many as 40–50% of cases [45].

The masking of intercurrent illness

It is important to remember that drug users do have a high morbidity and may be suffering from other illnesses besides their drug dependence. Septicaemia may be masked by the sweating that accompanies withdrawals, so it is important to exclude a high pyrexia.

Drug users may think that they are feeling unwell because of their lifestyle and drug use when in reality they are incubating hepatitis. They may think that their stomach cramps are caused by opioid withdrawal when they have appendicitis. Head injuries occurring during a state of intoxication with drugs or drink, or sustained during a convulsion, may not be remembered.

Drug users do need doctors to attend to their physical illnesses. Too often GPs see users as people who are asking for a prescription for drugs for their addiction and not as people who may be ill.

AIDS

The Acquired Immune Deficiency Syndrome (AIDS) is poorly named as it is only one of a number of acquired human diseases that provoke a deficient immune response. The causative agent is Human Immunodeficiency Virus (HIV), a retrovirus with the ability to convert RNA to DNA – the reverse of normal. It acts by preferentially infecting T-helper (T4) lymphocytes resulting in their functional depletion. Consequent to this the cell-mediated immune response becomes impaired, although T-suppressor (T8) lymphocytes remain virtually unchanged and the humoral system is relatively unaffected. The virus was discovered in 1983. More recently a new variant, HIV-II, has been isolated in patients with West African connections.

Routes of transmission and epidemiology

Like the virus that causes hepatitis B (HBV), HIV is found in body fluids and has been isolated from semen, cervical secretions, lymphocytes, cell-free plasma, cerebrospinal fluid, tears, saliva, urine, and breast milk. However, infection is less easily transmitted than with HBV although the routes are similar: infection by contaminated needles and sexual, particularly male homosexual, intercourse being the common routes of spread. There is no evidence that spread has occurred from saliva, by mosquitoes, lice or bed bugs, in swimming pools, by sharing cups and eating or cooking utensils, or by ordinary face to face contact. Among seropositive people, heterosexual spread from men to women has a slightly higher rate of transmission than from women to men but women with AIDS are still more likely than not to infect their male partner. Although the evidence so far is by no means conclusive and needs urgent clarification, it would appear that most heterosexual transmission occurs at two separate phases of the disease. The first is the initial phase just after a person becomes infected and while there is an accompanying viraemia. Then, following seroconversion, the virus hides within the cells out of reach of the body's immune defences. During this phase of being seropositive but well, heterosexual transmission is unlikely to occur. A recent study on the partners of a small number of seropositive haemophiliacs [46] suggests that heterosexual transmission then reoccurs with the development of the AIDS related complex (ARC) or AIDS. Presumably the failing immune system allows significant viraemia to be established and people become more infectious at this stage.

This however does not apply to all cases and it appears that sometimes heterosexual transmission can occur from the seropositive well. It may also be that, just as with hepatitis B, supercarriers for HIV can occur who are highly infectious. It would therefore be very unwise to abandon counselling safe sex to the well seropositive patient during the latent phase of infection. Further research clearly needs to be done as a matter of urgency.

Recent work published by Masters, Johnson and Kolodny in a book entitled *Crisis; Heterosexual Behaviour in the Age of AIDS* (publishers : Weidenfeld and Nicholson) suggests that heterosexual spread of HIV infection within the ordinary heterosexual community in America has occurred to a greater extent than has been hitherto recognised and that this community has not changed its sexual behaviour pattern to the extent that is needed to halt the rapid spread of the disease.

Vertical transmission from an infected mother to her baby can occur, both *in utero* and at birth. A few cases worldwide have been recorded where infection has occurred via the breast milk. Blood, organs and tissues from an infected person are also capable of transmitting the disease and anyone who has HIV antibodies should be warned neither to give blood nor to donate their organs and tissues.

In most countries, including Britain and the United States, heterosexual spread occurs through bisexual men, infected drug users and prostitutes. The role which drug misuse plays in the spread of AIDS is now being recognised as far more critical than was previously acknowledged. A study in New York [47] has shown that 87% of those who contracted HIV infection heterosexually did so from contact with drug users who inject. To some extent this reflects the fact that as in Edinburgh, HIV infection is mainly within the drug-using population of this city. In San Francisco, however where the epidemic among male homosexuals has dwarfed the epidemic among injecting drug users, very little heterosexual spread has occurred [48]. The risk of heterosexual transmission from seropositive bisexual men is said to be 14%

[49] whereas the risk to the wives of infected haemophiliacs is 6.8-9.5% [50, 51] and the risk to the partners of seropositive drug users 15% [52]. Although the risk of heterosexual transmission from seropositive drug users is difficult to define with any clarity. However, Moss points out [48] that three-quarters of those who have contracted AIDS heterosexually in the United States have done so from index cases who were injecting drug users. The main route of spread of HIV infection into the general heterosexual population in the United States is thus via those who inject drugs and it can be anticipated to be the same in Britain.

Spread within the general population has already occurred to an alarming degree in central Africa [49-52] and the male to female ratio of cases is virtually 1:1. This suggests that the main routes of spread are by heterosexual and vertical transmission of the virus. Surveys from some African countries show that the prevalence of infection is high among certain groups – 80-90% of prostitutes, 30% of their male clients, 30% of those attending departments for sexually transmitted diseases, 10% of blood donors, and 10% of women attending antenatal clinics [49]. Although these high levels of infection were originally confined to central Africa, the virus is now spreading out to involve the entire continent and the outlook is appalling to countenance. It has been suggested that the AIDS virus originated in Africa and was spread by European travellers [57, 58].

The American HIV epidemic had first of all been thought to originate in Haiti and this had unleashed a flurry of prejudice against Haitians. In a similar way prejudice was subsequently aimed against the African community. In this country a proposal was made that people from sub-Saharan Africa wishing to enter the United Kingdom should be screened for AIDS. National Front propaganda described black people as 'AIDS carriers', and there was a damaging loss of revenue from tourism throughout Africa.

Although the first recognised cases of AIDS occurred in 1981 in the USA, retrospective testing of stored blood has shown a specimen from Central Africa with HIV antibodies as far back as 1959. Clearly the disease remained unrecognised for several years. There is now recognised to be a worldwide pandemic and the World Health Organisation (WHO) is quoted as describing AIDS as 'the greatest public health disaster ever' [58].

Although in some areas, such as Scotland, the main source of HIV infection has been through injecting drug use, in general the first wave of infection in Britain, as in the United States, has occurred in male homosexuals. Injecting drug use is likely to be an important, if not the main route whereby a second wave of HIV infection will occur in the general heterosexual population.

There are at any one time 25 times more people infected with the virus than have AIDS and in this country the number of cases of AIDS doubles every eight months. The doubling time for drug users appears to be faster than for other groups. Although the doubling time has slowed in North America since 1981-2, this slowing should not detract from projected trends. By 1991 it is estimated that there will be 270,000 cases of frank AIDS in the United States [60]. In October 1987 there were 1123 cases of AIDS in the UK and worldwide there had been 60,000 cases reported with an estimation by WHO that five to ten million people had been infected. Projecting from this figure WHO have estimated that by 1992 half to three million deaths will have occurred from AIDS.

In Britain the epidemic started two to three years later than in the United States, but the number of cases reported to the Communicable Disease Surveillance Centre at Colindale (Table 3.2) shows a similar logarithmic rise to that in America.

The proportion of AIDS cases who are drug injectors has slowly risen in America and in September 1987 totalled 25% (8% of these

Table 3.2 AIDS UK: Cases and deaths by year of report to CDSC and CD(S)U. (Courtesy of the Public Health Laboratory.)

Year of report	No. of cases	No. of deaths
1982	3	3
1983	26	26
1984	77	73
1985	160	125
1986	305	212
1987	656	258
Total	1227	697

were also male homosexuals). In Britain it was still only 3% (1.5% being male homosexuals) at that time. This low level in Britain will almost certainly rise rapidly, for 16% of those with antibodies to HIV have a history of past or present drug use as did 58% of those tested in Scotland.

The proportion of drug users who are seropositive was 8% in England, Wales and Northern Ireland in August 1987 compared to 61% in Scotland.

There is a large regional variation in seropositivity. In New York up to 87% of drug users have been shown to have HIV antibodies [61] compared to 1.7% in California [62]. A study in Edinburgh from 1985-86 [63] showed a 52% seroposivity rate in drugtakers compared to 4.5% in Glasgow [64].

The high rate of prevalence among injecting drug users in Edinburgh was first demonstrated in blood samples sent from suspected injecting drug misusers attending the Edinburgh Royal Infirmary [65] when 38% were found to be seropositive. Then even higher figures were published from drug users attending an Edinburgh general practice. Robertson and Bucknall [66] did a retrospective testing of samples taken to look for evidence of hepatitis. They showed that the AIDS virus was introduced into a community of drug users in or around August 1983. By March 1985, 51% of 164 intravenous drug users were known to be infected. This steep rise from nought to over 50% within two years has also occurred in parts of Italy and Spain.

In Europe as a whole, the proportion of cases of AIDS in drug users rose from 2% in 1984 to 17% in mid-1987. At that time three countries – France, Italy and Spain – accounted for 85% of all AIDS cases [67]. In Italy and Spain 61% and 53% respectively of cases involved drug users. In these countries, serological surveys, often on a small scale, have revealed a prevalence of HIV infection among drug users of up to 70% although large regional variations can occur. There are many reasons for these variations including the date of introduction of the virus.

Vertical transmission is now occurring to a significant degree in many countries mainly to the children of drug users. At the time of writing (November 1987) 80 babies had been born in the UK with antibodies to HIV in their blood. The presence of antibodies in babies is not an accurate guide to infection but some of these babies have died.

The natural history of HIV infection

(1) Acute HIV infection (Group I)
Usually acute infection with the virus is asymptomatic but when symptoms do occur they are normally non-specific such as malaise, lethargy, myalgia, arthralgia, fever, sore throat, and lymphadenopathy. Rarely more serious symptoms do occur and an acute, but reversible, encephalopathy, meningitis, and neuropathy have been decribed. Seroconversion accompanies the phase of acute infection and HIV antibodies appear three weeks to three months after exposure to the virus. The presence of HIV antibodies does not

Table 3.3 New CDC classification of HIV infection.

Group	I	–	Acute infection
	II	–	Asymptomatic infection
	III	–	Persistent Generalised Lymphadenopathy
	IV	–	Other disease:
Subgroup		A	– Constitutional disease
		B	– Neurological disease
		C	– Secondary infectious disease
		C1	– As defined for AIDS
		C2	– Others
		D	– Secondary cancers
		E	– Other conditions

mean that the body has developed immunity to the virus and infection should be regarded as being life-long. For this reason it will be four or five decades before we know accurately the percentage of those infected who will progress to AIDS. Until recently it has been believed that up to 35% of seropositive people will develop the syndrome but some studies have now shown that given time the vast majority of patients will show deterioration in their immune system and it is possible that all may go on to develop AIDS at some stage.

(2) Chronic HIV infection (Groups II–IV)

Although the latent phase prior to the development of AIDS is often asymptomatic, signs of chronic infection with the virus do sometimes appear as recognisable syndromes prior to the development of AIDS. These are:

(a) persistent generalised lymphadenopathy (PGL);
(b) AIDS related complex (ARC);
(c) neurological manifestations of HIV;
(d) minor infections and skin conditions.

It is thought that apart from (d), up to 40% of seropositive people have these AIDS related conditions within 5 years of infection.

(a) Persistent generalised lymphadenopathy (PGL). The definition of this syndrome is 'enlarged nodes at least one centimetre in diameter in two or more (non-contiguous) extrainguinal sites that persist for at least three months in the absence of any current illness or medication known to cause enlarged nodes'.

These nodes are most commonly found in the head and neck region at the anterior border of the sternomastoid, in the posterior triangle, and in the submandibular region. Axillary nodes are also commonly found. Splenomegaly occurs in about one third of patients and up to 30% progress to AIDS within 5 years.

(b) AIDS related complex (ARC). Patients sometimes have the signs and symptoms of AIDS in the absence of the opportunistic infections or tumours necessary to make a diagnosis of AIDS. In order to diagnose ARC two or more symptoms and signs must be present for at least three months and be accompanied by two or more abnormal laboratory tests.

Symptoms/signs

- Intermittent or continuous fever of more than 38°C.
- Weight loss of more than ten per cent.
- Lymph nodes: PGL.
- Intermittent or continuous diarrhoea.
- Fatigue that reduces physical activity.

Laboratory abnormalities

- Lymphopoenia/leucopoenia.
- Thrombocytopoenia.
- Reduced T4/T8 ratio (>2S.D.).
- Reduced T helper cells (>2S.D.).
- Reduced blastogenesis.
- Raised γ globulins.
- Cutaneous energy.

ARC was of particular importance in helping clinicians make a diagnosis of HIV infection before a reliable test was discovered. The symptoms of ARC often cause as much distress to patients as do the symptoms of AIDS. The majority, if not all, of people with ARC go on to develop AIDS within 3 years. Weight loss of more than 10% body weight and persistent diarrhoea are now included in the Centre for Disease Control (CDC) definition of AIDS for surveillance purposes.

(c) Neurological complications of HIV infection. These appear to be common but because they are long term, taking several years to develop, tend to go unrecognised in the majority of patients. They may well be of increasing importance in seropositive patients who do not develop AIDS. They include subacute encephalitis, subacute vacuolar myelopathy, peripheral neuropathy, and chronic atypical aseptic meningitis.

Nearly a third of those with AIDS have been found to have a subacute encephalitis, and although a few have been found to be due to disseminated cytomegalovirus infection of the brain, the vast majority have been attributed to HIV itself. Subacute encephalitis is the most common complication of HIV. It has an insidious clinical onset with subtle cognitive changes but over a period of years progresses to a severe dementia associated with cerebral atrophy. HIV dementia has since September 1987 been included in the CDC classification of AIDS (Group IV).

Other neurological manifestations of HIV infection also occur. The next most common is subacute vacuolar myelopathy, which is found in 25% of cases of AIDS at necropsy. Clinical features of this condition include slowly progressive motor and/or sensory disturbances, often presenting as weakness of the legs and paraesthesiae and progressing slowly to eventual ataxia and incontinence.

Peripheral neuropathy and atypical aseptic meningitis are less common neurological complications of HIV infection.

(d) Minor infections and skin conditions. Viral, fungal, and bacterial infections are common in seropositive patients who do not fit into any of the recognised syndromes of HIV infection. They are a general sign of lowered host immunity. Hairy leukoplakia and seborrhoeic dermatitis are also sometimes seen.

(3)AIDS

There are two main clinical manifestations of AIDS: tumours and opportunistic infection. *Pneumocystis carinii* pneumonia is the commonest opportunistic infection in the UK, and Kaposi's sarcoma is the commonest tumour. The prevalence of the different presentations of AIDS in 1987 was as shown in Table 3.4.

Table 3.4

Disease category	Percentage of AIDS cases	
	UK	USA
Pneumocystis carinii pneumonia	46	64
Other opportunistic infections	24	22
Kaposi's sarcoma	21	14
Kaposi's sarcoma + *P. carinii* pneumonia	7	
Other tumours	2	

There is a higher frequency of Kaposi's sarcoma in homosexual men with AIDS than in injecting drug users. This may reflect the organisms latent in the host. It has been suggested that the high frequency of cytomegalovirus (CMV) infection in homosexual men, in whom CMV may be sexually transmitted, may account for the differing clinical spectrum of disease between these two patient groups. Although the evidence that CMV is the causative agent of Kaposi's sarcoma is at best circumstantial, we can expect our overall spectrum of disease in the British AIDS patients to change to become more in line with that of the United States as the proportion of AIDS cases who are injecting drugtakers rises.

Before the appearance of AIDS, Kaposi's sarcoma was a rare single vascular tumour generally found in elderly Jewish men. Its course was slow and patients often died of an unrelated condition. Occasionally it was also seen in immuno-suppressed patients, such as those undergoing renal transplant surgery.

In AIDS patients, Kaposi's sarcoma usually presents with multi-focal tumours which develop rapidly. At first these are small flat dusky red areas of skin discolouration, which progress over a period of weeks or months to painless raised nodules or plaques. They may occur anywhere on the skin. On the trunk they tend to be elongated and follow the skin cleavage lines. They also occur in the gastrointestinal tract and lung. Although generally accepted as being malignant, Kaposi's sarcoma does not appear to be spread by the blood stream or lymphatic channels, and the multi-focal way in which new lesions develop is not well understood. Very rarely haemorrhage from an intrapulmonary or intraabdominal tumour may be life-threatening, but apart from this, patients do not die from Kaposi's sarcoma. Rather, these tumours are an indication that the immune system has reached a stage where it has broken down. The mean survival time for those who have developed Kaposi's sarcoma is 21.2 months.

Occasionally other tumours such as non-Hodgkin's lymphoma and squamous carcinomas of the mouth and anorectum occur, but relative to Kaposi's sarcoma these are rare.

Pneumocystis carinii pneumonia (PCP) is by far the commonest opportunistic infection. It typically presents with breathlessness and dry cough, both of which symptoms persist for a six to eight week period. Commonly patients complain that they are unable to take a deep breath. There is invariably an associated fever, although the patient may not feel hot. A chest X-ray will confirm the diagnosis and the patient should be rapidly admitted to hospital. Thirty per cent of patients do not survive the first attack and the mean survival time in the UK for those with *P. carinii* pneumonia is 12.5 months. In those that do survive the initial attack subsequent attacks may be prevented by prophylactic co-trimoxanzole (2 tablets/day) or Fansidar (1 tablet/week). Recently nebulised pentamidine has shown promise as a prophylactic against PCP.

Although the number and type of opportunistic infections that can appear in AIDS is increasing all the time, the most common infections

Table 3.5. The most common infections occurring with AIDS. (From *ABC of AIDS* edited by M. W. Adler, 1987. BMA.)

Syndrome	Features	Common organisms			
		Protozoa	Viruses	Bacteria	Fungi
Lung	Cough, shortness of breath, fever, hypoxia Chest x-ray infiltrates	*P. carinii* pneumonia	Cytomegalovirus Herpes simplex virus	Mycobacteria* Gram positive *Str. pneumoniae* *H. influenzae* *B. catarrhalis* Group B streptococcus	Cryptococcus
Central nervous system	Meningitis/ encephalitis or focal signs	Toxoplasma	Cytomegalovirus Herpes simplex virus Progressive multifocal leucoencephalopathy (papovavirus)	Mycobacteria*	Aspergillus Cryptococcus Candida
Gut	Dysphagia High volume diarrhoea Bloody diarrhoea/colitis	Cryptosporidium Isospora belli Microsporidia	Cytomegalovirus Herpes simplex virus	*Mycobacterium avium intracellulare* *M. tuberculosis* Salmonella	Candida
Pyrexia of undetermined origin	Fever Weight loss± lymphadenopathy		Consider all pathogens and focal or disseminated infection		

M. tuberculosis and atypical mycobacteria.

that occur in this country are as shown in Table 3.5

Co-factors

What it is that makes some people with HIV infection progress to AIDS, while others appear to be well, is not clearly understood at this time. Nevertheless it is generally accepted that there must be a number of co-factors responsible. The current view is that the following are worthy of consideration as co-factors:

(a) Continued injecting drug use
Injecting high levels of street drugs has been shown by Des Jarlais [47] to be associated with increased rates of HIV-related immunosuppression (T4 cell loss) in seropositive drug users. Recent unpublished work by Brettle [68] in Edinburgh has shown that treating injecting drug users with oral methadone improves their immune status with the implication that frequent antigenic stimulus from injecting impure and unsterile drugs hastens the outset of AIDS. Low T4 counts in injecting drug users may well have adverse consequences for public as well as individual health, for there appears to be an increased rate of

transmission to the heterosexual partners of seropositive patients when the T4 count falls below 200/c.m.m. [46]. Thus prescribing oral methadone to opioid injectors not only reduces the risk of their contracting and spreading HIV if they are seronegative, but this evidence suggests that it will also reduce the risk of infectivity and the progression to AIDS if they are seropositive.

(b) Infections
Current research suggests that exposure of cells infected with HIV to other infectious agents leads to viral replication of HIV thus reactivating the disease. It would seem from this, that those seropositive individuals who take the trouble to look after their personal health are less likely to develop AIDS than those who neglect themselves. It is believed that those infections which of their own accord lower the T4 count are likely to be the most damaging. Infections that do this include the Epstein-Barr virus, CMV, viral hepatitis, and some sexually transmitted diseases [69, 70, 71, 72].

This combination of reactivating HIV infection at a time when the T4 count is low will also increase the risk of spread into the community by increasing the infectivity of the virus. Thus avoiding hepatitis by using sterile, or at least clean, injecting equipment and avoiding sexually transmitted disease by using safe sex techniques, not only protects a seronegative individual and improves the prognosis for those who are seropositive; it also protects the community at large.

Other factors
There are a number of other factors that in themselves cause mild cellular immunosuppression and depress the T4 count. Until recently the general advice was that anything that is likely to suppress the immune system should be avoided whenever possible on the theoretical grounds that this could accelerate the development of AIDS. However, the picture is now less clear. Pregnancy, which is well known to suppress the immune system, was originally thought to worsen the prognosis of a seropositive woman but the evidence is now conflicting. Cyclosporin A, an immunosuppressant, appears to have some beneficial effects on HIV infection. Thus, no definite statement can at present be made about factors that will mildly depress the T4 count but some of these are of considerable importance in relation to drug misuse and need urgent clarification.

Factors that are known to impair T-cell function include liver disease in general, anxiety and depression, chronic heavy drinking [73], cannabis and opiates. The inhibition of T-cell function by cannabinoids is relatively short-lived, returning to normal after 72 hours [74]. T-cell depression in opioid users is longer lasting and is present for at least three weeks following cessation of heroin use [75]. The mechanism through which this occurs is not completely clear but opiate receptors have been shown to be present on lymphocytes [76, 77] and lymphocyte populations are thought to be regulated by endogenous opiates [78] accounting for the impairment of T cell function in those suffering from anxiety and stress.

A number of chemicals have been shown to transform lymphocytes and this finding has been useful as an *in vitro* test of lymphocyte function. Brown *et al.* [79] have shown that lymphocytes from heroin users had impaired responsiveness to pokeweed mitogen. Lymphocyte transformation response to pokeweed mitogen has recently been shown to be a very sensitive short-term predictive marker for the development of AIDS and AIDS-related symptoms in homosexual men with HIV antibodies (80), but clearly this could not be used as a predictive test on heroin users.

White *et al.* [81] found no difference in the *in vitro* responsiveness to pokeweed mitogen between lymphocyte cultures from cannabis smokers and non-smokers, so this test is unlikely to be invalidated by cannabis smoking. This is just as well as cannabis smoking appears to be common in male homosexuals. An early study of homosexual AIDS patients in San Francisco found that more smoked marijuana than smoked tobacco [82]. Cannabis and opioids do not appear to summate in their effect on lymphocytes. It has been suggested that cannabinoids may be unable to impair further a response that is already maximally inhibited by opioids [75].

We then come to the question: does opioid use *per se* alter the prognosis of drugtakers with HIV antibodies? At present we do not know the answer to this. As noted above we do have evidence that a change from injecting heroin to oral methadone is helpful not only for the individual drugtaker but for society at large. Current work in America is looking at methadone itself to see whether it is deleterious or beneficial to HIV infection. If it is found to be more deleterious than abstinence then one way forward might be through the opioid antagonists as naxolone has been shown to reverse the opioid suppression of lymphocytes [72]. However, whether or not naltrexone also does this has yet to be determined.

Clearly there are many questions still to answer. Should we be counselling HIV positive drug users that taking cannabis and/or opiate drugs may increase their chances of developing AIDS? What is the position with regard to prescribed opioids and over-the-counter sales of these drugs, bearing in mind the fact that paracetamol, aspirin, and non-steroidal anti-inflammatory agents are the only analgesics that are not opioids? These are important questions and until they are answered it is reasonable to say in the light of Brettie's work that, both for their own benefit and for society at large, heroin and other opioid injectors should be encouraged to take oral methadone, but that abstinence should not be disregarded as a treatment goal.

Needle exchange schemes

In the light of the HIV epidemic and its importance in drug users, the government responded initially in two ways: first by an advertising campaign in 1987 with the message 'Don't inject AIDS' and aimed particularly at young people, and second by setting up 15 experimental needle exchange schemes around the country. Several unofficial schemes had already been set up following their apparent success in Amsterdam, one of the first in the UK at Dr Roy Robertson's practice in Edinburgh. Those that came within the government's scheme were researched [83]. Findings after the first 7 months showed that it was mainly the older age group of injectors that were attending and that the schemes were not generally attracting young injectors. Only 9% of clients were in the 15–19 year age band, although 32% were in the 20–24 year age band. The average time lapse between first injection and coming to the scheme was 7.7 years. This is more than twice as long as the average time lapse between the onset of heroin use and first attendance at a DDU for treatment.

The male to female ratio was approximately four to one. The schemes were attracting some amphetamine users and two-thirds of all attenders had no current contact with the treatment service. About one-third had *never* had contact with the treatment service and the schemes were clearly reaching a section of the drug using population that was not reached by other services. This in itself justified their continuation as part of the network of services designed to limit the spread of AIDS. Some schemes reported having to deal with an unexpected amount of primary health care and social work problems. One-third of all attenders admitted to sharing equipment in the last month and, as had been found in other services, greater changes in injecting practices away from sharing were reported than changes in sexual practice. Some schemes were clearly more attractive to clients than others. To some extent attractiveness depended on access and location but an atmosphere of 'user friendliness' appeared to be important.

For some schemes there were adverse local factors; for example, a continuing picket of local residents outside the Glasgow scheme clearly prevented many drug users attending. In Scotland, as there was some question as to whether syringe exchange would break the law, the Lord Advocate's office had issued a ruling to allow it but had stated that a maximum of three syringes only could be given at a time. This is thought by some to be the main contributory factor for the failure of the Scottish schemes.

Those needle exchange schemes that seem to be the most popular, such as the one in Liverpool, often give 20 or more syringes at a time and do not insist on counselling or a one-for-one equipment exchange. Rather they act as a needle and syringe bank with a flexible credit and debit system. Some schemes too have managed to achieve cooperation from the local police, with an agreement not to get involved with drug-takers in the vicinity of the clinic.

Recommendations for change

Two committees were set up to look specifically at the problems of drug misuse and AIDS in the UK. The first was the Scottish Committee on HIV Infection and Intravenous Drug Misuse, known as the McClelland Committee. Its report [84] in September 1986 stated the important principle that the threat to life of the spread of HIV infection is greater than that of drug misuse and the prevention of spread should take priority over any perceived risk of increased drug misuse. Among its recommendations were:

(1) Health Boards should ensure that all provisions in their area for dealing with drug users were adequate.
(2) They should actively promote syringe and needle exchange and substitution prescribing and encourage GPs to do this.
(3) A clinician should be identified in each Health Board with overall responsibility for drug misuse problems (for large Health Boards this would entail new appointments).
(4) Resource centres for HIV infection should be established.

The second committee on drug misuse and AIDS was set up by the Advisory Council on the Misuse of Drugs (ACMD) and prepared to make two reports. The first, completed in December 1987, was mainly concerned with the prevention of the spread of HIV infection through injecting drug use. The second is to concentrate more on the pattern and type of services needed when the AIDS epidemic has arrived.

The first ACMD report [85] stated a number of basic principles:

'(1) The spread of HIV is a greater danger to individual and public health than drug misuse. Accordingly we believe that services

which aim to minimise risk-laden behaviour by all available means should take precedence in development plans over those which seek solely to decrease drug misuse.
(2) We must therefore be prepared to work with those who continue to misuse drugs to help them reduce the risks involved in doing so, above all the risk of acquiring or spreading HIV.
(3) A change in public and professional attitudes is necessary as attitudes and policies which lead to drug misuse remaining hidden will impair the effectiveness of measures to combat the spread of HIV.
(4) We emphasise that prevention of drug misuse is now more important than ever before and in the longer run the success or failure of efforts to prevent young people from embarking on a career of drug misuse will have a major effect on our ability to contain the spread of HIV.'

Overall the report recommended a new approach to services. It emphasised that in the light of HIV, contact needs to be made not only with those problem drugtakers who are seeking help but also with the larger number of drugtakers who are not known to the treatment services. These include occasional users and those who still enjoy taking drugs. The term 'problem drug use' is now extended to include anyone who is at risk of contracting or spreading HIV through their drug use. Up to this time treatment services have concentrated almost exclusively on opioid users. Now those taking a wide number of other drugs by injection, including amphetamines, cocaine, benzodiazepines, barbiturates, and some others such as cyclizine, need to be reached.

This implies not only an expansion of existing services but also a change away from the standard approach of waiting for a drugtaker to be motivated to seek help. Outreach work is needed and because of the difficulties of making contact with the client group, prostitutes and former injecting drugtakers were recommended to provide information about HIV and safer practices.

The report recommended each Health District to have a community-based service for drugtakers with back-up support from hospital-based specialist services, these in turn to be backed up by further specialist support at regional level.

GPs were seen as playing a very important role. The report stated: 'We conclude that the advent of HIV makes it essential that all GPs should provide care and advice for drug misusing patients to help them move away from behaviour which may result in them acquiring and spreading the virus.'

GP involvement was already noted to be greater where support was available through community drug teams or other specialist drug services. Often GPs would also prescribe opiate substitutes if there was back-up counselling for the drug user through community drug teams. The report recommended that Health Authorities should ensure that appropriate support is available for GPs and that GPs should be made aware of it.

Training on the problem and management of drug use was recommended for all GPs at undergraduate level both during the three-year vocational training period and for established practitioners on a regular basis. Short-term clinical attachments to local specialist drug services were recommended to help build up a pool of general practitioners with experience. The White Paper *Promoting Better Health* had recommended a new postgraduate educational allowance for GPs and the report suggested that approved training courses should include the topic of drug misuse.

The advent of HIV forces prescribing to serve two wider purposes apart from direct treatment: first, to attract more drug misusers and keep them in contact with services and, second, to facilitate changes away from HIV risk practices. With this in mind there is now a hierarchy of goals in prescribing:

(a) a cessation of sharing of equipment;
(b) the move from injectable to oral drug use;
(c) a decrease in drug use;
(d) abstinence.

GPs have an important role to play in limiting the spread of HIV partly because of their capacity to prescribe, but also because of their accessibility, lack of stigma, and ability to provide a network of support and continuing care not only for the drug user but also for his/her family. They are well placed to intervene effectively at an early stage.

The place of the GP in relation to other services for drug misusers was clearly outlined in the report:

'... we see a clear analogy with other areas of health care. For example, GPs see it as within their remit to prescribe digoxin and propranolol to appropriate patients with heart disease, but require access to secondary level services for second opinions, investigations, and onward referral of more difficult cases. Thus we consider GPs should be equipped to deal with short term detoxifications and medium term withdrawal regimes in cooperation with Community Drug Teams or with support from voluntary sector agencies. More difficult cases may well require support from, or referral to, local specialist District provision including Community Drug Teams and the district psychiatrist with a special responsibility for drug misuse.'

This is a major change away from the Treatment and Rehabilitation Report of the Advisory Council which had only five years earlier stated that because hospital services could not be expected to provide a comprehensive service to drug users there was 'a possible role for some doctors outside the specialist services to play a part in the treatment of problem drugtakers ...'

GPs therefore are now seen as playing a central role in making treatment more accessible to drugtakers. Recommendations were also made in the AIDS and Drug Misuse report to improve accessibility to the specialist treatment services by reducing waiting times, changing opening hours, and shortening lengthy assessment procedures.

If the goals of prescribing are not being achieved then multidisciplinary teams should assess behaviour and behavioural changes. For GPs this would normally imply onward referral to a specialist. GPs should not normally prescribe injectable drugs. Cases where this is to be considered should be managed by, or with guidance from, the District or Regional specialist team.

It was recognised that if front-line services are to be successful in making contact with more drug users, the support available from hospital-based specialist services will need to be strengthened. If this more specialist support is not available the capacity of front-line agencies and GPs can be quickly sapped by a small number of the most difficult cases. The report cited evidence of this happening, with front-line agencies working under immense strain, in Scotland.

Scotland was seen as being in urgent need of major improvements in service provision and a separate chapter of the report was devoted to Scotland. The problems there were cited as: '... a dearth of psychiatric input'; '... of the few doctors willing to work with drug users only a handful are willing to consider the full range of treatment options, including prescribing ones ...'; there are '... major gaps in the provision of community-based services for drug misusers'; and pilot syringe-exchange schemes in Scotland were criticised in that they were '... hospital-based, medically supervised, have very limited opening hours, and will only issue up to three syringes at a time'.

In some areas of high seroprevalence, such as Edinburgh and Dundee, services were viewed as working under immense pressure. Growing numbers of drug misusers were attending these services, leading to more time being spent counselling individuals as a result of their seropositivity. Because of a lack of other facilities, the infectious disease unit was having to cope with the drug problems of seropositive patients, as well as their HIV infection but received no psychiatric support in doing so.

Another chapter of the report was devoted specifically to prisons. Prisons were seen as another area where major improvements were needed, all the more important because 'prison represents a unique opportunity to reach large numbers of drug misusers for the first time, educate them towards safer practices, and draw them into contact with a network of help'.

Two special factors relating to HIV infection apply in prison. First, if a syringe does get into prison it is likely to be widely shared, and secondly, there is evidence to suggest that homosexual acts occur on a significant scale among male prisoners. Men who are normally heterosexual engage in homosexual acts while in prison and return to heterosexual activity following release. Because of the high number of drug users in prison, HIV seropositivity is also likely to be high and become an increasing problem. Homosexuality in male prisons with a return to heterosexual activity following release is likely to be a significant way in which the virus will spread within the community if measures are not taken to reduce the risk of sexual transmission.

The report did not consider that exchange or provision of injecting equipment would be realistic in prison. However, a number of other countries have recently decided to make condoms available in prison and the report recommended that the UK should also do this. At present the possession of condoms by prisoners is not allowed on the grounds that homosexual acts are unlawful in prison because homosexual acts can only legally take place in private and nowhere in prison can be said to constitute a private place.

Many drugtakers conceal their drug use when they enter prison. Their identification becomes much more important in the light of HIV infection as adequate treatment for their drug problems will help to reduce the spread of HIV infection. There are a number of ways in which identification of prisoners with drug problems could be improved. Perhaps the most important is by providing incentives for drug misusers to come forward and minimising the deterrents for them to do so. The prospect of a comfortable withdrawal from drugs may be the best incentive that can be given but at present a prescription to assist withdrawal, although a matter for the individual clinical judgment of the prison medical officer, is not often given. Increasing the time spent with prisoners on reception and during their medical examination could also be helpful, as would the better training of prison officers generally, and prison medical officers in particular, in the problems of drug misuse.

The availability of advice and counselling in prisons remains patchy, and there appears to have been little or no improvement since 1979, which was the time when the heroin epidemic started in Britain. Considerable efforts have been made to educate prison staff about HIV infection and attention has now turned to educating the prisoners themselves, but in the words of the ACMD report: 'Education on AIDS/HIV for prisoners still has a long way to go'.

In conclusion, there is no doubt that this first report on AIDS and Drug Misuse by the Advisory Council is a starting point for a new look to the treatment of drug misuse where community services and GPs will play a central role. It is clearly a document of great importance. Many recommendations will be seen as contentious and controversial. Those whose minds are straight-jacketed by rigidly held attitudes – and there are many GPs who unfortunately fall within this category – will no doubt reject the report outright. Some other GPs will find it difficult to adapt and make the changes necessary within themselves to move forward and fully accept what is a new and difficult role. Treating and managing drug misuse effectively is difficult and time-consuming, but it is essential if progress is to be achieved in combating the forthcoming AIDS epidemic. Not to do so now will be catastrophic for the future. All GPs need to become involved.

Not only in regard to the specific problem of drug misuse and AIDS do GPs need to make changes within their own attitudes and develop new skills – such changes need to be made with regard to all aspects of HIV infection. Evidence regarding GPs' attitudes to HIV infection in general is now emerging [86, 87, 88]. There is still some prejudice and lack of knowledge, but it is encouraging to see that general practitioners who have experience of people with AIDS and HIV infection were more positive than the inexperienced about the job of the general practitioner in helping these patients and disagreed more with authoritarian measures to control the spread of HIV [88]. The new development in Oxfordshire of a GP facilitator to improve GP knowledge and skills in the management of HIV infection appears to be a promising way forward, and should be especially valuable for those GPs who do not attend postgraduate centres regularly.

Other infections

Tetanus

In 1968 Sapira reported [89] that the incidence of tetanus among drug users had consistently increased in America from the turn of the century. However, more recent reports failed to show a continuation of this phenomenon. Perhaps mass immunisations against tetanus contributed to the sudden decline in prevalence but one American detoxification unit was reported [90] as noting that 21% of men and 35% of women failed to display protective levels of antibody.

Candidal endophthalmitis

An epidemic of this rare infection was reported in 1985 in Glaswegian heroin users [91].

Tuberculosis

Drug users like heavy drinkers appear to be at increased risk of acquiring TB. A high rate of TB is also found in those with prodromal AIDS [92, 93] but the association with drug misuse occurred before the AIDS epidemic began [94].

Malaria

Malaria has been reported to occur in drug users as a result of sharing injecting equipment [95].

Drug misuse and its effect on immunity

Heroin

The effects of heroin on the immune system has been known since the mid-1970s. Humoral immunity is commonly stimulated in heroin users with hypergammaglobulinaemia, false positive tests for syphilis, and false positive latex fixation tests [96, 97]. This effect is almost certainly not a direct result of heroin use *per se*, but stems from the repeated antigenic stimulus obtained by injecting street heroin using unsterile techniques. In contrast, cellular immunity is mildly depressed by opioid drugs which may account for the increased propensity for drug users to develop TB and the outbreak of candidal endophthalmitis in Glasgow noted above.

Cannabis

There have been numerous studies on the effects of cannabis on the immune system but the results are difficult to interpret. Animal experiments suggest that both humoral and cellular immunity may be temporarily impaired. Human *in vitro* studies suggest that cell-mediated immunity is impaired after exposure to cannabis [74]. However, there is an absence of clinical evidence of greater disease susceptibility among regular cannabis smokers so that in healthy individuals this temporary mild impairment of the human immune system appears not to be of any clinical significance. But in individuals who are already immunocompromised it may be of greater clinical importance and this situation has already been discussed in the section on AIDS.

Vitamin and other nutritional deficiencies

These are probably common among the drugtaking population, particularly regular amphetamine users, although little research has been done in this field. Many drug users do not eat for several days at a time, or survive on chips and milk, or boiled sweets. Most regular drugtakers will benefit from vitamin supplements and a good meal.

Mortality and drug use

In 1984, at the same time as the Coroners' Rules were changed, removing the need for an inquest in cases involving alcoholism where there is no other reason for holding one, the Rules were also changed regarding drug misuse. It was suggested that the verdict 'Death from addiction to drugs' should be withdrawn and two new verdicts should be introduced: 'Death from dependence on drugs' and 'Death from non-dependent abuse of drugs'. Thus some deaths which would previously have resulted in other verdicts, e.g. deaths by accident or misadventure, could now be published as related to drug misuse.

It has been shown that published coroners' figures for deaths of drug users were considerably fewer than figures obtained by other methods. For example in a search of the Home Office Addicts Index, Hamid Ghodse *et al.* [98] found that of the 1,499 deaths between 1967 and 1981, 617 deaths had not been recorded in the published figures. Yet this in itself is almost certainly a considerable underestimate as the number of people on the 'Addicts Index' should be multiplied probably by a factor of at least five in order to obtain the true number of people misusing opioid drugs. Nevertheless, valuable information was obtained from this survey and Ghodse and his colleagues were able to calculate the crude mortality rate amongst drug users, finding that this fell from 23.5/1,000/year in 1968–70 to 18.4/1,000/year ten years later. The mortality rate for drug users under the age of 50 was 16 times that expected in the general population. They also found that over the 15-year study period there was a constant 15% of deaths in therapeutic drugtakers and over half of these were aged over 50, compared with only 5% of deaths in the non-therapeutic drugtakers. Most deaths of non-therapeutic users in which a drug was implicated were due to medically prescribed drugs. Barbiturates caused the majority of drug deaths in the early and mid-1970s – a time when illicit barbiturate misuse was frequent. Later, prescribed opioids such as dipipanone hydrochloride and dextromoramide were implicated. In spite of the known widespread use of illicit heroin amongst drugtakers, this drug was thought to be the cause of death in only 7% of cases.

With the exception of the frequency of death amongst drugtakers, these findings were essentially similar to the results of studies from Coroners' Courts. It is interesting to note that in one such study [99] 41% of deaths were of drug users not known to the Home Office.

In an earlier survey of Home Office statistics, Bewley *et al.* [100] reported in 1968 that accidental overdose and sudden death following opiate administration accounted for only 29% of deaths of heroin users. Suicides accounted for 23%, the remainder being either death by violence, septic conditions such as septicaemia, pulmonary infection and endocarditis or by natural causes.

Only one survey in UK general practice is reported in the literature. Bucknall and Robertson [101] surveyed a single group practice of 18,000 patients in Edinburgh and found a mortality rate of 9.72/1,000 heroin users/year. This is similar to the incidence of mortality of North American drugtakers of 1% per year. Bucknall and Robertson's figures included drugtakers in remission and so the mortality rate would be expected to be lower than those reported to the Home Office who by definition are actively misusing drugs.

In the future, AIDS-related illness is likely to be the leading cause of death among drugtakers and will almost certainly overtake all other causes.

Chapter 4

Legislation and The GP

The Misuse of Drugs Act 1971 and its subsequent regulations comprise the current legislation governing the control of drugs in the United Kingdom.

Various drugs are controlled under Schedule 2 of the Act. They are classified according to their harmfulness either to individuals or to society at large: Class A drugs (including the opiates and cocaine) being considered the most harmful while Class C drugs are regarded as doing the least harm. A few of these drugs are exempted from most controls in certain low dosages and in certain preparations under Schedule 5 of the Misuse of Drugs Regulations 1985. Schedules 1–5 of the Misuse of Drugs Regulations are listed in Appendix D.

The Advisory Council on the Misuse of Drugs (ACMD), comprising at least 20 members, was also set up by statute under this Act and it is their remit to give advice to Ministers on measures needed to counteract drug misuse and its harmful effects. It is a statutory requirement that at least one GP serves on the ACMD.

The international control of drugs is attained as a result of ratification of international conventions by individual countries. This imposes an obligation on those countries to introduce domestic legislation to control all the drugs cited in any particular convention. Apart from a few previously controlled CNS stimulant drugs, most of the drugs placed in Schedule 2 of the 1971 Act followed Britain's ratification of the United Nations Single Convention on Narcotic Drugs of 1961. This treaty, a codification of previous conventions, governs the control of opiate drugs, cocaine, cannabis, and cannabis resin.

Britain has now also ratified the United Nations 1971 Convention on Psychotropic Drugs, so there are obligations to control a number of other substances. This is one reason why 33 benzodiazepines and a number of barbiturates have been brought within the confines of the Misuse of Drugs Act.

The Misuse of Drugs Regulations

In 1973, Regulations were introduced obliging doctors by law to comply with certain requirements with regard to the drugs that are controlled under the 1971 Act. Subsequent updatings became so extensive that in 1985 new regulations were brought out. A working knowledge of these regulations is important for doctors as any doctor who contravenes them commits an offence under the Act for which he may be prosecuted. Furthermore, following a successful prosecution, the Home Secretary has the power to prevent the doctor from prescribing, administering and supplying either all or certain controlled drugs. This power also extends to cover those who are considered by a Tribunal to have prescribed controlled drugs in an irresponsible manner.

Possession, supply and production (Regulations 6–11)

All registered medical practitioners have authority to possess, supply and produce controlled drugs except those listed in Schedule 1 when acting in their professional capacity.

There is a further exception in the case of three drugs. A doctor must not administer or supply dipipanone, heroin, or cocaine, or any of their salts to anyone whom he believes, or has reasonable grounds to suspect, is dependent on any notifiable drug, unless he has a special licence to do so. This applies to doctors prescribing these drugs in order to treat dependence on a notifiable drug. Dipipanone, heroin, or cocaine may be administered or supplied if they have been authorised by another doctor who has such a licence. A doctor may, however, prescribe these drugs to a patient whom he suspects or knows is dependent on a notifiable drug if the prescription is for the treatment of organic disease or injury.

Prescriptions (Regulations 15–17)

The 33 controlled benzodiazepines are specifically exempted, (together with all drugs in Schedules 4 and 5). However, for all other controlled drugs in order to minimise the possibility of forgery or alteration of prescriptions, the prescription must be written in ink and

(a) be written entirely in the doctor's own handwriting, personally dated and signed;

(b) the form of the preparation (e.g. tablets or capsules) be specified, as well as the dose and (where appropriate), the strength of the preparation;
(c) either the total quantity or the number of dosage units must be written in words and figures;

Only (b) and (c) apply to phenobarbitone and phenobarbitone sodium.

Requisition of controlled drugs (Regulation 14)

With the exception of the controlled benzodiazepines and all drugs in Schedules 4 and 5, doctors may obtain a supply of a controlled drug by signing a requisition, which must state the recipient's name, address and profession, and total quantity and purpose of supply. In an emergency, a practitioner may obtain a controlled drug from a supplier even if he cannot immediately supply a signed requisition. He must, however, undertake to deliver a signed requisition within 24 hours of receiving the drug.

A person who purports to have been sent by a practitioner to collect a controlled drug from a supplier, cannot be supplied with that drug unless the requisition is accompanied by a statement signed by the practitioner that he is empowered to receive it on the practitioner's behalf.

Registers (Regulations 19–20)

Registers must be kept for recording all transactions for Schedule 2 drugs (see Appendix D). This does not apply to controlled drugs supplied to a patient on prescription and dispensed by a pharmacist. It does however, apply to stocks of controlled drugs as held by dispensing doctors and all GPs who have emergency supplies of controlled drugs in drug cabinets or cases. Registers should be laid out in the following way (see Fig. 4.1).

The register must be bound, not a loose leaf book, but it need not be printed. Any bound book is sufficient if it is appropriately ruled and the columns properly headed. Printed registers may be obtained at a cost of £17 from the National Pharmaceutical Association, Mallinson House, 40–42 St. Peter's Street, St. Albans, Hertfordshire, AL1 3NP or from Jordan Stationers, 13 Victoria Street, Liverpool, L2.

Entries in the register must be made in chronological order and should be made on the day on which the drugs are obtained or

Figure 4.1 Form of register.

Part I. Entries to be made in case of obtaining.

Date on which supply received	Name Address (of person or firm from whom obtained)	Amount obtained	Form in which obtained

Part II. Entries to be made in case of supply.

Date on which the transaction was effected	Name Address (of person or firm supplied)	Particulars as to licence or authority of person or firm supplied to be in possession	Amount supplied	Form in which supplied

supplied, or if this is not reasonably practicable, on the next day. No entry may be cancelled, obliterated or altered. Any correction must be made by marginal note or footnote and all entries must be in ink or other indelible writing.

A doctor must, on demand by any person authorised by the Secretary of State, give access to his register. In practice, such authorised persons will usually be Inspectors from the Home Office Drugs Branch or Regional Medical Officers.

A separate register must be kept for stocks held at each surgery premises. Registers must be preserved for two years from the date on which the last entry is made.

Although all Schedule 2 drugs are required under the regulations to be recorded in a register if stocks are held, only a few are in current general use in the UK. Taking those drugs that are currently listed in the British National Formulary, the ones that fall into this category are:

Class A
alfentanil (Rapifen)
* cocaine (cocaine eye drops)
dextromoramide (Palfium)
diamorphine (heroin)
dipipanone (Diconal)
fentanyl (Sublimaze, Thalamonal)
* medicinal opium (tincture of opium, omnopon, papaveretum)
methadone (Physeptone)
* morphine (Cyclimorph, Durmomorph, MST Continus, Nepenthe)
pethidine (Pamergan, Pethilorfan)
phenazocine (Narphen)
phenoperidine (Operidine)

Class B
amphetamine (Dexedrine, Durophet)
† codeine phosphate injection
† dihydrocodeine injection

These regulations do not apply to any Class C drug in general use.

---

* Some preparations of these compounds are exempted from most controls under Schedule 5 if:
(a) they are compounded with one or more other active or inert ingredients in such a way that they cannot be recovered by readily applicable means or in a yield which would constitute a risk to health and
(b) the strength of the preparation is low thus: for *cocaine* not more than 0.1% of cocaine calculated as cocaine base must be present and for *medicinal opium* or *morphine* the preparation must contain (in either case) not more than 0.2% of morphine calculated as anhydrous morphine base.
 Any powder of opium and ipecacuanha is excluded if it contains 10% opium in powder, 10% ipecacuanha root in powder well mixed with 80% of any other powdered ingredient containing no controlled drug.
† Codeine tablets and dihydrocodeine tablets are exempted from most controls under Schedule 5.

Destruction of controlled drugs (Regulation 26)

This applies to all controlled drugs including benzodiazepines.

Apart from the exception given below, GPs are not allowed to destroy any controlled drugs that they have in their possession, except in the presence of an authorised person. A record must be kept of the date of destruction and the quantity destroyed and this must be signed by a person authorised to do so by the Secretary of State. Authorised persons are:

- all police officers;
- inspectors of the Home Office Drugs Branch;
- inspectors of the Pharmaceutical Society of Great Britain;
- Regional Pharmaceutical Officers;
- Regional Medical Officers.

The provisions for supervision of destruction do not apply to drugs supplied to patients and retained in their possession after treatment has ceased. Thus patients or their relatives are allowed to destroy these drugs. GPs were originally unable to destroy controlled drugs which, after being prescribed, had become surplus and were handed back to them by patients or their relatives. However, a change in the regulations now allows GPs and pharmacists to destroy such drugs.

Notification

Under the regulations governing notification, a number of drugs are termed 'notifiable'. If a doctor believes or suspects that he is attending a person who is dependent on one or more of these drugs he is required by law to notify within seven days The Chief Medical Officer, Drugs Branch, Home Office, Queen Anne's Gate, London SW1H 9AT. In Northern Ireland the person to notify is The Northern Ireland CMO, Dundonald House, Upper Newtownards Road, Belfast. Failure to notify may cause a doctor to be brought up before a tribunal.

The notifiable drugs are:

- cocaine;
- dextromoramide (Palfium);
- diamorphine (heroin);
- dipipanone (Diconal);
- hydrocodone;
- hydromorphone;
- levorphanol (Dromoran)

- methadone (Physeptone);
- morphine (Duromorph, MST Continus, Cyclimorph, Nepenthe);
- opium (opium tincture, papaveretum, omnopon);
- oxycodone;
- pethidine (Pethilorfan, Pamergan);
- phenazocine (Narphen);
- piritramide.

The regulations state that a doctor is obliged to notify when he 'attends' such a person. Even if he refuses to accept the person as a patient or to prescribe any drugs, he must still make a notification and the following particulars should be given if available:

Name
Address
Date of birth
Sex
NHS Number
Name of Notifiable Drugs to which the person is addicted
Date of doctor's attendance
(Although not legally required, the Home Office also appreciate the names of any notifiable drugs the doctor prescribes)

If the patient is still attending the doctor, then there is a responsibility to renotify annually. Even if the doctor has grounds for believing that the person has already been notified, e.g. the person states that he/she has been attending a drug dependency unit, this does not relieve him of the responsibility to notify. Only if the person has been notified by another GP in the same practice within the past year is he exempted. Originally form H5 2A/1 was used in hospitals and no notification forms were provided for general practice use. However, in September 1987, a new notification form was implemented which could be used for general practice, hospital inpatients and outpatients, and by the prison medical service. This form includes an extra section on whether the patient injected any drugs and another section for details of any drugs prescribed. Supplies of these forms can be obtained from Family Practitioner Committees or from: DHSS Printing and Stationery Unit, Primrose Hill, Clitheroe, Lancs (Telephone: 0200-22187).

A doctor may obtain information about a known drug user – once the Home Office is satisfied that the call is genuine – by ringing 01-273 2213. General advice about subsequent regulations can be obtained by ringing one of the four Regional Inspectorates:

South Eastern, including Greater London, Home Counties, and East Anglia: 01-273 3530
Midlands, South West England and Wales: 0272-276736
Northern, including North of England and Scotland: 0274-727149
Northern Ireland: Belfast 63939 ext. 2874.

All notifications are compiled by the Home Office to form the Addicts Index which has two functions only:

(1) to form a basis for Home Office statistics;
(2) to provide information to doctors who are treating drug users (i.e. to help ensure that no one else is treating them at the same time).

The Addicts Index has been computerised so that up-to-date information is now readily available for doctors. It should be emphasised that the Index is *strictly confidential* and no other agencies (police, embassies etc.) have access to it.

Safe custody

With the exception of Schedules 3, 4 and 5 drugs, the regulations governing safe custody state that all controlled drugs must be kept in a locked receptacle which can only be opened by the doctor concerned or by someone authorised by him to do so. In practice, this applies to the same drugs that are required by regulation to be recorded in a register if stocks are kept. A previous High Court judgment has ruled that a locked car cannot be deemed to be a locked receptacle.

Although the security risks present in a dispensing practice are similar to those facing a pharmacist, dispensing practitioners are not required at present to conform to the detailed requirements laid down in the regulations for pharmacists. However, it would be prudent for all dispensing doctors to discuss their security arrangements with the crime prevention officer of their local police force.

Other aspects of security

All stocks of controlled drugs should be kept to the minimum required for routine needs and foreseeable emergencies. Blank prescription forms are of considerable value once stolen. All too often these forms are left in easily accessible places with little or no check being kept on the number in the doctor's possession. All practitioners should consider ways of improving the safekeeping of prescription forms.

It is a breach of paragraph 36 of the GP's Terms of Service to sign a blank FP10. Pharmacists have been urged to make every effort to verify prescriptions that are liable to be misused.

It is good practice never to leave a patient alone in the consulting room with an empty pad of FP10s. It is also wise to make a habit of putting a Z line through any unfilled space on a prescription ensuring this traverses the vertical blue lines on either side. If attempts are made to remove the Z line by chemical or mechanical means (e.g., by repeated pressure with a piece of sellotape), the vertical blue lines will also be removed and this can be spotted by the pharmacist.

If a prescription pad is stolen, both the FPC and the police should be informed as soon as possible.

Chapter 5

Prevention

In considering the prevention of drug misuse we should be looking at the whole spectrum of mood-altering substances. Some drugs, such as alcohol and tobacco, can be obtained legally, and the main thrust of preventive measures lies with fiscal policies that reduce their supply. Other drugs such as benzodiazepines, can only be obtained legally through a doctor's prescription. For this category doctors are in a prime position to influence preventive strategy. A further group of drugs cannot be obtained legally and this in itself is a deterrent to most people, although the very fact that they are illegal may encourage rebellious adolescents to experiment in drug use at a vulnerable period of their lives.

Many people have varying beliefs as to the causes of drug misuse. Views on aetiology are numerous, conflicting and usually supported in vehement terms. Poverty and disturbed upbringing are set against the excesses of those in the pop world who, idolised by many teenagers, indulge themselves in drugtaking. The pressures of life, the attitudes of adults towards tablets and alcohol are all often blamed. Many such beliefs are difficult to prove and some appear irremediable by the average doctor. So what does prevention cover?

Different classifications of prevention have in the past been attempted. The ACMD report on prevention [1] favoured two simple categories:

(a) reducing the risk of an individual engaging in drug misuse;
(b) reducing the harm associated with drug use.

Other reports such as a report of the London Boroughs Working Party on Drug and Alcohol Problems [2] have applied Professor J. Morris's classification of primary, secondary and tertiary prevention to alcohol and drug misuse. For the purposes of this book it is easier to consider prevention under a number of separate headings.

Education

Complete prevention of any drug use is of course an unrealistic goal, but it is hoped that the government's initiative in 1986 to ensure education about drugs in all secondary schools will have the effect of reducing the numbers who experiment with drugs. GPs and the police are sometimes asked to go into schools to give a talk on drug and solvent misuse. Any GP who gets such an invitation would be wise to refuse it. There is evidence that young people can be educated to become more resistant to pressures placed on them, but this task is best carried out by those with teaching skills who are known to the young people concerned. In the past, talks by specialist visitors have often concentrated on the dangers of drug misuse in a way that, far from discouraging engagement in drug misuse, may actually have been attractive to certain groups of young people. This was highlighted in the Advisory Council's Prevention report [1] which stated:

> 'Whilst we accept the need, in appropriate circumstances, for education to include factual information about drugs and their effects, we are concerned about measures which deliberately present information in a way which is intended simply to shock or to scare. We believe that educational programmes based on such measures on their own are likely to be ineffective or, at worst, positively harmful; there may, however, be scope for the use of such measures, where appropriate, in individual counselling.'

Teachers may, however, wish to consult specialist workers in particular fields, and so doctors with experience may find unobtrusive ways of helping to prevent young people engaging in drug misuse. Generally speaking, health education about drugs in schools is best kept at low key and should be taught within a broad framework of positive health including regular exercise, healthy diet, no smoking and moderate alcohol consumption.

One of the best ways that GPs can provide health information about drugs for their patients is by displaying materials in the surgery waiting room. Posters, DHSS leaflets and information about local self-help groups, local counselling and treatment services are a good way of spreading information either to drug users themselves, or indirectly through a friend or relative.

GPs are sometimes invited to talk to other professionals or lay workers involved with helping drugtakers. Youth workers, Samaritans, trainee GPs, nurses and voluntary groups all need to have good information and it is a good principle to write to ISDD beforehand for a pile of free booklets entitled 'Publications on the misuse of drugs'.

Even in a full hour one cannot hope to cover the essentials of such a wide subject, but one's enthusiasm may generate a desire to study further. People can then order the inexpensive leaflets and booklets from this list. Even without such a stock, one can read out the ISDD address, tell the audience to send for the booklist and ask them to jot down a selected few numbers to order. A good choice might be the following which at present cost no more than £1.50 each: *Drug Abuse Briefing; Drugs: what every parent should know* and *How to help – a practical guide for the friends and relatives of drug users.*

Changing attitudes

Central to any educational campaign must be the establishment of attitudes that will make drug use discredited and unfashionable to young people. The acceptance of such an attitude by any individual will be considerably easier if his or her peer group have similar attitudes already established. Thus the government's decision to campaign against drug use both in schools and via the media may well have been correct, even though, at the time, it was done against the advice of the Advisory Council on the Misuse of Drugs.

In the past, attitudinal change has been known to be successful in helping to overcome dependence. A change in attitudes due to the Methodist Revival which swept the country in the eighteenth century was, at least partly responsible for ending the gin epidemic of that period. Similarly the communist revolution in mainland China in 1951 played a large part in ridding that country of its opium problem.

Recovery for any individual who becomes dependent on drugs and the prevention of subsequent relapse also depend very much upon an attitudinal change encompassing a new set of values. In short, the change from spending 95% of time obtaining, using and thinking about drugs to one of a drug-free existence necessitates the acceptance of a new identity. The attitudinal changes required to do this do not occur suddenly, but usually slowly and are brought about by the increasingly disastrous happenings that can be the result of drugtaking. Loss of friends, loss of employment, imprisonment, marital disharmony and breakdown, all in themselves may help to convince the drugtaker that he or she needs to change.

The attitudes of many of those professionals to whom drug users turn for help also need to change if this country is to prevent a continued escalation of its huge drug problem and the rapidly expanding AIDS epidemic. GPs are often rightly criticised on this point, but it is frequently overlooked that there is just as much prejudice against drug users from psychiatrists, social workers and probation officers, all of whom have key roles to play in the treatment of drug misuse.

Cultural attitudes can be regarded as very strong influences that either promote or inhibit drug misuse. For example, it appears that the West Indian community in Britain did not get involved with heroin taking on any scale until the mid-1980s. In an article in *DrugLink* published in 1984 [3] Hartnoll wrote: 'There is little evidence of heroin use amongst Black and Asian communities. This is a very interesting contrast to the United States.' However, in 1985 the situation had changed and one survey [4] concluded: 'It would appear that heroin use amongst young black people is largely a fairly recent phenomenon, having begun to accelerate in the last eighteen months or so'.

By contrast, marijuana smoking has traditionally had a high prevalence amongst West Indians and for the Rastafarian community smoking cannabis is part of their religion where it is used 'not so much as a recreational drug but as a sacrament and a tool to aid the process of individual and group awareness' [4].

Restricting supplies and thoughtful prescribing

Restriction of supply is a matter for the authorities, but a GP can make a significant contribution by trying to ensure that no legal drugs reach the black market from medical sources. As a general principle, prescriptions for drugs of dependence should be kept to a minimum and where possible these drugs should be avoided. In the case of benzodiazepines, whether or not minor affective disorders actually need psychotropic medication is a matter of debate [5]; simple counselling may be equally effective.

When prescribing is undertaken, it may be possible to find an alternative drug with a low or negligible dependence potential and therefore unlikely to be misused. Unfortunately this is not always so. For instance, it may cross the mind of the GP that the reason a particular patient is asking for strong analgesics might be because he or she is dependent on opioids. Unfortunately, all of the more powerful analgesics are opioids capable of producing dependence, and there are no suitable alternatives. Another difficulty is that it is impossible to determine objectively the degree of pain that a patient is experiencing and therefore heavy reliance is placed upon the history given. Some drug users have an exceptional ability to persuade doctors that they are in severe pain. Pethidine misusers are not as frequently encountered nowadays but many doctors will recall the remarkable ability of some to mimic classical renal colic. Dihydrocodeine, Palfium (dextromoramide), and Temgesic (buprenorphine), now appear to be much more commonly misused than pethidine. Suspicions should be raised by those patients who have no clinical signs, particularly if they state that their pain is only controlled by a specific opioid drug (even though many drugtakers will misuse any drug of the opioid class and frequently interchange them).

With particular regard to the benzodiazepine group of drugs, the best way of avoiding dependence is by thoughtful prescribing [6]. Prescriptions should be kept under regular review, non-pharmacological alternatives should be considered, and the doctor should make it clear from the start that prescriptions will only be given on a short-term basis.

Special care should be taken when prescribing for anyone with a history of dependence. In a study of a large sample of women drinkers, one-third were found to misuse the benzodiazepines that had been prescribed for their disorder [7].

Thoughtful prescribing also entails the avoidance of possible harm to the patient. A prescription for a long-acting benzodiazepine hypnotic such as nitrazepam, or a long-acting tranquilliser such as diazepam can impair driving skills and lead to road traffic accidents and, if given to an elderly person, may precipitate falls and dementia.

As a general rule, short-acting drugs are more liable to induce dependence and thus to be more sought after than long-acting drugs of the same class. It is not clear why this should be so, but it may be related to the simple fact that the more often a drug is taken, the more readily a subject becomes conditioned to take it again. Thus, from first principles, lormetazepam should have a lower dependence potential than temazepam and methadone, if given to a subject in the same conditions over the same period of time, and should cause a less severe opioid dependence than the equivalent dose of heroin which needs to be taken more frequently.

Certain drugs, because of the way they are formulated, are readily injectable. This applies in particular to temazepam, which is in liquid form inside the capsule, and Temgesic (buprenorphine) which is easily dissolved in water. These drugs should not be prescribed to anyone who is considered to be at risk of misusing them.

Other drugs such as Valoid (cyclizine), Phensedyl and Heminevrin (chlormethiazole) may not be immediately recognised by doctors as drugs of misuse. A great deal of drug misuse remains hidden and it is prudent to retain a high level of suspicion. Additionally, all doctors should make a habit of minimal prescribing, both for the total amounts given at any one time, and the total length of time for which prescribing is undertaken. This maxim should apply to all prescribed drugs as it has been shown that the more parents take medicines for both physical and psychological problems, the more likely their children are to misuse drugs [8].

Care with prescriptions

If a doctor suspects that a patient might be tempted to alter a prescription, for example for benzodiazepines or dihydrocodeine, he would be wise to write the total amount to be dispensed in both words and figures as he would for a controlled drug with handwriting requirements.

All the major points about the security of NHS prescriptions were covered in the last chapter, but private prescriptions are more difficult to protect than NHS ones. They are easy to photocopy and it may be impossible for the chemist to distinguish between photocopies and the original. Ordinary headed notepaper is normally used for writing private prescriptions and it is not unknown for drugtakers to have printed a large supply of the headed notepaper of a doctor of their choice.

Screening for substance misuse

It is good practice, when a patient first attends after registering with a GP, to include a history of smoking, alcohol consumption in units per week, and drug use. This breaks the ice for anyone who wishes to discuss their drug problem, and also allows the doctor the opportunity to give some health education about smoking and safe limits of alcohol, which are: for women less than 14 units per week and for men less that 21 units per week [9,10,11]. Time is usually limited at first interview and questions are probably best confined to:

(1) *Do you smoke?*, and if so *How much?*
(2) *Do you drink alcohol?*, and if so *How much per week?*

one glass of wine	
½ pint of beer/cider	each equals
one measure of sherry/fortified wine	one unit
a single measure of spirits	
1 standard bottle of wine	7 units
1 litre bottle of wine	10 units
1 bottle of sherry or fortified wine	12 units
1 bottle of spirits	30 units

(3) *Do you take drugs of any kind?*

This latter question, encompassing both prescribed and non-prescribed drugs is a useful opener as, although most people will lie about their illicit drug use, it will allow those who feel they need help to either come forward or at least to recognise that their GP is someone who is willing to discuss their problem with them in the future.

Most people are fairly honest about their smoking habits but alcohol and drug problems are often concealed for long periods of time, sometimes several years. Research into the efficacy of prevention exercises in any field is always fraught with difficulty. In the field of drug misuse, this problem is compounded by the known heterogeneity of drug misusers [12] and the fact that so little is known about natural history of drug use patterns of those that do not attend clinics. For these reasons it is not even fully known how effective our treatment services are. Nevertheless, what evidence there is does suggest that measures in prevention are likely to be worthwhile attempting. One study [13] of those attending treatment clinics has shown that those who were abstinent at follow-up were at intake likely to be younger and have a shorter history of heroin use before coming to the clinic. Another study [14] has confirmed that opiate users treated earlier in their drugtaking careers (less than 18 months use) are significantly more likely to be abstinent from opiates at both one and five years after treatment than the group who had been using them for more than 18 months.

Actively seeking out drug misusers may be helpful, not only for the more effective treatment of drug misuse, but also for the opportunity it provides to help reduce the harm engendered by drugtaking practices. This message has been brought to the forefront by the emergence of the AIDS epidemic and the crucial role that injecting drug users play in spreading this disease into the general heterosexual population. It is no longer acceptable to stand back and wait for an injecting drugtaker to be motivated to seek help. Those who are indulging in recreational drug use and sharing needles or syringes, including recreational injectors of amphetamine, cocaine, benzodiazepine, barbiturate and opioid drugs, need to be actively sought out if any headway is to be made in reducing the spread of HIV infection. GPs have a role to play in doing this.

At a subsequent interview with the patient, when the doctor-patient relationship is more firmly established and there is an atmosphere of mutual trust, the GP could re-explore the issue of drug misuse in a more sensitive way. One way of doing this might be to say:

'Can I ask you confidentially, have you ever, even in the past, tried any illegal drugs such as cannabis, speed or heroin, or misused any other drugs for example barbiturates or tranquillisers?' If the answer is yes, then the question should be asked: 'Have you ever injected a drug, and if so, have you ever shared needles or syringes even once?' Those who have used drugs but have never injected may still be in a high risk group because of their social circle. They may have had a sexual experience with someone else who has unwittingly contracted HIV infection either sexually or by sharing injecting equipment. They may be worried that they might have contracted the AIDS virus and might wish to discuss these fears. The opportunity to provide information on safe sex and the hazards of 'sharing works' should never be lost. Such information is best given verbally with leaflet back-up. Some useful leaflets are available through the Terrence Higgins Trust. HIV testing should in all cases be done only if the individual wishes it and after comprehensive pre-test counselling fully understands the implications of such a test and still wishes to proceed. Practical advice over counselling for harm reduction and HIV testing is given in Chapter 6 of this book.

Screening for drugs by urine testing without the patient's consent is certain to seriously damage the doctor/patient relationship and should never be considered in general practice. In addition, in view of the reversal of the BMA's decision on HIV testing without consent, it is now almost certainly unethical to do this. There is also the practical problem that hospital laboratory methods for drug testing are not 100% accurate. Even when a positive test is confirmed by a second test using a different technique and the results are known to have an accuracy of at least 99%, there is still a margin of error in current routine hospital laboratory testing.

One way of obtaining 100% accuracy is by using mass spectrometry. Mass spectrometers are extremely expensive, but because of the consequences of a wrong test result, they are now used in all the forensic science laboratories in Britain.

Urine screening for drug misuse in the workplace is a rapidly growing field. Unfortunately, in North America it took off in a big way before much thought was given to the potential consequences.

In a blaze of publicity Ronald Reagan and all the White House staff presented their urines for testing. Further official encouragement was given when the President instructed the head of every federal agency to test for drugs, which potentially affected 2.8 million people, although the Supreme Court has yet to rule whether this is constitutional. In 1987, the National Institute for Drug Abuse estimated that 30% of all large companies were screening for drugs and a further 20% would begin over the ensuing two years.

The ethics of screening where the benefit is not to the individual but to others is controversial. It is important that all employees are protected at their place of work by well thought out policies on drug and alcohol use.

Heavy use of alcohol and other drugs does correlate with an increased risk of accidents, but it is not clear what, if any, increased risk can be attributed to moderate alcohol or drug use away from the workplace.

However, studies are emerging from the United States and these suggest that drug monitoring is having a beneficial effect, especially when combined with employee assistance programmes and further evidence indicates that it is reducing accidents in the workplace. There is no doubt that the drug use of some employees, for example airline pilots, poses a risk to others. A strong case can be made for screening other employees working in dangerous situations.

The Addiction Research Foundation of Toronto has issued the following recommendations [16] which seem to be reasonable guidelines:

- mass or random drug screening for all employees and/or applicants for employment should *not be implemented*;
- drug screening should be considered for employees who show deficits in job performance and whose behaviour in the workplace is judged to constitute a safety risk to self or others. All such cases should be referred to a qualified medical practitioner, the decision to test for drugs to be made by this individual;
- pre-employment and continued random drug screening should be considered for employees in jobs that pose risk to co-workers and/or the public and that are unsupervised for periods such that evidence of impairment would not normally be subject to observation;
- if drug screening is instituted, the following procedures should be followed to guarantee valid, accurate and confidential results:
  - samples should be collected by qualified staff under medical supervision and be forwarded to a qualified laboratory;
  - the individual being tested should have the right to provide and to have recorded a statement of current medical or other drug use;
  - all positive results should be confirmed by gas chromatography/mass spectrometry. The laboratory should not forward positive test results unless the results have been confirmed by this method;
  - the laboratory should communicate test results only to the licensed medical practitioner who forwarded the test samples to the laboratory; and,

- the practitioner should report back to the employer on the results of the testing and his/her interpretation of the same in accordance with standard medical ethics and any applicable company policies and collective agreements;
- if drug screening is instituted, employees with confirmed positive test results should be referred to an employee assistance programme for assessment and, if needed, counselling and rehabilitation;
- if drug screening is instituted, it should be preceded by a formal employment policy stating the rationale for the testing and the consequences of confirmed positive test(s) results in relation to continuation of employment.

Harm reduction

Although harm reduction has been recognised by research workers for many years as a positive outcome of therapy, it has only recently, with the advent of the AIDS epidemic, been generally accepted as a useful therapeutic approach. The difficulty has always been that the promotion of harm reduction methods can also be viewed as an official endorsement that it is all right to carry on using substances as long as this is done in a less harmful way.

In 1981, ISDD attempted to promote harm reduction among those sniffing glue and other volatile substances [17]. Over 40% of deaths from this activity in the previous decade had been due to indirect causes, such as accidents and injuries due to sniffing in dangerous situations, or suffocation from plastic bags [18]. ISDD were criticised for stating that some solvents were relatively safer than others and for suggesting to health educators that children should be advised not to sniff from large plastic bags, nor to sniff alone or in potentially dangerous places like railway embankments. It was seen to be encouraging an occupation that was harmful.

With the emergence of HIV infection, harm reduction programmes have now become respectable. The ethic, first proposed in this country by the McClelland Committee [19], that 'the prevention of the spread of HIV infection should take priority over any perceived risk of increased drug misuse', has gained national acceptance and was endorsed by the working party on AIDS and Drug Misuse set up by the ACMD.

Harm reduction programmes are aimed at those drug users who are not motivated towards abstinence and who may still be at the stage of enjoying their drug use. In order to make contact with this population, in some countries outreach workers have been used with some success. Apart from providing information on safer injection techniques and safe sex, harm reduction has also included in some places, needle and syringe exchange schemes, advice on the cleaning of injection equipment, the provision of free condoms, and methadone maintenance. These are discussed in greater detail in the sections on AIDS in Chapters 3 and 6.

An interesting new development in harm reduction is the attempt to introduce a single use syringe. At the time of writing two such devices are currently being tested; one with a ratchet inside the barrel of the syringe, and the other with a 'J' valve in a side arm. Both of these appear not to have fully overcome the difficulties presented by the need to be able to draw up a liquid into the syringe before it is injected. Clearly when these problems are surmounted, the single use syringe will be a major contribution towards harm reduction.

The disposal of used needles by drug users has caused some media attention recently. Children playing on rubbish dumps have been pricked with dirty needles [20] and it has been suggested that a needle clipper, like the B-D Safe-Clip for insulin-dependent diabetics should be made for injecting drug users.

Part 2:
Practical Managemenet

Dr A. Banks

Chapter 6

Initial Care

A field worker in a northern city told one of the authors he was in touch with two drug users who had been giving him their views on doctors. They said they had met only two kinds. First, those who if drugs were asked for, just didn't want to know. Such doctors felt that dependence was the drug user's own choice and it was up to him or her to get out of it. Second, those who were an easy touch. The two men had a hit list of six doctors whom they could con into giving them regular scripts as temporary patients. There were no threats but the two admitted expertise in removing prescription pads and other surgery items.

There are, however, doctors of a third kind who may constitute a majority. These have never had to deal with problem drug users. Their attitudes may vary, but until presented with the opportunity of helping a drug user, they cannot tell how they will react. Finally, come those doctors who while being firm and cooperating with other workers in a team effort, do their best to assist in the long-term goal of a patient becoming drug-free.

In the world of drug misuse treatment choices vary widely, from hospital and medical models to social and entirely non-medical models of management. The ideal approach at this juncture appears to be the 'cafeteria' system where the drug worker has as many options as possible to offer individual drug users. Within this framework a doctor may only be called on to take an active role in certain circumstances. For instance, a doctor may be asked to help with a detoxification programme (detox) for someone who has applied to an advice centre, to arrange for him/her to go to a drug-free rehabilitation (rehab) house, or the doctor may offer general medical care to someone waiting one or two months to be seen at a hospital unit. Hopefully the doctor will keep in touch with the person for a year or two after the process of coming off drugs when relapses may occur.

On the other hand, an experienced GP may initiate both detoxification and rehabilitation of a drug user in the community, if the GP has some kind of a back-up group to work with, such as a Community

Drug Team. If the GP manages a few such cases a year, then understanding of drug problems will rapidly increase. Provided one follows the DHSS *Guidelines*, this can be done without too much aggravation to oneself or the practice. This means setting limits to what one can do and sticking to them.

First, as in other branches of medicine, the drugtaker should be viewed as a whole person, not just a drug problem. The DHSS *Guidelines* put it thus: 'The aim of treatment is to help the individual deal with the problems caused by, as well as causing, his drug misuse and eventually to achieve a drug-free life'.

This means helping users to clear up the chaotic state of their lives, to develop trust and confidence in the doctor and others dealing with them and build up a relationship in which they seriously consider ending dependence on drugs.

The ultimate aim is to restore the drug user to being a person who is no longer relying on chemicals to solve problems. As Rowdy Yates of the Lifeline Project has said: 'Recovery is dependent on fundamental change in the addict himself ... the individual can never be seen as the victim of addiction and must be encouraged to take responsibility for his attitudes and actions in order to understand the possibility of and need for personal change'. Management on such lines is not likely to leave one at the mercy of a flood of drugtakers.

More recently, the thinking of some GPs and drug workers is moving towards an aim less rigorous and clear-cut than total abstinence. They remember that drug addiction can be a relapsing condition, and that in some cases the ultimate target of a drug-free life may never be reached. One can encourage the drug user to move gradually toward less damaging levels of drug use, one can help to pick someone up after a relapse and not speak of it in terms of failure – but rather like a 'dry run' or a trial situation from which they can learn for the next time. Problem drug users can be helped gradually to think of themselves as achievers, not failures. The drug worker is then perhaps less disappointed and frustrated by numbers of failures and as an aim of treatment this can still bring a measure of satisfaction when one looks back over two or three years and sees someone slowly improving despite the setbacks.

The advent of AIDS has consolidated this approach. Treatment is now seen as occuring in stages with a hierarchy of goals – the move away from shared injecting and reducing the risk of sexual spread of HIV being the initial and most important goals. The drug user should then be aided to move on through the hierarchy – moving from injectable to oral drug use and finally achieving abstinence.

Social care

When other facilities are available, a fair number of drugtakers manage to overcome their addiction without seeing a doctor or hospital. Some are actually frightened of going to a doctor because they know they will be notified, and they misunderstand what this means. However, where there is a well established advice centre, the non-medical specialist staff can arrange both detox at a clinic and rehab at one of the therapeutic houses. The family doctor in this situation can refer a drug user to this chain of care, offering only to provide general medical attention. He can test for hepatitis B or HIV status with appropriate counselling, and treat complications or health problems.

Similarly, where the drug user first approaches a parents' or users' self-help group whose total care and concern enables him or her gradually to come off and stay off drugs, the family doctor may only need to supply the normal GP care to the user and any family he or she may have. Some chronic drug users become rootless wanderers whose way of life has discouraged doctors from taking them on permanently. So when they do pluck up courage to approach a doctor, they tend to remain temporary residents and outside the full range of health care to which they are entitled in the National Health Service. Because no one has ever explained the confidentiality entailed in notifying them to the Home Office they may even give false names and addresses. Some do this, of course, to get a free and legal supply of controlled drugs in a crisis, but they should nevertheless be persuaded to take a long-term view.

Finally, there is always a small proportion of drug users who decide to 'kick the habit' entirely on their own. Then, with perhaps only help from a friend, they withdraw from drugs without any medication, or they may go and buy methadone on the black market and successfully give themselves a solitary detox. A much greater number try these options and fail, but they may try again a few times or use other avenues later.

Hospital care

A brief history of the development of hospital care has already been outlined.

In the 1960s and 1970s, in some cases there was a policy of maintaining difficult drugtakers on heroin and later methadone for certain periods of time or even for life. In recent years, many of the maintained patients have been brought off or denied further prescribed drugs, and instead are offered support in coming off. Sister Mary Sharp of University College Hospital DDU, London, writing in the *Nursing Mirror* in March 1983 described the new policy as follows:

> 'The new method of treatment concentrates on getting an addict off the drug in a short space of time. He is then given a plan of four weeks or six months after which treatment will stop. It is the short, sharp shock on a reducing prescription of methadone which, with counselling, group therapy and discipline must be adhered to or else the patient is shown the door mid-treatment. A urine sample must be left for testing each week and the patient must be on time for appointments or he will be out. Many fail to get off the drug in a short time or even after several sessions. We then advise them to apply to one of the residential communities.'

Certain drugtakers, and those with severe problems will be offered an inpatient detoxification or, in some centres like the Bethlem Royal and Bexley, they may be given 6 or 12 months rehabilitation. Where staff and time permit, and if recovering users are willing to keep returning, follow-up will be done.

The drawbacks to hospital treatment are:

(1) The fact that among today's drug users there is a low incidence of psychiatric morbidity which means that some people are reluctant to attend a mental hospital. A drug user for whom one of the authors found a hospital bed said: 'I'm not a nutter; I'm not going in with that lot'.

(2) The long waiting lists. These may vary from four weeks for an initial appointment to three months for an inpatient bed with wide regional variations. This means that, at a crisis point in their life, drug users have to remain on black market supplies and will have urine tests to estimate their drug use. The GP may be needed to encourage motivation and it is reasonable to prescribe oral substitutes during the waiting period, particularly to regular or occasional injectors, but this should only be done in collaboration with the unit involved.

(3) The fact that some drugtakers prefer to deal with a single doctor who is known to them as opposed to an anonymous team. GPs, however, should never work with a drug user in total isolation and community drug teams in particular are invaluable as extra support.

To get a place one can telephone the clinic, if the patient can claim to be within the catchment area. Very little help is available for non-opioid drug users as the DDUs have tended over the years to concentrate almost exclusively on opioid users, although advice will be given. When it is difficult to get hold of the consultant, much may be gleaned from talking to registrars, the sister in charge, or other drug workers on the phone – even at night. The same applies to non-medical drug centres.

Private care

The Association of Independent Doctors against Addiction (AIDA) is very critical of the hospital set-up, maintaining that a large proportion of drug users seeking treatment either do not go there at all or break away when they find out what the policy is. AIDA seeks to maintain standards in the private sector, particularly in London where psychiatrists are in turn critical of the Harley Street approach. A *Lancet* leader (27 March 1982) said of private practitioners prescribing opioids:

> 'Their rationalisation is that the patient is thereby saved from the black market; however, since most addicts can only finance their private consultation by selling part of their prescription, knowingly or (with a stretch of the imagination) unknowingly the doctor is prescribing sufficient drugs for this purpose.'

The fact remains that so long as patients desire private treatment it will be available.

Where long-term users with a family and steady job are concerned, or in the wealthier sectors of the population, there is usually the ability to pay for consultations which start at about £25 a time plus the chemist's dispensing fees. AIDA members are urged to look into their clients' ability to pay and to reduce spillage on the black market by demanding to see empty containers or foil papers etc. before further prescriptions are given. The advantage of private treatment is the one-to-one relationship with a single doctor, convenient hours for those who are working, and a more flexible approach to drug regimes including maintaining patients on a fixed dose for a longer or shorter period.

Outside London there are few such private doctors practising but certain GPs will prescribe more flexibly and take on private patients, or see drug users on behalf of neighbouring practices. Others prescribe large amounts unwisely or purely for gain and bring the profession into disrepute. Thanks to the friendly vigilance of the Home Office Inspectors such instances are becoming fewer. The DHSS *Guidelines* provide useful advice for doctors who are in doubt.

The other area of private management is the nursing home or private clinic. There are perhaps 15 or more of these, with weekly charges ranging from £400 to £1500, but they do have a certain number of 'assisted places'. Patients on social security can make use of these, but finances need to be looked into very carefully to make sure the patient is not committed to a long-term instalment payment which cannot be maintained later. The clinics take patients from six weeks up to six months and have ample resources and psychiatric expertise. Several are based on the Minnesota Method, a system used in America but not widely described or evaluated in the medical literature. It has links with Alcoholics Anonymous and uses Narcotics Anonymous for follow-up in the community, working on the same 12 principles. Protagonists rather assume there is no other worthwhile treatment in the country, whereas drug workers in other fields are dubious about some of the Minnesota attitudes and about providing services to drug users for a fee.

General practice care

Like family practice in any other field like geriatric or child care, this is an amalgam of single-handed management and referral to other sources of help. It is a good idea *before* being approached by drug users, to find out what other resources there are. You should also decide, with your colleagues what the response would be in certain situations and the limitations of your personal help or involvement. If you are looking after, or prescribing for a certain number of drug users you have to decide how much extra time in the surgery list you can afford, and as with maternity cases, who will cope when you are away. Remember that some drug patients are unpredictable, unreliable and demanding, although most are pleasant to deal with. They try to cooperate, but are under extreme pressures which the ordinary person or doctor finds hard to understand, so while being firm, you have to know when to be flexible. This experience can only come gradually, with advice from others, and as much contact with drug users as possible. It may be better to deal with only two or three clients in depth, and tell the others 'I'm sorry I can't help with your addiction problem at present. Here are some telephone numbers. I will look after your medical needs, but I'm not geared up to getting you off drugs.'

If this policy leads to arguments, implying that you are uncaring, you can keep a copy of the *Guidelines* handy and, without showing people chapter and verse, say that you are trying to help a certain number of drug users on those lines. This means that though you would like to help, you can only manage a few patients at a time. If the reply is then 'Well, Doc, just give me a script and I'll be on my way', explain that you have agreed, with your partners, to follow the *Guidelines* and not do this.

Half a dozen drugtakers a year treated on these lines will keep you busy but it will be a tremendous contribution to the country's drug problem.

At the same time, your practice will not become overwhelmed and chaotic in an effort to meet too many needs. There are exceptions, where an epidemic of drugtaking has arisen within a practice, as in Edinburgh and the Wirral. Some doctors here have taken on 50 or more users and have still managed to run their ordinary practice, with cooperation from partners and the community.

General medical care

When family doctors have no experience or knowledge of the treatment of drug addiction, or if they already have their own quota of users, they should not attempt addiction treatment if a drug user comes to them. Instead they should offer, if possible, general medical care under the NHS both to the user and their family. This is a great service in itself, but it may not be smooth going.

If a clinic is not already doing tests the doctor should arrange for tests of hepatitis B status, liver function, and normal blood count. HIV status may be determined if requested and if pre- an post-test counselling is undertaken. If drug workers request it and with the agreement of the user, a random urine screening can be done. A general physical examination is important at an early stage, and drug complications should be dealt with, remembering they may be obscured by any analgesic taken. Normal conditions should also be dealt with, especially as a user may be in a weak, run-down condition. A state of pregnancy should be handled extra carefully in a user, and in view of an irregular lifestyle, make sure any children in the family have their normal injections brought up to date. Follow-up over the years, even after absences is a desirable feature of this care.

Referral to other facilities

If you decide not to treat the drug problem yourself, the best way to help is to refer the drug user to other facilities in the area. Even if the user's request is only for a supply of tablets, you could have some local telephone numbers to hand so that a refusal to supply an immediate prescription can be followed by an offer of alternative help.

Referring may not be easy if facilities are overstretched, so if a drug user has relatives or friends where he can stay within the catchment area of a DDU or voluntary drug centre, it would be better to go there. Hospital referrals may be through a doctor's letter, but if a letter is requested for a private specialist, you should stipulate that a case history and examination should be undertaken. Voluntary centres usually accept self-referrals, but using the SCODA Directory *Drug Problems – where to get help* (see Appendix B) the doctor can supply names and addresses of facilities, indicating which places might be suitable.

Where a drugtaker is cooperative and seems motivated, the doctor may telephone more distant facilities to enquire about waiting periods and the suitability of the patient.

Practical management

Part of this section refers to the *Guidelines of Good Clinical Practice in the Treatment of Drug Misuse* issued by the DHSS in 1984 and sent to all doctors.

(1) Temporary residents

Some drug users are homeless and have not registered with a GP. If they ask for psychoactive drugs doctors who refuse to have them in the surgery may be at medico-legal risk if the drugtaker is suffering an undiagnosed fracture or head injury, pneumonia or appendicitis masked by drugs. There is no obligation to take them on as permanent patients later but if they agree, blood and urine tests can be done to exclude hepatitis B or screen for drugs, and a full examination should be done. If they are insistent on an immediate prescription for a legal drug and nothing else, you should suggest other possible sources of help together with an AIDS warning about injecting.

Those who present with spurious symptoms usually give the game away by asking for a specific drug, like dihydrocodeine, diazepam, dipipanone or a barbiturate. You should attempt to treat them like any other patient by investigation of the 'backache', 'dysmenorrhea', or 'epilepsy' before prescribing. If they argue or refuse examination they may not even be a drug user, but a dealer seeking supplies, or a journalist looking for a juicy story. On the other hand, drugtakers who are short of funds may seek milder drugs to sell and obtain their own particular illicit drug.

If you have not treated drug users much before, you can learn a good deal from these encounters, not least about yourself. Such tussles therefore need not always be avoided; it depends on how the surgery list is going and how much rumpus the patient creates. The thing is to know what you can offer, stick to certain limits and politely terminate the argument when it is clear that nothing will be achieved. It is helpful to keep an eye on the descriptions sent to each surgery of persistent offenders who 'do the rounds' of doctors under various aliases. Further information can then be sent to the Family Practitioner Committee to warn other doctors. Notification should also be done within seven days. Threats or violence should not force you into writing a prescription just to get rid of them as it may then happen again. If a weapon is used, don't go to extremes; most people value their lives more than a prescription. Such violence should be reported to the police as soon as the offenders have left the surgery.

(2) *The consultation*

The DHSS *Guidelines* speak of a 'first consultation' and a 'diagnostic consultation'. These are extremely variable and must be adapted to the circumstances. A patient coming with a drug problem should be given the same reception as any other patient. The family doctor has the required skills to deal with this kind of problem and if he treats the user as he would any other patient, he may be the first person to have accorded the user such respect. The problem does require longer than the usual five to ten minute appointment, so once you have got a brief picture of the situation, the patient should be asked to make a longer appointment or even two in the next few days. You should explain the reasons and be firm but sympathetic.

However dramatic, opioid withdrawal symptoms are not normally dangerous, but the serious effects of other drugs or masked illness should be looked for and treated appropriately with hospital referral when necessary. Otherwise the doctor can explain that, before discussing treatment, he needs to check with the patient's previous doctor, wait for the results of a urine test to confirm that he is taking drugs and make a full assessment including a blood test to see if he has, or has had, hepatitis B. Section 5 in chapter III (p. 8) of the *Guidelines* says:

'We strongly recommend that the general practitioner should

explain clearly and sympathetically at the first interview that treatment will not necessarily involve prescribing of opioids or barbiturates, and will certainly not involve long-term maintenance prescribing.'

(3) History and examination

Those who have to see several drug users may be able to save time by using a duplicated form such as the one devised by Dr Mike Ross, who has kindly allowed us to reproduce it in Fig. 6.1 (and any doctor to use it). The questions give an excellent idea of the sort of information you are seeking and the drug user can take it away to fill in.

Dr John Strang has written, 'In my view drug use should be seen as a 'presenting symptom' like abdominal pain, and appropriate management depends on the aetiology, the presenting symptoms and the personal and social characteristics of the patient. In assessing the problem it is necessary to establish not only the substance being used but also the pattern of use and the causative (or perpetuating) factors' [1].

The assessment process should be continued beyond the initial consultation bearing in mind that users may minimise or exaggerate their drug intake and may conceal information.

(4) Assessment

(i) Is there a problem at all? For example, a teenager experimenting with drugs may be brought to the surgery by an anxious parent, but is not dependent and a medical response would be inappropriate. A warning may be enough.
(ii) The term 'problem drug user' indicates that medical problems are not the only difficulties a drug user may face. Are there any social, financial or emotional problems? Are any legal proceedings pending?
(iii) What kind of drugs are being used? What amounts and by what route? What is the drug history? Have there been any changes? Are there any medical complications? What is the daily cost and how is it funded?

Reassurance about confidentiality may be needed and prompting about prostitution (male or female) should be tactful. This could be important, in someone who sniffs or smokes their drugs. They might avoid contracting AIDS from injections, but may still

Initial Care 177

This information is for my use only. It is to help me help you.

Please fill in this form:

Name:
Date of birth:
Address:

Tel:
Name and address of your GP:

Medical problems any time in the past: Y/N. Please list with dates:

Psychiatric/emotional problems any time in the past: Y/N. Please list:

Do you take any prescribed tablets: Y/N. Please list:

Are you: Single/Married/Separated/Divorced/Living with parents/
Living with girlfriend/boyfriend/Living with other friend.
Does anyone at home use heroin/other opiates/other illegal
drugs? Y/N Who?............ What?............
Have you got a job? Y/N. If so, what?............
Have you got a trade/qualifications/exams/training? If so,
what?............
Is there anyone close to you who will give you support as you are
coming off?
Y/N   Who?............
Can you briefly give the reasons why you want to come off?
(1) Heroin/Methadone/Morphine/Diconal/Opium (please circle drugs
used)
(a) When did you first take heroin/others............
(b) How long have you been dabbling?............
(c) How long have you been strung out?............
(d) Have you ever been off? Y/N
     If so, how long for, and what were the circumstances of your
     coming off and then restarting again afterwards.

Occasions off:

	Date	Time off	Why off?	Why restart?
(i)				
(ii)				
(iii)				
(iv)				
(v)				

How much are you using each day nowadays?.............
What is the maximum you have used each day?.............
What is your normal method of administration: Smoking/Injection/Medicine by mouth/Snorting
What methods have you used in the past: Smoking/Injection/Medicine by mouth/Snorting

(2) Other drugs:
(a) Alcohol: Never/Moderate/Heavy drinker (Now)   Y/N
            Never/Moderate/Heavy drinker (In the past)   Y/N
(b) Cannabis: Joints per day   0 ... 1-3 ... 4-10 ... 10+ (please circle)
(c) Cigarettes per day: 0 ... 1-5 ... 6-15 ... 16+ ... (please circle)
(d) Speed   Never/Occasionally/Often/In the past only
(e) Acid   Never/Occasionally/Often/In the past only
(f) Cocaine   Never/Occasionally/Often/In the past only
(g) Glue/Gas   Never/Occasionally/Often/In the past only
(h) Other   Please give details:
(i) PS   How many sugars taken in your tea/coffee?.............

Thanks for your help. This information is absolutely confidential.

Figure 6.1 Drug History Assessment Form (courtesy of Dr Mike Ross).

become antibody positive through promiscuous sexual activity or prostitution.

(iv) What previous treatment has been given, if any? What efforts have been made by the user to come off? Why did these fail?

(v) What does the drug user want the doctor to do and what reasons do they have for wanting help at this stage?

(vi) What is the family background and social history, education, relationships, skills, work, accommodation, present circle of friends? How many of them use drugs? Do they have 'straight' (non-using) friends whom they could see more of? This is very important in prognosis, or in deciding whether to undertake treatment.

(vii) Who is available to give support in detoxification and over the next year or more in rehabilitation? There should be a social worker or probation officer, parents, spouse, lover or friends who can be firm yet resilient and who care enough to keep taking it on the chin. They will need to spare a lot of time especially at the beginning.

Few, if any, general practitioners have time to cover all these points themselves. Just to look at them might put you off the effort. Unlike the psychiatrist or social worker who may have spent two to three hours assessing the patient, the GP will only be able to acquire information in a piecemeal fashion, in shorter bursts and over a longer period of time – and then pick out salient points according to individual cases. With experience you will choose your own approach.

In addition to this, there should be other members of the team who will gather some of this information, and hopefully share it with the doctor. You may involve a health visitor, CPN, voluntary or statutory workers and other members of the local Community Drug Team. The two doctors featured in the DHSS video, *Working with Drug Users* provide us with excellent examples of interviews covering the important aspects of drug use (see Appendix C for details).

Until trust has been built up, the doctor is the type of establishment figure that drugtakers have had to deceive in all sorts of situations. Covering up from parents, or police to preserve continuity of drug supplies and avoid consequences of illegal use becomes a way of life. When speaking to the doctor, the amount of drug use may be minimised or more often exaggerated so as to achieve better bargaining power and start detoxification at a higher level than the doctor would otherwise wish. The drug user may misunderstand 'notification' and the confidentiality of records and so withhold information. However, the possibility of information being withheld means that wherever possible doctors should double check. On weekdays, a phone call to the Home Office where the Drugs Branch will ring back to make sure they are talking to a doctor, may elicit information on former medical contacts. This may be treatment from a drug clinic, a GP, private doctor or prison medical officer.

When asking about recent treatment, you may glean the name of other doctors who have seen the drug user. But an accompanying telephone number particularly from a temporary resident should be treated with caution in case there is a bogus doctor at the other end.

Drugtakers must be informed that you can only help them fully if you can speak to relatives or supporting friends in their presence about their history, present drug use, or future hopes. Unless the supporter shares confidentiality and the drug user agrees to let him/her advise, or even hold the drugs in a planned methadone reduction, life will be difficult for both doctor and client. ('Kevin's Story' in module three of the *Working with Drug Users* video covers this point.) If permission is given to seek information even when the user is not present, you can then check the story with statutory or voluntary workers and supporters later. You may also share ideas on treatment. This is in addition to seeking advice from the drug clinic or voluntary centre of your choice as to how to manage the user; even a family doctor experienced with drug users may benefit by confirming certain ideas with a colleague, or the Community Drug Team.

(5) *Preventing HIV and hepatitis infection*

GPs have a responsibility to their staff, their patients, hospital workers and themselves to ensure that no one is exposed unnecessarily to the possibility of infection with AIDS and hepatitis viruses. To ensure that the chances of cross infection are reduced to a minimum, clinical procedures should be undertaken in a way that assumes that all patients are carrying these viruses.

Any procedure that involves the handling of body fluids, particularly blood, must be undertaken with great care and gloves should be routinely worn by the handler. Gloves should also be worn to clean up any spilt blood, which should be treated with bleach diluted 1:10 before removal. In addition, thick gloves should always be worn by any doctor, nurse or anyone dressing an open wound such as an ulcer, cut or graze or doing a vaginal or rectal examination and, for the protection of others, no wound should be left exposed. When attending to dressings or other potentially dirty procedures, disposable plastic aprons also help to protect against contamination.

Biohazard labels should be attached to the containers of pathological specimens and their accompanying forms if the patient is considered to be in a high risk group. All dirty sharps should be placed as soon as possible in a sharps box and when this is full it should be sealed and arrangements made for its incineration. In the event of a needle stick injury, local toilet should be applied as soon as possible to the wound. Blood should be eluted from the syringe and needle, and arrangements made to test it for hepatitis B virus and antibody to HIV. While awaiting these results and within 48 hours of the needle stick injury, hepatitis B immunoglubulin should be given, unless the person concerned is known to have good immunity following a course of hepatitis B vaccine or prior injection with the virus.

The hepatitis B vaccine, a course of three injections, gives good immunity in over 90% of cases. It is prudent to ensure that immunity has been established by testing for antibodies to surface antigen (HBsAg) following injection of the third vaccine. The vaccine should be offered to all doctors and nurses working in GPs' surgeries, and uptake should be particularly encouraged in areas of high prevalence of drug misuse.

Protection of other patients from cross-infection needs to be reviewed with regard to human immunodeficiency virus (HIV), the hepatitis viruses, and human papillomavirus. *HIV* is probably inactivated by heat at 56°C for 30 minutes and should be inactivated by a temperature of 80°C for one minute. Chemical disinfection also inactivates the virus and should be substituted when heat cannot be used. Activated 2% glutaraldehyde solution of hypochlorite (10,000 ppm available chlorine) for 60 minutes will effectively kill off the virus.

For *hepatitis B virus* the chemical method for disinfection is the same as for HIV. The virus is also thought to be inactivated by 'moist heat' at 98°C or more for one minute, 'dry heat' at 160°C for one hour and by boiling water for at least ten minutes.

Human papillomavirus is also recently causing concern with regard to disinfection of vaginal specula and 'trial-caps'. Transmission is via virus-infected cells, rather than free virus, and there is very little 'virus-load' in the lesions. The virus is very heat labile, with boiling water (100°C) for five minutes more than adequate for inactivation. However, because the virus is cell-associated, preparation of instruments is very important, requiring thorough cleaning with hot water and detergent to remove cells and mucus, prior to the disinfection process. Heat is preferred to chemical agents because the latter may not reach the cell-associated virus.

In the document circulated to all general practitioners in one Health District [2] the following conclusions were made:

'Thorough cleaning in hot water and detergent is important in the preparation of any article for the sterilisation/disinfection proocedures. Cleaning in hot water and detergent alone is suitable for items such as earpieces of auroscopes.

The most predictable means of sterilisation is an autoclave. For example 121°C at 15 lb/square inch for 15 minutes will destroy all bacteria, spores and viruses. The equipment is expensive and needs proper maintenance.

A hot-air oven is also suitable for sterilisation but the higher temperatures required may harm some instruments and the cycle time is much longer.

Boiling water does not sterilise but is adequate for disinfection of some equipment, and when used correctly will inactivate HIV, hepatitis B virus and papillomaviruses within ten minutes.

Chemical agents are sometimes useful for heat-sensitive equipment. Prolonged immersion in 2% glutaraldehyde is suitable for sterilisation. Contaminated surfaces should be disinfected with 1% hypochlorite solution (10,000 ppm available chlorine) which is left for 30 minutes. Isopropyl alcohol (70% v/v) or 0.1% hypochlorite solution should be used for general disinfection of work surfaces.'

Further information is available in:

- *Aquired Immune Deficiency Syndrome*, Booklet 3. DHSS, April 1986. Guidance for Surgeons, Anaesthetists and Dentists.
- *Decontamination of Equipment, Linen or other Surfaces Contaminated with Hepatitis B or Human Immunodeficiency Virus*. DHSS circular HN (87) 1, Jan 1987.
  BDA Dental Health and Science Committee Workshop, 1986. The problems of cross-infection in Dentistry. Br. Den. J., Feb 22, 131-134.
- *Sterilisers: Health Technical Memorandum 10* (HTM 10). DHSS, March 1980.
- *A Guide to Hygienic Skin Piercing*. CDSC, 1983. Dr N. Noah, (currently being updated).

(6) AIDS considerations

Measures to help prevent the spread of infection are outlined above and a detailed exposition of HIV and AIDS can be found earlier in the book. Here we look at the GPs role in relation to HIV and AIDS.

Testing for HIV antibodies

This should only be done with informed consent and with both pre- and post-test counselling. Although such counselling is available elsewhere, particularly through Genito-Urinary Medicine (GUM) clinics, every GP should know how to counsel a patient for the HIV test. Testing and counselling drugtakers is best undertaken when their drug use is stable and it is often wise to extend the counselling period over the course of two or three consultations. Testing without any prior counselling must never be undertaken in any circumstances. There have been several recorded cases of suicide when this has been done.

HIV testing is best confined to high risk groups. Testing the 'worried well' may be counterproductive. At present the likelihood of a false positive result is 250 times greater than the likelihood of a true positive. The ratio of false positives to true positives is always high when the prevalence of HIV infection is low in the population being tested. Currently this is the case in almost all general practices. The sensitivity and specificity of tests for antibodies to HIV are about 99.5% and the current prevalence of HIV infection in Britain in 1988 is about 0.002%. If general practitioners nationally perform 50,000 tests on this population there will probably be one true positive, 49,749 true negatives, and 250 false positive results. Thus positive results found by general practitioners, especially in cases where there is no major risk factor for HIV infection, should be treated as false positives until confirmed by specialised tests.

Confidentiality as to the result of the test is of course essential but it is regrettable that GPs are often unaware of the result of a positive test done by other medical sources on the basis of confidentiality. In every other circumstance the GP is normally notified of confidential medical matters with the knowledge that this is in the interests of the patient and that medical confidentiality will be maintained. However an exception is generally made with HIV testing on the grounds that this will interfere with his or her life insurance rating. This is to the patient's detriment as much future physical and psychological morbidity will be related to the emotional distress and anxiety surrounding a positive test result, and if the GP is aware of this result then much of this morbidity can be prevented. Also, at a later stage the GP may well need to become involved in providing terminal care at home, and it is therapeutically helpful if he has the opportunity to cement a good relationship with his patient at an early stage before adverse symptoms appear.

(1) *Pre-test counselling.* This should include all those things that are necessary to say if the test is positive as a positive result is likely to 'blow the mind' of the patient, making it impossible to take in important information. For a drug-using patient the news is likely to precipitate a bout of chaotic drug use, making counselling even more difficult and putting the patient and others around him at risk. Pre-test counselling should include:

(1) Advice that a positive test does not mean that you have AIDS. Only a minority of people with a positive test result go on to develop AIDS. A positive test means only that the body has come into contact with the virus. The fact that antibodies have been formed against the virus does not imply that the virus has been rejected by the body. The virus must be considered to have a continuing presence within the body with the capability of infecting others and causing disease. Nevertheless, on current knowledge, most people with a positive test will not develop AIDS.
(2) Advice that if a person is seropositive they can spread the virus

sexually, by sharing injecting equipment or, if they are women, the infection can be spread to a baby that is born to them (vertical transmission) and possibly also by breast feeding. It is therefore important to give advice on ways of reducing the risk of spread by discussing in particular safer injecting, safer sex, availability of injecting equipment and in some cases the cleaning of such equipment. This advice is so important that it is best given on first encountering a drug user as this may be the only time he/she attends. It can then be repeated both before and after the HIV test. It should be given to all drug users as those who never inject may progress to doing so and other 'non-injectors' may inject occasionally.

(a) *Advice about injecting* should stress that because the virus is so easily and rapidly spread by sharing needles and syringes this must never occur and is of the utmost importance both for the patient and for others.

Advice should also be given that the virus is spread by any form of injecting: intravenous, intramuscular, or subcutaneous (skin-popping), not, as some people believe, purely by intravenous injecting. The availability of clean injecting equipment through local needle and syringe exchange schemes and local pharmacies should be discussed, and information should also be imparted on how to clean syringes. As hot water causes blood products to coagulate, injecting equipment is best rinsed first with cold water alone by drawing up the cold water into the needle and syringe and then expelling it. A jug should then be filled with cold water, given a squirt of washing up liquid, and a second rinse given by drawing this up. After a final rinse with cold water alone the needle and plunger should then be removed from the barrel of the syringe and all three should be boiled in water for 5 minutes. Bleach was originally recommended for cleaning syringes and in some places, for example San Francisco, bleach has been dispensed to drug users on a large scale. However it is not recommended in the UK because bleach itself increases clotting and the virus can 'hide' behind the clot and be protected by it. Bleach also has possible toxic effects and varying strengths are available.

Generally speaking the advice should be: Don't inject, but if you do don't share, but if you do clean your needle and syringe.

Cleaning equipment is thought only to provide a minimal degree of protection and is no substitute for sterile equip-

ment, either purchased or obtained free at a needle and syringe exchange scheme.
(b) *Advice about safer sex* should aim at reducing the risk of transmitting HIV by the avoidance of medium and high risk sexual activities. The various risk categories are.

No risk
Solo masturbation
Massage away from genital area

Low risk
Mutual masturbation
Dry kissing
Body rubbing

Medium risk
Wet kissing
Fellatio (sucking)
Urination (water sports) external only
Anilingus (rimming)

High risk
Anal and vaginal sex
Fisting (insertion of hand or fist into the rectum)
Sharing sex toys
Any sex act that draws blood

Fellatio may be safe if it is stopped prior to ejaculation. Anal and vaginal sex may be safe if a condom is used. Condoms have been shown to give a degree of protection against the transmission of HIV [3]. Many spermicides give additional protection: HIV is inactivated in vitro in 60 seconds by 0.05% nonoxynol [4], an ingredient present at concentrations of 5–12.5% in several British spermicides, e.g. Duragel, EMKO foam, Ortho-form and Staycept pessaries. Condoms should only be used with water-based lubricants (e.g. KY jelly) as oil based lubricants can damage the rubber. General practitioners cannot at the time of writing prescribe condoms.

Even with good and thorough counselling on safer sex, drug users as a group do not appear to change their sexual behaviour away from high risk activities as readily as do male homosexuals and they may need repeated counselling in this area. Additional problems revolve around the fact that many specialist drug workers and doctors find it embarrassing or difficult to discuss sexual habits and special training may be required to overcome these problems.

(3) Explanation of the risks of vertical transmission. The risk of a seropositive pregnant woman transmitting HIV to her unborn child is thought to be about 30–50%. Testing new born babies is difficult as they have their mother's antibodies and will therefore be seropositive whether or not they carry the virus. Full discussion about pregnancy, contraception, and sterilisation may prevent the tragedy of a young child with AIDS. Seropositive and untested, high risk women should be advised not to breast feed.

(4) Exploring the patient's possible reaction to a positive test result. This is important. If, in answer to the question 'What would you do if the test was positive?', the patient replies 'I would probably kill myself', then either further counselling is required or the test should not be done. It is important to elucidate who would be supportive to the patient over the first few days of knowing a positive result. Some drug users are very isolated, having little in the way of social support, and these people are also probably best not tested unless there are strong reasons for doing so, such as the need to make a diagnosis, or because the drugtaker is pregnant and would want a termination if she was seropositive. In such cases testing is best done in a contained environment (e.g. inpatient treatment unit, rehabilitation house, prison etc.) where a lot of support can be given from professional carers.

(2) *Post-test counselling* For all patients, whether or not they are drug users, the knowledge that they have a positive HIV test is shattering, however well they may have been prepared. Most will not hear or remember any counselling or advice that is given so that written handouts as a supplement to oral advice are invaluable. There are a number of good handouts available. One, *Advice for people who are HIV Positive* by Dr Charles Farthing was published in the November 1986 issue of *Maternal and Child Health* and is reproduced in Appendix F. Another handout compiled by the Terrence Higgins Trust and entitled *Advice for People who are Antibody Positive* is also useful. For copies, telephone 01-831-0330.

Drugtakers, on finding they are HIV positive, usually respond by indulging in chaotic drug use, and intentional or semi-intentional overdoses may occur. It is therefore of great importance that as much support as possible is available over the first few days. The telephone number of the surgery, the local Samaritans and the Terrence Higgins Trust Helpline: 01-242-1010 (open 3 pm – 10 pm, 7 days a week) should be given to the patient for use in times of crisis. The doctor should attempt to make himself as available as possible. Further telephone numbers can be given for more information and advice about HIV infection. These are the local health education department the National AIDS Helpline: 0800-567123 (which is free); Healthline telephone service: 01-981-2717; 01-980-722 or 0345-581151; the Welsh AIDS Campaign 0222-464121; the Scottish AIDS Monitor 031-558-1167 and the Northern Ireland AIDS line, Belfast 0232-226117. The local GUM clinic may also be a useful resource for information about AIDS.

The seropositive drugtaker should be advised that his/her chances of avoiding AIDS will be best if he/she leads as healthy a life style as possible. Adequate nutrition, sleep, exercise and the avoidance of sexually transmitted disease, excessive alcohol use and illicit drugs, particularly cannabis and opiates and especially any street drug that is injected, are all probably helpful in preventing progression of HIV infection to AIDS.

The advice given in the pre-test phase regarding injecting and safer sex should be repeated, and the drug user should be reminded that treatment for his/her drug problem (as it clearly is a problem now even if it was not thought by the drugtaker to be a problem before) is available should he/she wish it.

Up-to-date information about local self-help groups such as Body Positive and the Women's HIV Group is available through the Terrence Higgins Trust.

In the immediate phase of knowing the result of a positive test patients should be advised against telling others, particularly employers, who are unaware that the test was being done, as negative and hostile reactions can make this phase much more difficult to cope with. A follow-up appointment, where possible in the company of a lover, spouse, relative, or parent is helpful. About 5 days after hearing the test result is a useful time to do this. If the sexual partner accompanies the patient this provides an opportunity for counselling him or her about safer sex techniques, otherwise the sexual partner needs to be sought out to do this. In almost every case the partner will also wish to be tested, and if he/she is on the GPs list, the GP is responsible for arranging for this to be done together with full pre- and post-test counselling. It should not be forgotten that some partners of drug users may also use drugs themselves and may be in need of advice and treatment about this as well.

Treating and coping with AIDS in a drug user is proving to have special difficulties in North America. Providing a service to homeless drugtakers with AIDS has been a major problem. Those that have homes are often too unstable through their drug use to take AZT (Zidovudine), which has to be taken 4-hourly even through the night.

From the point of view of treatment, drug users present as a very difficult group compared to homosexuals with AIDS, who are generally well motivated and responsible with good social back-up. Dr J.A. Cohn from the Bellevue Hospital, New York, lists the following lack of innate resources available in drug-users:

(i) Physical and economic resources – functioning household, employment, regular income, provision for dependants.
(ii) External emotional support – family and friends in a position to provide comfort and to help with out-of-hospital care.
(iii) Personal emotional resources – the ability to deal with the stress of a severe prolonged and fatal illness.
(iv) Knowledge about AIDS – consciousness of having been at risk, awareness of the implications of the diagnosis, understanding of one's past and future role in transmission.
(v) Interactive style – the interactions between the patient and providers impact on the quality of care, effect of the patient as 'good' or 'demanding' or 'manipulative', effect of bias by providers, such as homophobia and negative feelings about drugtakers.

(7) Urine testing

Principles
Where no opioids are to be prescribed by the doctor, there is less need to screen urine for drugs. The test may be used initially to confirm drug use, and as a later check on whether the drugtaker is really serious about giving up on all drugs. The chromatography test will reveal if, having abjured heroin, there is continuing use of amphetamine or cannabis.

During methadone detoxification, however, urine tests are essential:

(i) To see on first contact with the drug user whether or not the story of current drug use is correct. Since the test is qualitative but not quantitative you cannot check on the amount of each drug being taken, but if you ask for a 'total screen' you may be surprised at what you get. If a drug user protesting that he/she only takes 'smack' (heroin) comes up with phenobarbitone in the blood, for example, he/she may not be lying as some illicit supplies of heroin are laced with phenobarbitone powder. Sometimes when a drug user has obviously been injecting, the test comes up negative, which means the last injection may have been several days ago. At other times, it may be loaded with a variety of drugs: amphetamines, largactil and cannabis plus heroin (or rather the metabolites) despite protestations that only one drug is being taken. The user should then be informed of the test results and urged to be frank with the doctor if there is to be any hope of a useful relationship.

(ii) because random urine tests are needed every few days, or every week or two to test what the pharmaceutical companies love to call 'patient compliance'. Negative results might indicate that the patient no longer required methadone but was selling it; whereas if the urine showed that the patient was taking other drugs in addition to methadone, after one or two lapses the course should be terminated. Then, one could either suggest an inpatient detoxification or a second try when the patient is more motivated.

Practical points

(i) The urine should be passed ideally in the presence of a doctor or nurse. While this is embarrassing and increases the atmosphere of suspicion, one should explain that in other places drug users have made use of doctored urines, and so the rules have been made accordingly. A cold false urine specimen may be warmed in the hands to simulate a fresh sample, or even more ingeniously a small tube is strapped to the underside of the penis. Of course, as police surgeons well know, some people cannot urinate on demand or under the eagle eye of a medical supervisor, so common sense must prevail.

(ii) Some enquiry should be made beforehand at the hospital as to what facilities are available for a urine screen. It is frustrating, to say the least, to be landed with a vital specimen, near the weekend, and not to know where to dispose of it. Increasingly local hospital laboratories are doing the chromatography, but even if they don't, they are duty-bound to send it on for you. This may take a week or more, so it is useful to discuss the situation with the pathologist in charge. On the NHS this service should be free to the GP, but privately it may cost a few pounds. Established laboratories like the Guys Hospital Poisons Unit at New Cross Hospital, Avonley Road, London SE14 have special forms you may request, or they may give advice (01-407 7600, extension 4014 – the Addiction Screening Unit). If you are sending off specimens on an irregular basis, it is a courtesy to ring up and say you wish to do this. Normally the result comes in three to four days. This is crucial if you make the rule, as some doctors do, not to prescribe opioids until you have seen the result of the test. A test positive for opioids in itself may not be a true guide to the patient's user status. Learning through the grapevine of the doctor's habits, a user may have loaded the bloodstream with heroin previously in order to obtain a script.

(iii) Now the patient has gone and you are standing there with a kidney dish of warm urine. What to do next? Any plain 30 ml specimen bottle will do, without preserving powder. Preferably have a member of staff trained to take over at this stage with all the kit ready to hand. The bottle should be labelled and wrapped with enough absorbent material e.g. paper towelling or wool, to soak up the urine should the bottle break in transit. This is then put in one or two sealed polythene bags. To be quite safe these should go into a path-style cardboard box or a plastic tablet jar about five inches tall. A few drug injectors are hepatitis B positive, and since this is much more infectious than AIDS, you are sending a somewhat hazardous substance through the post. You may have had the wisdom to take the three HB Vax injections yourself but if your staff member is not inoculated he or she should be even more carefully instructed to do everything over the sink with polythene gloves and wash down thoroughly. If you are sending the bottle away by post and not by hand across to the local laboratory, one of the old strong glass bottles may be adequate with the absorbent wrapping in a jiffy bag. If it is in a box, wrap it up as a parcel, labelling it clearly and affix a yellow 'Biohazard' or 'Danger from infection' label, from your local laboratory. Where you have obtained the right lab. form, enclose it with the bottle, or write the details on headed notepaper. These include name, age, address, sex and what drugs are expected to be found, and you should request a total addiction screen. If you are sending the bottle to your own laboratory, ring up and warn them that it could be a hepatitis B positive specimen and affix a warning label to the bottle.

All this rigmarole may sound enough to deter you from doing urine specimens at all, but if you can work out the procedure with your staff, it will become an almost painless routine in time.

Treatment of Opioid misuse

To prescribe or not to prescribe opioids?

Until recently it was very generally true that the further North you travelled from London, the less likely you were to find clinics prescribing methadone even on a short-term basis. This is still broadly valid (with the exception of Liverpool), but in Scotland, where the most hard-line approach to prescribing methadone has prevailed, the attitudes of some clinicians have been modified by the need to attract more users to the clinics and away from injecting.

Before going on to detail the non-medical resources, we will describe two typical medical approaches which may be adopted by the general practitioner – opioid detoxification both with and without the use of methadone.

Opioid detoxification without methadone

With a non-methadone treatment regime, one does not have the inducement of a regularly given drug to keep the user coming. Some patients will try elsewhere or not be motivated enough to try coming off yet.

(i) *The principle.* Those who do come avoid the drawbacks of methadone detoxification. They no longer need to be monitored carefully; there is no call for urine tests to see if they are cheating; no arguing about the dose or about breaking contracts and less emphasis on security and leakage to the black market. You get away from the suspicion and manipulation which can avoid the tacit agreement that drugs are *the* important thing to talk about, so there is more freedom to talk about other problems. You also avoid the use of a highly addictive drug.

The non-prescription of methadone relies on the fact that withdrawal from opiates is not dangerous. Heroin users can and do withdraw safely without medical cover. For the user to know that he will not endanger his life by withdrawing even though at times it may feel like that, and for this to be reinforced by either lack of prescription or symptomatic prescription, actually reduces the problems experienced as does a sympathetic environment and understanding care.

(ii) *Indications.* Obviously, the non-prescribing approach is ideal for the young, recent drug user or heroin smoker, or habitual experimenter with a variety of drugs and alcohol. It is also used in Scotland for the long-term opiate user. Dr Roy Robertson, whose studies include large numbers of young drug users, describes the alternatives [5]:

> 'There may be attendance at a hospital outpatients' or a family doctor's surgery followed by contact with community psychiatric nurses experienced in drug treatment. Among facilities in Scotland there are self-help groups; some have an open door approach and group discussions or individual work. Other drug users attend voluntary centres and are involved with non-specialist social workers. Few are suitable or able to get to rehabilitation centres nearly all of which are in England'.

In view of the high proportion of positive HIV antibody tests among intravenous drug users (over 60% in 1986), Dr Robertson supported a policy of supplying sterile syringes and needles to injecting users, which has now been taken up in other areas of the country. At the time of writing, 15 needle exchange schemes (12 in England and 3 in Scotland) are being evaluated through DHSS-funded research. It is easier to put a non-prescribing policy into action where there is a variety of flexible resources and the doctor has more time himself for counselling.

(iii) *Symptomatic prescribing.* Those who use symptomatic prescriptions of diazepam are wise to limit it to a two or three week course and a decreasing dose of up to 40–50 mg given at night to help the sleep problems. Temazepam should never be used because it is so readily injected. Also, because it is so short-acting, it will cause rebound insomnia and anxiety after 3–4 hours. Loperamide (Imodium) or Lomotil (diphenoxylate and atropine) though mild opioids can help diarrhoea in the first week or two but no longer. Other symptomatic medicines mentioned in the DHSS *Guidelines* are thioridiazine (Melleril) and propanolol (Inderal) to control anxiety, but the *Guidelines* recommend that they 'should not continue for more than two weeks following a last dose in an opioid detoxification regime'.

(iv) *Antagonists and clonidine.*

CLONIDINE. Family doctors are familiar with clonidine in two of its formulations; as Dixarit in 25 microgram doses it is indicated for the prophylaxis of migraine and the prevention of menopausal flushing and as Catapres in 0.1 or 0.3 milligram tablets, it can be used for all grades of hypertension. Although it is an alpha-adrenergic agonist rather than an antagonist, clonidine is also finding a place in the treatment of opioid withdrawals. The area in the hind brain known as the locus coeruleus is modulated by endorphins, the body's natural opioids. These exert a presynaptic inhibition on the synapse in the locus thus regulating the release of noradrenaline in normal amounts.

In opioid dependence, the following processes take place, as illustrated in Fig. 6.2.

'The differences in the mode of action of opiates and clonidine in the locus coeruleus are greatly simplified in Fig. 6.2. The acute opiate effect (1A) results in stimulation of the opiate receptor by exogenous opiates, with subsequent inhibition of noradrenaline (NA) release.

In opiate addiction there is a continuous stimulation by exogenous opiates, resulting in a reduction of endorphin activity and at the same time a relative inhibition of central neuronal activity. However, the development of opiate tolerance leads to a gradual normalisation of NA release (1B). In opiate withdrawal there is no longer any stimulation of the opiate receptors or inhibition of neuronal activity and consequently there is no inhibition of NA release; there is an

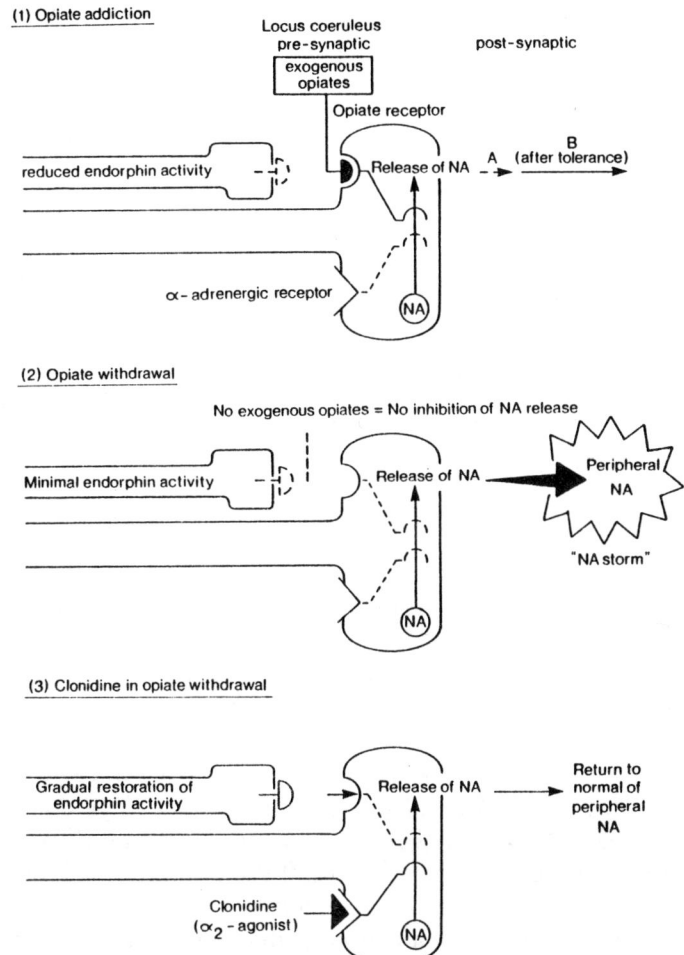

Figure 6.2 Differences in the mode of action of opiates and clonidine in the locus coeruleus. (Source: Mortality and Morbidity Weekly Report.)

overshoot release of NA, a peripheral 'NA storm', which accounts for most of the symptoms of opiate withdrawal. Clonidine, a pure agonist, is able to normalise NA release without stimulation of the opiate receptor, thus inhibiting many of the symptoms of opiate withdrawal.'[6]

(1) SIDE EFFECTS OF CLONIDINE

Less desirable features of clonidine treatment when used alone (i.e. without naltrexone) are as follows.

(1) There is a risk of postural hypertension during detoxification. Dr Mike Ross, a GP in Liverpool whose outpatient regime is

mentioned below, has found this effect to be less troublesome in practice than in theory, provided his protocol is followed.
(2) Rebound hypertension is a risk at the end of clonidine treatment but in doses of 0.5 mg over the 24 hours, this does not seem to be a problem.
(3) Other side effects include insomnia, lethargy, bone pains and headaches, and after 5 days of treatment 50% of patients may start to feel depressed. The ongoing reduction of dosage and plenty of reassurance will mitigate this.
(4) A clonidine course gives less relief from withdrawal symptoms than methadone.
(5) It is not popular with some patients simply because it lacks any dependence potential and is useless on the black market.

Two examples of its current use are given.

(a) The inpatient regime
At Guys Hospital, London, a series of opiate addicts were treated with clonidine instead of methadone before passing them on to a rehabilitation centre. Those who were followed up in a general psychiatric clinic only, tended to relapse. The following regime was used.

After admission, assessment and blood pressure measurements, clonidine is given in a dose of 0.1 mg qds for five days and is then tapered off, to complete the course in seven days. The nurses check blood pressure before giving each dose. If the diastolic is below 60 mm Hg the next dose is omitted. Where withdrawal symptoms are more severe up to 0.8 mg per day of clonidine may be used. For methadone users, the course usually requires 10 days instead of seven. This contrasts with dosages in America where up to 1–2 mg daily were given, probably maintaining patients supine to avoid postural hypotension. In the UK, patients prefer to be ambulant, but even when the diastolic blood pressure was at the arbitrary limit of 60 mm Hg fainting was not a problem.

Of the side effects, insomnia was the most troublesome for which a benzodiazepine hypnotic was prescribed. Diarrhoea was not worrying and was controlled by imodium, nausea by maxolon, headaches or bone pains by paracetamol [7].

A letter in the *British Medical Journal* concluded:

> The only significant limitation to the usefulness of clonidine is its hypotensive effect ... Lofexidine, a clonidine analogue with much lower hypotensive potency has proved effective in open trials ... Our own experience has convinced us of the value of a clonidine

detoxification and we have now used it successfully for almost three years.'[8]

(b) The outpatient regime
Many authorities still disagree with this but Dr Mike Ross has used clonidine for several years in Liverpool and has built up a series of well over 200 cases. He has produced a typed protocol for other doctors which he is willing to supply, along with a page of instructions for the patient. He is willing to supply these papers or answer telephone queries at The Princes Park Health Centre, Bentley Road, Liverpool L8 0SY (telephone 051-728 8313).

The course is suitable for the milder cases of heroin dependence, especially where the patient is well motivated and wishes to avoid methadone treatment. For users taking a gram or so of heroin daily, or over a long period, or coming back for the second time Dr Ross now uses methadone detoxification, but still finds clonidine helpful for others.

His present regime is to give clonidine 0.1 mg, one tablet during the day and three tablets at night. He starts to cut down daytime doses after five days. To counteract insomnia he gives diazepam 10 mg, two to three tablets at night, for a period of two weeks, or longer if necessary. Patients are warned about driving or using machinery and about taking extra tablets to quicken the course. They are watched for postural hypotension and side effects. They are asked to bring a friend or relative to help them manage the course. Each patient monitors his own withdrawal symptoms and adjusts tablets accordingly after a few days [9].

(2) NALTREXONE WITH CLONIDINE
Opioid antagonists like naloxone, used in overdose crises, have to be given by injection and cause distressing side effects, only tolerable in a life or death situation. In the USA, because of the need to detoxify safely certain patients on the methadone maintenance programmes there, a modification of naloxone, named naltrexone, was developed in the early seventies which was long-acting, relatively safe, available in tablet form and without euphoriant (agonist) properties. One drawback remained: naltrexone still required a period of 5-10 days (in methadone users – less with heroin) for the opioids to leave the system. To cover this crucial period when relapses would occur, clonidine was employed as a useful bridging method. The protocol is complicated in the USA and still requires a hospital setting, usually an inpatient course. The theoretical dangers of hypotension and bradycardia have not proved in practice to be much of a drawback in the USA and the programme has continued successfully.

A further development was to continue naltrexone on a supervised basis to prevent relapses, arguing that it could play a similar role to that of Antabuse, in alcoholism. This proved of value in a prison work-release programme.

In this country a modification of the American protocol has been undertaken by Dr Colin Brewer. The opioid withdrawal period has been reduced to about 3 days, and with almost 100 cases completed, a report of 60 of these is in preparation (1987).

> 'Although (naltrexone) causes severe withdrawal symptoms if given in full dosage to patients still using or withdrawing from opiates, smaller doses (1–5 mg initially) given every 3 or 4 hours with clonidine reduce the duration and severity of withdrawal symptoms very significantly compared with clonidine alone. After only 3–4 days patients' can be given full doses of naltrexone thrice weekly. This technique is suitable for day patient use and means that expensive inpatient detoxification can be reserved for those addicts who clearly need it.'[10]

Up to now (1987) other clinics have not attempted the naltrexone course in the UK and the three day course in a private hospital costs several hundred pounds.

On Dr Brewer's course, a naloxone challenge is now given at the outset to determine how severe the withdrawals might be, along with diazepam if required to relieve it. A test dose of clonidine (0.2 mg) is also given after admission, and a brief preliminary cardiovascular examination. The withdrawals are modified partly by the sedating effect of the clonidine, and by the addition of diazepam over 2 or 3 days, at an average rate of 70 mg per 24 hours. On the first day the average dose of naltrexone given is 14mg. For severe distress the drug may be stopped for a few hours. For vomiting an injection of hyoscine or maxolon suffices.

In the follow-up naltrexone is continued wherever possible, and is particularly effective in probation cases. 'By the third day most patients can tolerate the normal daily dosage of 50 mg and naltrexone is then continued at a dosage of 100 mg on Mondays, and Wednesdays and 150 mg on Fridays which simplifies the supervision and prolongs the action.'

Dr Brewer compares the effect of supervised long-term naltrexone with that of Antabuse in alcoholism, pointing out that the lack of pleasurable result if a user does try some opioid deters further experimentation. Not all would accept this comparison. The difficulty lies in the supervision of the drug, where the parents, friends or voluntary groups are concerned but the drop-out rate appears to be no more than with other long-term treatments and may be better. (Certainly, drop-outs during the three day course rarely if ever occur.) Cooperation with general practitioners has been good in general. The drug which has not yet (1987) received a general licence, can be obtained on private or NHS prescriptions, if the words 'Named patient basis' appear on the prescription. The manufacturers, Du Pont, can usually supply it within 24 hours. Certain cases are now managed as day-case detoxification.

The treatment has been criticised from various angles, partly by non-medical workers who see it as an 'easy option' bypassing the psychological need for change. A medical comment warned of the dangers of regarding naltrexone as a drug of low toxicity, especially in liver function, and possible effects on endocrine systems. GPs who undertake prescribing with naltrexone should ensure that the liver function is regularly checked. The same letter quoted the manufacturer's warning of the 'dangers should the patient attempt to override naltrexone blockade with large doses of exogenous opiates'. Similar problems arise if potent analgesia is medically indicated due to intercurrent illness and trauma.

If a comprehensive, well-researched follow up scheme can be combined with the NHS treatment, either inpatient or outpatient, there will be an increasing demand for this alternative to a methadone detoxification.

(v) *Helping 'cold turkey'.* 'Cold turkey' (abrupt withdrawal) can take place in a number of circumstances: when the drugtaker goes into police custody or prison, or it may be a course decided upon by the drug user voluntarily. It is much feared by opioid drugtakers, but may not be as drastic as they anticipate.

Why should any doctor's help be needed? Occasionally the drug user or his friends or family may feel that advice or guidance is needed on the health hazards or methods of withdrawing or doing 'cold turkey', so that the procedure has the best chance of succeeding. If a doctor therefore wishes to help a particular drug user or family not just to come off drugs but stay off he may advise as follows.

The health hazard is negligible in a straightforward case. Where several drugs are being used (particularly barbiturates), withdrawal can be more dangerous with convulsions and fits.

Regarding the method of going through withdrawal, drug users and their friends should be advised to send to ISDD for two booklets produced by the Blenheim Project – *How to Stop* and *How to Help* (95p each). These suggest that if the drugtaker is working he should ask for a certificate, 'a tactful sick note' for perhaps two but no more than four weeks off work. The booklets recommend a comfortable place in which to get over the physical effects of withdrawal – a bed, warmth, fresh air, books, TV, records, games etc., a stock of food and drinks, and general care as for 'flu. A supportive friend or family, who can encourage the drugtaker during the hard times, and keep a strict eye open for temptations, is a great asset. Plans for the future should be made for the business of staying off drugs. Once withdrawal is completed, arrangements for avoiding relapses and perhaps moving to a new environment should be considered.

(vi) Neuroelectric therapy. Like the philosopher's stone, a physical method of aiding withdrawal from drugs which avoids the use of chemicals has long been sought. Electro-acupuncture was used in San Francisco but without enough success for the programme to be adopted generally. A study is being conducted in Merseyside at present (1987) into the use of electro-acupuncture by the Society of Biophysical Medicine, but this too will require the completion of controlled outcome studies to be accepted widely.

Many hopes, therefore, have been pinned on the controversial NET (NeuroElectric Therapy) developed by Dr Meg Patterson after her experience with addicts in Hong Kong while she was Head of Surgery at the Tung Wah Hospital. A neurosurgical colleague Dr Wen, recently back from China having learned about 'electro-acupuncture' was using it for pain relief. He discovered in November 1972 that some of his patients who happened to be heroin or opium addicts had experienced relief in withdrawing from these drugs. Dr Patterson then started to experiment and analyse the effects of the electrical stimulus itself. This did not involve acupuncture or its applications and the stimulus was mediated through two electrodes placed behind the ears. She then went on to develop a new apparatus capable of delivering the necessary complex electrical signals, popularly known as the black box.

It was given a year's trial in Sussex at the Pharmakon Clinic from January to December 1980. 102 patients were treated and the results added to those patients treated from 1973 onwards to make a total of 186 cases, described in an article in 1984 [7].

Patients treated over the years have included a number of well known rock musicians like Pete Townshend and most recently Boy George, who took a course of NET but also other treatment. This led to a great deal of publicity and media claims for its universal efficacy. In the summary of the 1984 paper, Dr Patterson writes:

> 'Neuroelectric therapy (NET) is a 10-day treatment with a transistorised stimulator, which rapidly reduces both the acute and chronic withdrawal symptomatology of all chemical substances without

drugs and with no negative side effects. It is hypothesised that NET acts by specific electrical frequency stimulation of endorphin production that has been decreased due to chronic substance abuse. This has been demonstrated using NET in rat models; corticosterone levels and hepatic enzyme activity were also significantly altered. Of 186 patients 98.4% were successfully detoxified, with marked feeling of well-being and no craving (in 95%) or anxiety (in 75%). Detailed assessments of abstinence syndrome in NET are given. Of a 50% response to follow-up, 78.5% were addiction-free (80.3% of drug addicts) one to eight years after NET, although the average time in (inpatient) rehabilitation was only 16 days. Alcohol, marijuana and cigarette use were decreased in 64%. Diminished substances use was reported in 76% of recidivists.' [11]

In the meantime, before publication of the total results and without consultation with Dr Patterson, an independent three month trial was conducted in 1981 at the Bethlem Royal Hospital, in London. Dr Gossop *et al.* in their summary, stated:

'A group of 24 opiate addicts admitted to an inpatient drug dependence unit received either electrostimulation or gradual oral methadone withdrawal. Addicts treated with electrostimulation showed high levels of withdrawal symptoms during the first week of treatment: these reached a peak on day three. In this respect, electrostimulation was markedly inferior to methadone withdrawal treatment. However, although progressive methadone withdrawal quickly reduced symptoms to a moderate or low level, there was no reduction in symptomatology as late as one month after admision (i.e. after ten days without methadone).' [12]

Dr Patterson complained that the 'so-called independent trial only peripherally resembled her NET, that the frequencies used in the black box were wrong, and the methodology unsound'. She quoted the Gossop paper: 'only seven out of ten electrostimulation patients stayed for the ten-day ES period and nine out of twelve patients completed the twenty-day methadone withdrawal treatment'. (*Guardian*, 25 February 1980). Dr Strang, one of the authors of the paper, however, commented that he went into the trial with high hopes but after persuading authorities and enthusing staff he felt a personal disappointment at the outcome. [13]

Since that time NET has continued to be employed but the models used hitherto have required six months training for a nurse, who would then stay with the patient for most of the ten-day period – a requirement beyond the reach of many GPs or hard pressed DDUs. A computer-programmed model has now been developed which, with a handbook requiring 20 minutes to read, will enable anyone who can learn to operate, say, a videotape recorder to work the machine which the patients carry with them. This will be cheaper to purchase and more suitable in general practice.

Three independent trials in the USA in leading universities are now being started, under the Food and Drugs Administration regulations. One will also be conducted by an experienced English general practitioner. The outcome of these will be keenly observed by the medical profession on both sides of the Atlantic (1987).

Both Dr Patterson and Dr Strang stress the importance not just of a painless detoxification but of a long-term change in lifestyle, and agree that coming off drugs is not the major problem. The problem for drug users is in staying off.

ELECTROSTIMULATION IN FRANCE. A remarkable study at the Centre Carrière was conducted on work proceeding since 1979 which may add a corroborative flavour to the work on NET. This time it was the anaesthetists at the centre who thought of transferring the undoubted benefits of electrostimulation in anaesthesia during operations to the withdrawal process for drug users.

During long operations the 'ANESTHELEC' apparatus had reduced the amount of opiates needed, and a well planned study was mounted for the 500 patients treated with it for heroin withdrawals since 1979. This was to determine whether they received genuine benefit from ES rather than a placebo effect. The anaesthetists working with psychiatrists were able to devise double blind procedures which might well be emulated in the objective assessment of the widely varying treatments of today. No follow-up studies after the five-day detoxification course were attempted. The conclusions on the physical detoxification by ES were as follows:

> 'Our first experiement shows that there is a specific positive effect of electrostimulation treatment on the withdrawal for opiate users. The treatment is *not* a pure placebo.
>
> The second experiement shows that 24 hours of continuous stimulation is not always sufficient to ensure a lasting comfortable level of the withdrawal syndrome and that after 48 hours of continuous stimulation, the effect is such that the subsequent stimulation can be left under patient control.'

The doctors stressed that the course was only a beginning for long-term rehabilitation.

Naloxone was used with all patients studied to prove objectively whether full detoxification had taken place. This brought out another fact: 15% of those who said they were addicted to opiates proved indisputably to have no physical addiction. A similar approach to that of this study could be used in outcome studies of drug treatments in this country, where claims for efficacy do not always achieve full evaluation or long-term follow-up [14].

Opioid detoxification using methadone
The method may be suitable for:

(i) long-standing chronic (up to ½ gram daily) heroin injectors;
(ii) where doctors are working in isolation with few nearby facilities, but where they have telephone contact with a DDU or other experienced drug workers;
(iii) well-motivated heroin users who are working or have a family and cannot attend more than once or twice weekly for psychosocial support;
(iv) heroin users who have some illness, pregnancy, legal or other crisis which contra-indicates immediate or rapid withdrawal from opioids.

The actual method of detoxification is described in the following pages, along with general points of assessment and management which apply to opioid detoxification by other methods, and even to the treatment of other drug dependencies.

The general principles as outlined in the DHSS *Guidelines* are a helpful introduction to this procedure:

> 'Withdrawal syndromes differ according to the particular drugs involved, the daily amounts taken, the duration of use and individual sensitivity.
>
> Physical dependence is characterised by the development of tolerance, and in addition a physical withdrawal syndrome when the daily dose is stopped or abruptly reduced. Psychological dependence is most evident when drugtakers fear cessation of supply of their drug. They often have an exaggerated view of the severity of withdrawal symptoms such that anxiety about withdrawal precedes actual physiological symptoms.
>
> The severity and management of withdrawal symptoms is greatly influenced by psychological factors present in the treatment setting. Thus, drug withdrawal regimes have optimal clinical impact when doctor and patient have got to know each other, and a basic contract about the regime has been mutually agreed. Doctor and patient must therefore be in clear agreement about the need to reduce the drug dose and the timescale of the regime. In general, it

is best to respond to a patient's own determination and timescale to withdraw from drugs, rather than the doctor imposing a too speedy or protracted regime. If a patient is eager to come off drugs quickly or abruptly, it may be better to support this clinically so as to reinforce motivation. If, however, the patient finds speedy withdrawal too stressful, the doctor can adjust the regime to be more gradual. Very long protracted withdrawal schedules, e.g. for opioids, in excess of six months, are too close to a self-perpetuating maintenance type schedule and are to be avoided. All regimes should keep in the forefront a clear management strategy of eventual drug abstinence.

During any reduction regime the patient requires encouragement and reassurance. The need for psychological support provided by the doctor, friends and family members, or an associated counselling agency, cannot be over-emphasised.

Both during and after withdrawal the need to anticipate longer term treatment and rehabilitation is essential.'

Opioid detoxification means the prescribing of methadone mixture BNF or DTF in decreasing doses over a fixed period of time in order to diminish or remove the symptoms of withdrawal.

The detox may be done as a hospital inpatient procedure or out in the community. In hospital, a titration of the dosage against withdrawal symptoms is done to determine the level of methadone at which to start. In general practice, this is not practicable and the doctor must judge, by what he can confirm of the history of drug using, the level of the starting dose.

The advantages of detoxification in the community are that the drug user is coming off opioids in a home setting despite the pressures of drug using friends and the easy availability of illicit drugs. The detox therefore is more liable to stick, if successful, than if he comes back drug-free suddenly into the pressures of his former life. Also, frequent visits to his family doctor may build up a trusting relationship which can then continue more easily over the next year or two than if he has been away during the crisis. Community Drug Teams are available to help GPs organise home detoxification where appropriate.

It is not possible to convert directly the effects, time duration and addictive potential of opioid-based drugs to a fixed equivalent of methadone. Table 6.1, based on information from City Roads Projects, London, is a rough guide only. (The heroin street prices are those in London 1987.)

---

*If heroin is smoked, or inhaled ('chasing the dragon'), rather than injected, the methadone equivalent can be reduced by one third.

Table 6.1 Opioid equivalents for prescribing.

Drug		Methadone equivalent
Street heroin*	1 gram at £80–90	80 mg (should not be attempted as outpatient)
Street heroin*	½ gram at £40–45	40–60 mg
	¼ gram at approx. 2 × £20 'bags'	30–40 mg
Pharmaceutical heroin*	10 mg tablet	10 mg
	10 mg freeze-dried ampoule	10 mg
	30 mg freeze-dried ampoule	25 mg
Methadone	Physeptone ampoule 10 mg	10 mg
	Mixture (1 mg/1 ml) 10 ml	10 mg
	Linctus (2 mg/5 ml) 10 ml	5 mg
	Suppository 50 mg	30–40 mg
	100 mg	80–100 mg (should not be attempted as outpatient)
Morphine	10 mg ampoule	10 mg
Diconal (dipipanone)	10 mg tablet	0–5 mg
DF118 (dihydrocodeine)	30 mg tablet	0–3 mg
Palfium (dextromoramide)	5 mg tablet	5–10 mg
Pethidine	25, 50 mg tablet	3–5 mg
	50 mg ampoule	4 mg
Temgesic (buprenorphine hydrochloride)	0.2 mg tablet	2.5 mg
	0.3 mg ampoule	4 mg

Fortral (pentazocine)	50 mg capsule	4 mg
	25 mg tablet	2 mg
Codeine linctus 100 ml	300 mg codeine phosphate	10 mg
Codeine phosphate	15 mg, 30 mg, 60 mg tablets	1,2,3 mg
Actifed compound 100 mg	200 mg codeine phosphate	6 mg
Gee's linctus 100 ml	16 mg anhydrous morphine	10 mg
Dr Collis-Browne's Compound 100 ml	1.4% opium	10 mg

Table 6.1 contd

The Guidelines of Good Clinical Practice in the Treatment of Drug Misuse set out the following specific prescribing regimes:

'(i) Two-week methadone detoxification
In general practice this regime is only suitable for a recently confirmed opioid misuser, with less than one year's use, and a daily use of not more than 40 mg equivalent methadone. The patient should have stable accommodation, with strong support from family or determined friends. Motivation needs to be high and can be encouraged by daily contact at the surgery or at the patient's home to support him through any panic or anxiety and to plan further rehabilitation. Symptomatic non-opioid drug prescribing is useful but adjunctive use of benzodiazepines and similar tranquillisers should not be longer than four weeks and whenever possible should be avoided.

As daily prescription and dispensing will be necessary to control the dose, it is useful to write out daily prescriptions for a week's supply, and to send the prescription directly, or by post, to a pharmacist who has agreed in advance to dispense. When the regime covers Sunday, a two-day dose must be dispensed on Saturday.

25 mg of methadone (25 ml) should be given initially and may follow prior reduction from a higher starting level. If possible, the pharmacist should maintain the volume of liquid base at 25 ml per day, but for safety reasons the actual dose of methadone must be clearly stated on each bottle. A typical course might be: Methadone

Mixture (DTF) 25 mg (three days); 20 mg (three days); 15 mg (three days); and 5 mg (three days).

(ii) One to two month detoxification

This is suitable for a rather more entrenched drug misuser with a higher daily dose, less personal and domestic support, but adequate motivation. The patient should be assessed as above, and during the detoxification regime seen once or twice weekly at home or at the surgery, to provide support and to assess progress and motivation. Where possible, occasional random urine drug screens should be sent to a local laboratory. Counselling from a social worker or other agency is recommended. Daily, or with exceptionally stable cases, twice weekly, dispensing should be arranged through the pharmacist.

A 28-day regime might be as follows:

Methadone Mixture (DTF) 30 mg (four days); 25 mg (three days); 20 mg (four days); 15 mg (three days); 10 mg (four days); 6 mg (three days); 3 mg (seven days). The volume of dispensed methadone base liquid should not be less than 20 ml throughout.

A two-monthly regime might be:

Methadone Mixture DTF) 40 mg (seven days); 35 mg (seven days); 30 mg (seven days); 25 mg (seven days); 20 mg (seven days); 15 mg (seven days); 10 mg (seven days); 5 mg (seven days). The volume of dispensed methadone base liquid should not be less than 20 ml throughout.

Adjunctive use of benzodiazepines and similar tranquillisers is to be avoided.

(iii) Three-to-six month detoxification

Longer term detoxification regimes may be more suitable for patients with five years or more drug use, (of up to 0.5 g a day illicit heroin or equivalent), or without complicated or chaotic multiple drug and alcohol misuse. These regimes should only be used for patients who are domestically stable, e.g. with a family and a job, where daily attendance or a long period away at a rehabilitation residential community is not convenient, or might place the domestic situation in jeopardy.

For some patients it is useful to maintain a stable dose for one or two months to allow them to make adjustments in their personal life, and to tackle problems related to illicit drug use. This maintenance period should not be prolonged and it should be made clear from the outset that it is only a prelude to a detoxification regime such that prescribing will terminate within a three or six month period.

Assessment, prescribing and dispensing arrangements are exactly as in shorter term regimes with an emphasis on daily dispensing.

During the contracted regime the doctor should see the patient at least once a fortnight, and arrange additional supportive counselling for him and his family with a social worker or community agency. Where possible, occasional random urine drug screens should be sent to a local laboratory. Some patients find the last doses very difficult to come off and may require a short hospital admission for the final reduction.

For a baseline dose of 60 mg Methadone Mixture (DTF) the reduction regime might be as follows: Methadone Mixture DTF 60 mg (two weeks); 50 mg (two weeks); 45 mg (two weeks); 40 mg (two weeks); 35 mg (seven days); 30 mg (seven days); 25 mg (seven days); 20 mg (seven days); 15 mg (seven days); 10 mg (seven days); 5 mg (seven days). The final volume of methadone base liquid should not be less than 20ml.

Adjunctive use of benzodiazepines and similar tranquillisers is to be avoided.

Failure to cooperate in a long-term reduction should not be allowed to develop into the fixed prescription of long term maintenance.'

Such patients should be referred on to secondary level care, e.g. a local DDU, when a full multidisciplinary assessment can be made.

Indications for the various regimes. In general, the shorter courses starting at a smaller methadone dose are suitable for recent injecting drug users or those heavily smoking heroin. Someone may actually ask for a short course, but the advisability must be looked at with each patient. If the user is trying to come off before going to rehabilitation then post-detoxification support will be given during the time spent in the rehab unit. But if the purpose is to come off before a court case, when the situation changes after the verdict, support may be lacking. That might be a case for two-three weeks maintenance rather than reduction.

Explanatory notes on these regimes.

METHADONE. This drug has been chosen because it can counteract the withdrawal effects of heroin or other opioids in a single daily dose. Instead of having to inject or smoke heroin three to five times daily to prevent withdrawals, the long-acting nature of methadone maintains an effect over 24 hours. It must be explained to the drugtaker that he will not experience the same effects as from injecting heroin, but it will definitely relieve the symptoms of withdrawal. Only liquid oral methadone mixture BNF (or DTF) 1 mg per ml strength should be used, as tablets can be ground up and injected and have a high resale value on the streets. This is a green mixture, containing chloroform and tartrazine dye and if a drug user thinks he will try injecting it he is in for a shock. Methadone linctus (2 mg in 5 ml) is a yellowish sweet cough mixture and this can, with difficulty, be injected, so should not be used for detoxification. In addition, working out doses while an anxious drug user is breathing down your neck is much more difficult at 1 mg in $2\frac{1}{2}$ ml.

DIHYDROCODEINE. Some reputable doctors dealing with large numbers of young heroin smokers or with other opioid users who do not wish to start on methadone, sometimes give tablets of dihydrocodeine (up to six or eight daily) in a short detoxification course, believing they are less addictive than methadone. The DHSS *Guidelines* disagree with the use of any tablets, DF 118 are just as saleable on the black market, just as addictive, and were they to be crushed up and injected, just as harmful as other tablets. They are a popular request with those temporary patients who feign backache or dysmenorrhoea to get a legal supply of drugs and may be sold to buy heroin later.

The prescription

Hospital doctors are fortunate in being able to prescribe on a pink two-page prescription form – FP10HP(ad) – by which two weeks' supply can be written out, but the dose be given out daily and recorded on the script. The DHSS is in the process of bringing out a similar prescription form for controlled drugs for family doctors' use, but until this happens, we must continue to write out each day's prescription on a separate FP10 if the chemist is to dispense daily.

Many experienced doctors believe that one should expect the drug user on a detox to pick up the prescription every day at a fixed time. The user should also be seen by the doctor or a team member daily at least in the early stages, to check closely on his/her compliance and reactions. Other doctors, also experienced, feel they do not have time to help more than one or two drugtakers in this way, and if the patient appears reliable, with good support, they will see him/her twice a week after the first few days and therefore write a prescription for either three or four days. It must be made clear that if the patient loses or breaks the bottle or finishes it in one day no extra will be prescribed. On a six-month detox the prescription might be given out weekly. Leaving a repeat prescription at reception to be collected, or given to a friend is most unwise, but apparently some doctors do it.

Delivering the prescription
One of the commonest causes of friction between doctor and patient is the possibility of something happening to the prescription *en route* to the chemist. Apart from the risk of alteration and forgery in a few cases, the chaotic lifestyle of drug users does render them liable to accidents. If they are homeless or living in a squat, with careless or unscrupulous friends the script may be stolen, or destroyed (one or our patients in a squat had his belongings set on fire). So excuses like the script being washed out in the laundry or being eaten by the dog can be true. To avoid this, it is much better to write out two or three prescriptions, carefully dated in advance, and have them delivered by hand or post to the chemist of your choice. For daily prescriptions this is somewhat tedious, especially with the importance of getting every detail right on a controlled drug prescription. Even when the drug user is not present to confuse or distract you, the wastepaper basket may benefit more than he does. The same applies when you are due to go on holiday. Unless a partner is well versed in seeing your drug patients and writing their scripts, you may find it wisest to write out the one or two weeks' prescriptions in advance and make sure they are delivered. Nothing is more agonising to drug users on detox than to find when they go along to the chemist in the evening the script is not ready. They are tempted either to ring the practice doctor on call or use the black market. For weekends, those on a daily prescription should be given a double dose on the one prescription to cover Saturday and Sunday.

The pharmacist
In these days when pharmacies are liable to be broken into, the pharmacist prefers not to keep stocks of methadone in the place and some are not even keen on having drug users coming in daily. So it is best to inform the pharmacist that you wish to send a drug user on a regular basis for methadone mixture. You may agree with him that if the drug user fails to turn up or causes trouble, the pharmacist will inform the doctor and if there is to be any change, or cessation of the programme the doctor should remember to tell the pharmacist what is happening. When the dose of methadone falls below 20 mg in 20 ml daily, the final bottle containing one or two teaspoons of precious liquid is hard for some drugtakers to bear. One way to overcome this

is to keep the amount of liquid prescribed daily at 20 ml and ask the pharmacist to reduce the dose. For this he will need to order from his stockist a 500 ml bottle of methadone mixture base without the methadone unless he wishes to concoct it himself. He may then dilute the daily amount as required. A typical prescription might then read:

Methadone Mixture BNF (1mg/1ml)
15mg (fifteen) daily in 20ml methadone base, for three days.
Total 60ml (sixty millilitres)
Total dose 45mg (forty-five milligrams)

The contract
Opinions vary about this way of persuading a drug user to stick to a programme of methadone detoxification by signing an agreement or contract. The Association of Independent Doctors against Addiction, representing mainly private practitioners, feel that it spoils the relationship between doctor and patient, and that as practised by DDUs it is too harsh and rigid. Those who prefer detoxification without methadone, of course, do not require a contract. Doctors who use methadone, whether in hospital or general practice vary in their policies; a few wait until a detox has got going, and only introduce a contract if compliance appears to be bad or lapses frequent. The majority start off with a contract at the beginning.

Our own opinion is that for those who are starting to treat drug users themselves and use methadone, it is best to begin with a contract and keep everything cut and dried. Rather like those general patients who are very talkative or full of their symptoms, drugtakers tend to dominate the interview because of the pressing nature of their needs. They hope to influence the treatment rather than passively wait for the doctor to give his opinion. In the face of this, if you have little experience of dealing with drug users you need to have your options clear, a limited programme which you can offer without being pushed out of your depth. Later, with experience, you can be more flexible or experimental, increasing your commitment if you wish. If you are pressed to vary your treatment you may take refuge behind the DHSS *Guidelines* or quote a local policy worked out with your partners.

In this setting, a contract actually brings stability into the relationship between doctor and drugtaker.

What kind of contract?
On the doctor's side, you are agreeing to start a methadone reduction course, give or arrange support and regular examinations, help the drug user in his long-term aim of a drug-free life, and continue the

course to its conclusion. That can prove to be *some* commitment! On the drug user's side, he or she should undertake to follow the mutually agreed reduction programme (without constant argument); to attend regularly at the surgery and the chemist's without lateness or hassle to others; and to take only the drug prescribed, in the correct way, without resorting to the black market for it or other drugs. You are asking them to be honest if any lapses do occur, but you have to say that if they are unable to stick to this contract, you may terminate it and possibly consider another course in the future when they feel more motivated. The punctuality and honesty are very important things to be relearnt by the drugtaker as part of the process and they may not come easily.

Counselling during detox
A family doctor is experienced not only in handing out prescriptions but in giving all manner of advice to patients, and encouraging patients where possible to find their own solutions to the problems they bring to him/her. We have an advantage in that the situation has probably been met with often before, in the surgery, and a few words in the right direction may set the patient on the right lines. These skills and the same authority may be exercised to advantage with the drugtaker. The doctor does not have to be trendy and identify with the patient to the extent of using the same jargon, or being of the same age group, to be accepted by even a punk-style user. A doctor's willingness to listen, to find out what certain phrases and ideas mean, and to appreciate the dilemmas which the drug user is faced with, go a long way. When the doctor's natural authority and experience is backed up by knowledge of the drugs field and the pressures likely to be both felt and exerted by the drug user, he or she is in a good position to give the right kind of counselling.

Counselling during detoxification means checking to see how the process is going (also checking with supporters in the presence of one's patient). It means giving encouragement and praise when he or she has done well and reproach or warnings if there have been lapses. There are decisions as to whether to continue if a contract has been truly broken. It also means urging the patient to set himself a succession of goals (outlined below) and encouraging him each time to reach those goals. It implies often an entirely new process for the patient of looking ahead, planning for the future, deciding how, after detoxification he is going to stay off drugs and avoid the various pitfalls and pressures which will make him fall back. The same applies in obesity treatment and giving up smoking. It means, on the one hand, giving hope to one who appeared beyond hope, and sustaining that encouragement in the succession of setbacks or unexpected events which always seem to afflict drug users. On the other hand, one has to deter false optimism when a drugtaker is kidding himself that everything will be all right despite lack of effort or perseverance – he may also be kidding you!

Counselling starts before detoxification and continues long afterwards, even if the patient has been away a year or more in residential rehabilitation. One must probe to find out what is really happening, be sceptical without cynicism, and once decisions are made, it is better in most circumstances not to go back on them. This particularly applies to prolonging or altering detox courses 'mid-stream', which may lead to a manipulative attitude on the part of the drug user. It can mean drifting into a 'maintenance' situation which should be avoided, unless thoroughly agreed upon by a drug centre for special reasons.

Before starting to prescribe
(1) Confirm the facts of drug use. Take a good history from the patient and where appropriate from relatives or partners. Look for fresh and old injection marks on arms, hands, legs and feet and in genital regions. Check on motivation and support. Collect a urine specimen for analysis for drugs. In view of the increased importance of getting drug users into treatment quickly in the light of HIV, it is no longer always necessary to wait for the result of urinalysis before starting to prescribe. This is particularly so in the case of injectors and it is not unreasonable to start prescribing within 24 hours in some cases.
(2) Give advice concerning HIV infection. Enquire if HIV testing has ever been done but if the patient is asking to be tested put this off until his or her drug use has stabilised. A positive HIV test at the start of a detox is a certain way of ensuring the failure of any treatment plans as the patient will almost certainly go through a period of chaotic drug use.

Ensure that HIV harm reduction advice is given at the first interview with the drug user, as this may be the only time that he or she attends. Such advice should stress the importance of never sharing injecting equipment; indicate the availability locally of sterile equipment from pharmacies and needle exchange schemes; and give information as to the correct way to clean injecting equipment should this be necessary. Counselling about safer sex also needs to be done and may need to be repeated later or in treatment several times before the required changes take place.
(3) Where possible involve relatives and/or partners or intimate friends if they are non-users. If they are living with the drugtaker they

are likely to be more important as a form of help and support than any professional and in addition they may be in need of help themselves. Involvement of the family in treatment has been shown to improve the success rate for the drug user.

(4) Consider making a contract with the patient. A contract is likely to be particularly helpful where a rigid abstinence-orientated detoxification is being planned. The less complicated patient who is suitable for detoxification in a general practice setting often falls into this category. What goes into the contract is a matter between the drugtaker and the doctor, but usually the doctor outlines certain conditions that he feels should be met if the drug taken is accepted into treatment. Commonly there is a dated programme of reductions and stipulations about lateness for appointments, failure to attend appointments, using drugs on top of the prescription, and expectations about attendance for regular extra counselling with, for example, the community drug team or other local resource e.g. social worker. It is often useful to stipulate one attendance at a Narcotics Anonymous meeting as some drug users find this self-help group extremely helpful and this 'breaks the ice' for them. Regular attendance at NA should not be stipulated as this would be against their philosophy and could be counter-productive. The doctor should make it clear at the outset which, if any, of the conditions and expectations of the contract will result in the prescription being terminated if they are not fulfilled.

(5) Telephone the Home Office (01-273 2213) to ensure, as far as is possible, that no one else is prescribing for the drug user. If any doctor has prescribed opiate substitutes over the past year valuable information about your patient may be obtained by ringing them directly.

(6) Notify your patient to the Home Office if this is legally required. It has to be done within seven days and there are special forms HS 2A1(rev) for this, which can be obtained from your Family Practitioner Committee or from DHSS Printing and Stationery Unit, Primrose Hill, Clitheroe, Lancs (Tel 0200-22187).

(7) Discuss your plans with all those whom you wish to be involved in the network of support for your patient in the community (community drug team, social worker, health visitor, probation officer, youth worker etc.) and elicit their cooperation.

(8) Ensure that the patient's environment is as ideal as possible for detoxification. Attempting to detoxify someone who is living in a squat where everyone else is using drugs is unlikely to be successful. Such patients should be encouraged to stay with relatives or friends who do not use drugs and who would be supportive to them during detoxification. The other thing that is particularly helpful is to encourage the drug user to avoid all drugtaking friends and to start

developing friendships with people who do not use drugs. Peer group pressure appears to be an important cause of relapse when the patient maintains contact with the wrong peer group. Conversely, peer group pressure from non-using friends can be an important aid to recovery.
(9) Write out several prescriptions in advance and arrange with the patient and chemist when they should be picked up. Ask the chemist to notify you if he/she does not attend to pick up any of the prescriptions.
(10) Arrange with the patient the date and time he or she will next see you.

From the start of a prescription
The frequency of attendance is of course up to the individual doctor's discretion but it will also depend to a certain extent on the length of prescribing envisaged, any prior experience the drug user might have had of detoxification, and the amount of support he or she has both at home and in the community.

At the beginning and end of detoxification the patient should be seen more frequently and double length appointments are usually needed. Some doctors prefer to see patients twice a week at these times, others may even see them daily, but if a good network of other professional support is available in the community and utilised at these times a very intensive commitment from the GP should not be necessary. The following is a method that the author used successfully when there was no community drug team and very little in the way of additional support for the patient.

Day one. The patient picks up his supply, decides whether to take the day's dose in one swallow, say 40 ml methadone mixture, or spread it out. He should have something, television, music etc. to occupy his mind.

Day two. Either an appointment, or a home visit to assess withdrawal effects and cooperation. If the dose is obviously too little or too much, 5 or 10 mg methadone may be adjusted, and the programme altered. For severe side effects, diarrhoea etc., symptomatic medicines may be prescribed, but aching, etc. should be met with reassurance, warm baths, massage of the limbs, etc. rather than medication.

Day three onwards. See the patient every two or three days; give encouragement; check with the drug user and relative on compliance, doing an occasional random urine test and checking all the injection sites for possible fresh use. Try to establish enough rapport for the user to tell you if he has failed, without fear of instant termination of the course. Complications of drug use, or other complaints, must be dealt with, but not by giving any addictive analgesics.

Day ten onwards. You may now be giving a prescription twice a week, on fixed days. Some doctors prefer daily prescriptions in the first month. Remind the user of the final date of the course, but also get him thinking forward to rehabilitation. Encourage him to make several goals, punctuality, self-discipline, honesty with self and others and trust, most of which have been submerged in his recent existence. Where possible he should be seeing one or two of the support team on a regular basis, health visitor, community psychiatric nurse or probation officer.

Day twenty onwards. There should be a good rapport by now between the drug user and the medical team unless the programme looks like failing. If the user cannot stand the pace, is failing to cooperate, it may be that the detox or the timescale was misjudged, the motivation inadequate, or rather the drug user not yet ready for this exercise. With one or two real failures in cooperation, one must decide at what point to terminate the contract and make this crystal clear to the drug user. As mentioned before, cessation of the course should not be regarded as a failure, but as a 'dry run', a practice effort, which may be tackled again later on. It may have proved to the drugtaker that people are willing to help and that the withdrawals are not as bad as feared.

Day thirty onwards. By this time the drug user's tolerance to opioids will have been reduced as he moves towards being drug-free. If he is tempted to take another illegal dose of heroin, particularly an injection, what would have been safe for him a month ago could now be an overdose. Some sort of warning needs to be given by the doctor himself, without implying one expects him to fail. Dr Chang has suggested that one uses the passive tense or speaks in general terms, giving the following example: 'Unfortunately many addicts die of overdose if they relapse after they come off drugs, since they don't realise that their tolerance has altered'. Some doctors might regard this as too strong a statement, but when the risk is a matter of life and death in a weak moment, the position must be made clear. The largest number of deaths from overdose occurs within a few days of a drug user leaving prison, having lost tolerance.

Day forty onwards. Of course with the shorter programmes, these phases will be telescoped. By this time the drug user may be below the 20 mg a day level and one will have given him the choice of having the dose made up to 20 ml daily with methadone base, or taking it 'neat'. The last 10 and 5 ml are often the hardest to come off, and sometimes require admission to hospital.

Perhaps the main reason for the difficulty is the prospect of soon being without drugs after perhaps years of dependence upon them. Dr

Anne MacDonald has compared it to a bereavement, and says much of her psychotherapy is directed towards this. Some drug users are addicted not so much to the drug as to the mystique of the 'needle' and the way of life which keeps them keyed up all the time. There may be much emotional pressure by drugtakers on doctors at this stage to prolong the course. Often some crisis looms up and repeated postponements can lead to a sort of maintenance. Where the decision is not easy, the doctor may bring in other members of the team, so that whichever way it goes, the action is a joint action to present to the drug user, and not one doctor's arbitrary judgement.

'Freedom' day plus one. Once the user is drug-free, he or she will come under more pressures, especially from drug-using friends or from sheer psychological misery, and may demand other psychoactive drugs to help with sleep etc. In most cases this can be resisted, but should be accompanied by maximum encouragement from the team and the doctor, with continued weekly appointments.

Follow-up should now go on for at least a year, spreading out appointments to once a month, but using the team or relatives to keep an eye on progress. Make it clear that even if the drug user goes to rehabilitation or moves away, you would like to hear news, whether good or bad, over the next year or two. In no other way can one evaluate the results of all the effort that has been put into such detox programmes.

The snags
Since our first publication appeared, the DHSS *Guidelines* have emphasised some of the pitfalls awaiting the GP who decides to try and help those whose drug use has become problematic.

If a doctor makes a move towards helping rather than avoiding the occasional drug user, he will need certain warnings, as clearly shown in Dr Bewley's paper 'Conning the general practitioner' [15].

(i) *Demand.* In case it appears that all drug users are awkward customers, one must say that the majority are friendly, peaceable and cooperative patients. They may indeed be your own patients wishing to reduce psychoactive drugs. The pressing need for renewal of the drug, however, makes them among the most demanding and manipulative of clients. They will use emotional blackmail and stress what suffering will occur if you do not prescribe.

(ii) *Dishonesty.* Some drugtakers are on the lookout for prescription pads, headed notepaper, MIMS, BNF, doctors' bags, syringes, needles, drugs and any samples lying around or in drawers. They acquire 'epileptic' cards from OPDs to show a need for barbiturates, diabetic cards to prove they need slimming pills and DDU cards to show they are attending a clinic but have run out of supplies.

Drug users have been charged with breaking into doctors' cars, drug cupboards and premises – so strengthen your windows. At lunchtime they may wander into unguarded rooms looking for prescription pads, so tighten your security.

(iii) Deception. GPs are familiar with the circularised notices of users giving various names and aliases, and the alteration of prescriptions or forgery are well-known. A carbon copy is a useful precaution for prescription writing and careful recording will ensure one partner is not played off against another. It also provides authentication in enquiries by police or HM Coroner.

Yet some of the stories drug users tell are extremely convincing like that of the 'soldier' in battle dress 'on leave from Northern Ireland', who, when Diconal was less strictly controlled, went to three doctors in one morning. His convincing performance would have fetched – at £4 per tablet for 3 × 100 tablets – £1,200 for a morning's work.

Prescriptions may have 'got lost in the laundry', 'been eaten by the dog' or 'been stolen' from the drug user. Symptoms are simulated convincingly and even needle marks in veins can be recent artefacts.

Bewley found that 43% of the drugtakers questioned had sold some or all of what was prescribed, some was given or exchanged and only 30% of the users used it for themselves [15].

Your 'addict' also could be a disguised reporter from a Sunday newspaper, seeking a story. Remember there is not and never has been any such thing as a 'registered addict'.

(iv) Disruption. A few drugtakers will choose a busy time in the surgery, preferably with children present, to pressurise staff by arguing, shouting, or, as one of our patients did, sitting on top of the reception desk.

We have heard of an isolated elderly doctor who works alone and will yield regularly to threats of being 'done over' rather than inform the authorities. Some drug users work in pairs to divert attention, or so that one prevents the doctor ringing the police while the other demands the prescription. A knee button beneath the desk will solve this. A few users will go on creating havoc till they get their demands or are removed by the police. One should try to avoid leaving the consulting room with a drug misuser in it.

Treatment of non-opioid drug misuse

Cocaine

Because cocaine misuse in this country is not a major problem, the treatment of chronic use has mainly been documented in the USA. Those dealing with large numbers of cocaine misusers (and some who are on very heavy doses, freebasing, injecting, or using 'crack') now accept that cocaine is also physically addictive. Much of this section reflects the writing of Herbert D. Kleber MD, Professor of Psychiatry at Yale University Medical School, and his colleague, Frank H. Gawin, who has been quoted as saying, 'We think cocaine addiction is a physical addiction whose expression is occurring in parts of the brain that have to do not with physical regulation but with psychological' [16]. Treatment programmes for heavy users need to recognise this.

In the last few years, treatment in America has begun to include pharmacological as well as psychological therapy. Historically, two main approaches have been tried in the last decade, the first relying on inpatient treatment. This was for heavy cocaine smokers who 'may have been incapable of combating cocaine craving without hospitalisation and seclusion from cocaine sources' [16]. It used frequent supportive psychotherapy sessions, self-control strategy, exercise therapy and liberal hospitalisation during the initial detoxification. Nowadays, other types of inpatient treatment or rehabilitation programmes combine the confrontation groups long in use at residential communities for narcotic users such as Day Top Village with strong Narcotics Anonymous emphasis.

Outpatient programmes have been developed mainly in two directions.

Self-help groups
NA or Cocaine Anonymous provide structure and limits as well as group support, a religious background and a round-the-clock helping network. They employ both behavioural therapy and supportive techniques. Telephone advice networks such as Cocaine-800 cover the country and are widely used. As well as being counselled, users are directed towards local recovery programmes.

Medical programmes
Medical programmes on an outpatient basis mainly use three types of psychotherapy and outcome studies have been done on much of this work.
(1) Behaviour therapy techniques. These include what is called 'contingency contracting' [17] in which there is application not so much of the carrot as the stick. The drug user agrees to join a urine monitoring programme and also agrees that if his or her urine shows cocaine or the sample fails to arrive, an 'adverse effect' will be applied, such as

sending off a previously deposited letter to an employer admitting the use of cocaine. However, milder contingencies may be applied first or even some kind of carrot for a clean urine. Desensitisation and assertiveness training may also be used.

(2) *Supportive treatment.* This can include increasing the contacts with non-using friends, eliminating drug paraphernalia and secret hoards or stashes, avoiding dealers (in some cases the user must stop dealing himself), and changing telephone numbers or even addresses. There is also counselling for spouses and psychotherapy for problem cases.

(3) *Psychodynamic treatment.* This helps the user to understand the functions which cocaine served in their lives and to acquire an increased sense of control. This is one of the commonest lines of approach in America.

A more experimental but hopeful development is the use of chemotherapy. If indeed in chronic cocaine use there are definite signs of a physical dependence with withdrawals and tolerance now well demonstrated, then this 'neuro-adaptation' may respond to pharmacological agents. The main ones being tried are tricyclic antidepressants (especially desipramine), lithium carbonate and dopamine agonists such as amantadine and bromocriptene.

The depression following abstinence from cocaine, as with amphetamines, can be long-lasting or intermittent, and does not necessarily respond to antidepressant drugs. The experimental use of tricyclic antidepressants is mainly directed towards the reduction of the craving for cocaine. Supportive therapy, therefore, is especially needed, whether from the doctor or other members of the multidisciplinary team.

Kleber and Gawin write [16]:

'Our clinical impressions gained in work with severe abusers lead us to favour outpatient treatment. The cocaine abuser must resume his or her everyday life at some point and hospitalisation merely defers this inevitability. Studies of animal behaviour as well as clinical work highlight the importance of environment in conditioning drugtaking behaviour. We have observed that a period of abstinence akin to a period of 'extinction' within the context of everyday stimuli and stressors is necessary before long-term reduction in craving occurs. The current, almost ubiquitous, presence of cocaine in many areas of American life makes it unlikely that former users will be able to simply *avoid* temptation. Like the former cigarette smoker or alcoholic, the person attempting to give up cocaine must make the drug 'psychologically' unavailable because it is almost impossible to make it physically unavailable.'

Table 6.2 Possible future guidelines for cocaine abuse treatment.

Cocaine abuse severity	Psychotherapeutic approach	Pharmocotherapeutic approach
Mild.	Behavioural with or without psychodynamic.	None.
Moderate.	Supportive and psychodynamic with or without behavioural.	Only if psychiatric diagnosis is present. Choice of agent based on symptoms. If no treatable diagnosis exists, general treatment (desipramine) may be usefully tried in difficult cases.
Severe	Supportive with or without hospitalisation for acute phase, then as in 'moderate'.	General treatment (desipramine) indicated unless diagnosis dictates another treatment choice.

The course and prognosis of treatment
Withdrawal from cocaine misuse follows three stages. First comes the 'crash' when there is agitation and craving followed by fatigue and depression going on to somnolence and lack of craving. In one study this lasted from nine hours to four days, then came a space of up to ten weeks with low anxiety and low craving, followed by a third stage of anhedonia (inability to feel pleasure), anxiety and high cocaine craving. If cocaine is obtained, the cycle begins again. The greatest danger of relapse is in the period of anhedonia. The course of care may follow this cycle of therapy, abstinence and relapse, with increasing intervals between the relapses until the drug user comes off altogether. Even then, like the alcoholic, he may always be at risk of relapse.

Cocaine addiction is often combined with the use of other drugs or alcohol. An effort must be made to obtain abstinence from all mood-altering substances, even cannabis, as advocated in AA-related programmes, because the continuation of other drug use may bring back the craving for cocaine.

It may be thought that for the average family doctor who is unlikely to see a cocaine user, this amount of detail is unnecessary. It is a fact, however, that most drug centres are geared to the heroin user, although rehabilitation centres are willing to accept stimulant users once they are drug-free. With some idea, therefore, of possible lines of treatment, particularly in the self-help groups, a GP may find this background information helpful for his own team, for referral or for pressing for facilities should the need ever arise.

Treatment for other stimulants

Far more common in this country than cocaine misuse is the misuse of amphetamine sulphate or 'speed', a drug which can be injected but is generally sniffed like cocaine. Heavy users of the drug often lead chaotic, frenetic, exhausting lives without much food or sleep. For the user motivated to come off, the family doctor is in a good position to supply the necessary support.

Acute stimulant poisoning
Cocaine or amphetamine poisoning needs emergency treatment and transfer to hospital. Artificial respiration and cardiac massage may be the initial demand, but usually the onset is not so clear. The stimulant abuser can be alert and over-anxious, with volatile behaviour, or if lacking sleep and food, may be fatigued and malnourished, with skin excoriations, chewed tongue or worn teeth from bruxism. Dilated pupils, dry mouth and hyperactive reflexes may be accompanied by tell-tale needle marks or with sniffers, nasal septum ulceration. Hyperthermia and convulsions can lead to coma, or respiratory depression and cardiac irregularities may supervene. Emptying the stomach may help in early cases if large oral doses have been taken. Diazepam intravenously will help the convulsions.

Treatment of chronic misuse
Since the cessation of amphetamines leads the patient to 'crash out' into a long sleep, for milder cases no further action is required other than building up the patient physically and giving psychological support. Anxiety may be calmed by reassurance and the presence of friends in a quiet place. Chlorpromazine 25-50 mg intramuscularly counteracts the dopaminergic and peripheral noradrenergic effects of amphetamines. Over the succeeding months, the same sort of support as described for cocaine users will be of value for amphetamine users.

A reassessment of prescribing habits in the light of HIV infection has led the Advisory Council on the Misuse of Drugs to recommend short detoxification for some amphetamine injectors using dexamphetamine over a period of one to two weeks. The availability of such chemical help may encourage some amphetamine users to come forward for treatment when they would not otherwise do so. All amphetamine and cocaine drugtakers should be given HIV harm reduction counselling at the first interview.

The very long-term amphetamine user may suffer from an intractable severe depression if withdrawn. Those who have been using amphetamines daily for fifteen years or more are best referred for a second opinion as to whether they should be maintained on amphetamines.

Treatment of psychosis
This can be similar both in cocaine and in amphetamine users and is marked by paranoid delusions, hallucinations and bizarre behaviour. It tends to follow chronic drug use over several months or reappears with further doses. With cessation of amphetamine the hallucinations decrease fairly quickly, but may linger on vestigially. Neuroleptic drugs, haloperidol etc., can improve florid psychoses rapidly. Hospitalisation may be necessary to obviate further drug use, risk of suicide, and to provide a reassuring framework during the frightening recovery phase.

Continued episodes of depression after discharge must be watched for, as the temptation to resume drug use is greatest at these times and tricyclic antidepressants may help to shorten the period of anhedonia.

Barbiturates

Whereas the GP when faced with someone withdrawing from opioids or stimulants may say there is no particular danger in such withdrawals and may decide not to treat them, he cannot afford to take the same line if someone is addicted to barbiturates or large doses of chlormethiazole (Heminevrin). Too rapid a withdrawal from either may lead to convulsions and sometimes death. It is important, therefore, to recognise whether and how much barbiturate use has occurred. Barbiturates may be used with alcohol or to come down from prolonged stimulant use. Heroin users running low on supplies may substitute barbiturates. Chronic barbiturate users tend to be more chaotic and careless of their own safety and appearance than heroin users.

Where inpatient facilities, either at hospitals or specialised treatment centres, are available these should be used. In the Greater London area, the City Roads Crisis Centre, Islington, is an option, but outside London there may be no special facilities at all. In these circumstances, an experienced GP may use the following detox regime, as set out in the DHSS *Guidelines* – we are talking here of the young drug user who has become addicted to barbiturates, possibly with other drugs, not the elderly lady who is dependent upon two tablets of Seconal every night. For each 100 mg of short acting barbiturate previously taken by the drug misuser, 30 mg of phenobarbitone is substituted, subject to a maximum of 300 mg phenobarbitone daily: e.g. a drug misuser who takes 9 × 100 mg pentobarbitone (Nembutal) daily will require 9 × 30 mg phenobarbitone = 270 mg phenobarbitone, as an initial daily dose. The daily reduction regime would then be:

Day 1 Day 2	Tabs phenobarbitone 90 mg t.d.s.
Day 3 Day 4	Tabs phenobarbitone 60 mg t.d.s.
Day 5 Day 6	Tabs phenobarbitone 60 mg b.d.
Day 7 Day 8	Tabs phenobarbitone 30 mg b.d.

The addition of other anticonvulsant medication such as phenytoin (Epanutin) is unnecessary, complicates withdrawal, and has a potential for misuse. Phenothiazines such as thioridazine (Melleril) should also be avoided as they lower the threshold for epileptic convulsions.

Detoxification should only be given to prevent withdrawal convulsions and not for the psychological well-being of the drugtaker who has difficulty in coping with withdrawals. It is best to use a long-acting barbiturate such as phenobarbitone as drug users do not seem to get a 'buzz' from this preparation.

There are various points to look for in such a withdrawal regime, which are well described in the section on barbiturate abuse, in the book *Treatment Aspects of Drug Dependence* (available from ISDD: quote accession number 35126). Such background information and advice from those already experienced should be sought before attempting withdrawal treatment in general practice.

Chlormethiazole

Dependence on high doses of chlormethiazole (Heminevrin) commonly leads to epileptic seizures on withdrawal. At doses of 5 g/day or

Table 6.3 Phenobarbitone equivalents for prescribing.

Drug	Oral sedative dose	Equivalent phenobarbitone dose
Amylobarbitone (Amytal)	100 mg	30 mg
Butobarbitone (Soneryl)	100 mg	30 mg
Cyclobarbitone (Phanodorm)	200 mg	30 mg
Heptobarbitone (Medomin)	200 mg	30 mg
Quinalbarbitone (Seconal)	100 mg	30 mg
Quinalbarbitone and amylobarbitone (Tuinal)	50 mg + 50 mg	30 mg
Pentobarbitone (Nembutal)	100 mg	30 mg
Glutethimide (Doriden)	250 mg	30 mg
Methyprylone (Noludar)	200 mg	30 mg
Methaqualone (illegally imported varieties)	250 mg	30 mg

more a prolonged and serious delirious state may occur as part of the abstinence syndrome. Hospital admission is essential for drug users dependent on chlormethiazole to enable gradual withdrawal using chlormethiazole itself together with benzodiazepine or phenobarbitone anti-convulsant cover.

Following detoxification, the patient is said to be likely to experience irritability and sleep disturbance for up to 3 months.

Benzodiazepines

(1) Dependence on prescribed benzodiazepines

The abrupt cessation of a prescription for benzodiazepines to a long-term user may precipitate rebound anxiety, insomnia, the specific benzodiazepine withdrawal syndrome, an acute confusional state or even, occasionally, grand mal convulsions. To avoid these complications most authorities recommend slow withdrawal and some advise changing the benzodiazepine to diazepam because of its long elimination half-life. Gradual withdrawal lasting several weeks is also recommended even after only short-term treatment because of evidence that dependence can develop after this length of time.

The withdrawal regimes following long-term benzodiazepine use described in the literature vary in length from 4–16 weeks. This is at variance with regimes recommended by Tranx and most other self help-groups who advise on average about a year to completely withdraw from the drug.

In his book *How To Stop Taking Tranquillisers*, Dr Peter Tyrer describes two withdrawal regimes, one rapid, the other slow. The major difference between the two is that the slow withdrawal regime is decided by the patient rather than the therapist. Personal responsibility by the patient is often an important factor in overcoming dependence successfully and in a primary care setting, the patient's cooperation is often best enlisted by making a combined decision as to the most suitable rate of reduction. As a result, many general practitioners take longer than 16 weeks to withdraw their patients from benzodiazepines and reduce at a rate at which the patient feels able to cope with. Few GPs impose a rigid withdrawal regime or consider using a contract with the patient, yet the anecdotal evidence of those who have an active policy to withdraw their patients from long-term benzodiazepines is that they are usually successful. It is generally reported to be hardest to wean people off the last ¼ tablet of 2 mg diazepam (or a similar sub-therapeutic dose of another benzodiazepine) indicating the importance of psychological dependence. Most doctors recommend that this final tiny dose be kept going for a period of time before complete cessation. Other methods that have been used to overcome this final stage of withdrawal include having the drug only on alternate days or giving the patient a small reserve supply for particularly difficult times. Many doctors say that it is harder to wean patients off benzodiazepine hypnotics than tranquillisers.

Table 6.4 Roughly equivalent doses of benzodiazepines.

Long-acting	Short/medium acting
Diazepam 2.5 mg	Lorazepam 0.5 mg
Chlordiazepoxide 5 mg	Oxazepam 7.5 mg
Nitrazepam 5 mg	Temazepam 5 mg
	Triazolam 0.125 mg

Thus there are considerable variations of opinion as to which method of withdrawal is the most suitable. Basically, there seem to be two different approaches. Those who advocate the shorter regimes tend to concentrate solely on overcoming the physical side of benzodiazepine dependence (indeed some authorities recommend titrating the reduction in dose against the appearance of physical withdrawal symptoms). Those who advocate these shorter regimes often talk of 'prolonging the agony' if withdrawal takes place over any period longer than 16 weeks. Self-help groups, on the other hand, tackle the problem of psychic dependence first; attenders of the groups usually reduce their drugs when they feel psychologically prepared to do so, although it is to be assumed that both hidden and overt pressures from other group members also play a role. The process of overcoming psychic dependence to a point where the benzodiazepine taker feels confident enough to face life without the drug in their system seems usually to take from 12-15 months. It is interesting to note that this is about the same period of time that most of the rehabilitation houses expect a confirmed heroin user to take to reach a stage where he or she can cope in the community without drugs.

What then happens to those people who are withdrawn from benzodiazepines in 16 weeks or less? Most of them seem to do quite well, but the temptation to borrow a supply from relatives or friends, or to find a substitute such as alcohol, cannabis or another drug is sometimes high. Sometimes, patients get into more trouble with a substitute they have found than they did with the original drug itself. Those who do carry on without substitutes no doubt overcome their psychic dependence at a faster rate than those attending self-help groups. Nevertheless, this will not be without a certain amount of stress in a group of patients who were probably prescribed benzodiazepines in the first place because they had trouble coping with anxiety.

It is usually helpful to explore the reasons why a patient needed to take benzodiazepines. A frequent confidential consultation with the family doctor while a slow withdrawal takes place may be an ideal setting to help the patient resolve conflicts that have been impairing his or her social functioning for many years. It is probably as much for this reason as for any other that many GPs prefer not to have a fixed withdrawal schedule for benzodiazepines and to strike a bargain with the patient about the speed of withdrawal as the opportunity arises. This middle of the road approach may not suit all GPs but is more in keeping with a policy of treating the whole person rather than just the symptoms. The withdrawal regime used can be tailor-made to suit the needs of each patient.

Alternative therapy using relaxation treatment or training in anxiety management skills, although helpful, is only moderately effective. However, a recent development using cognitive therapy seems to be a promising approach.

With cognitive therapy, the aim is not to treat the anxiety itself, but the cognitive processes that are linked with it. Many cognitive processes such as perception, memory or attitudes have been clearly shown to be linked to emotional states. The therapist sets out to correct misperception, misinterpretation, incompatible attitudes, and counterproductive styles of thinking. This is usually done with the aid of a diary and recordings are made of distressing physical symptoms and the thoughts that accompany them. If possible, the sequence of events, thoughts and sensations leading to a worsening of symptoms is recorded, to be discussed later with the therapist.

By this means, panic attacks, which appear to be spontaneous, can often be shown to be related to hidden cognitive events. This method of therapy, although well-established in the treatment of depression, is still at a fairly early stage of development in the treatment of anxiety, but shows signs of being an effective and valuable method which could be adapted for use in general practice.

Drugs, particularly clonidine and β-blockers, have both been used as adjuncts to withdrawal, but their benefits can at best be described as moderate. Most of the work done on use of β-blockers as an adjunct during withdrawal has been with propranolol. β-blockers in general lessen some of the bodily symptoms, but do not alter the frequency or the psychological aspects of the withdrawal symptoms.

Sometimes withdrawal from benzodiazepines may precipitate a frank depressive illness which may itself require treatment. One-third of all patients undergoing benzodiazepine withdrawal are said to benefit from an antidepressant treatment. However, if an antidepressant is used, it should not be given in high doses or over a long period of time, for antidepressants themselves can provoke a withdrawal syndrome if suddenly stopped. The withdrawal syndrome from tricyclic antidepressants has both cholinergic and adrenergic components. The former leads to abdominal cramps, sweating, nausea and vomiting, but increased adrenergic activity may mimic symptoms of anxiety and cause spontaneous panic attacks. This adrenergic component can make withdrawal from benzodiazepines extremely difficult.

Thus, there are various aids to benzodiazepine withdrawal which, if used properly, can be helpful in a difficult case. When the withdrawal regime has started, patients should initially be seen at least weekly and enquiries should be made, particularly regarding depression, increased alcohol consumption, and relationship difficulties.

Generally, the symptoms of increased sensory perception attributable to the specific benzodiazepine withdrawal syndrome, can be dealt with by sympathetic reassurance that they will go away and an explanation that they are a temporary withdrawal effect of the drug.

It is often surprisingly easy to withdraw people from benzodiazepines even though they have been taking these drugs every day for several years. Indeed, the majority of patients do not have significant withdrawal symptoms when they stop their drugs. The literature suggests that about 55–60% of these patients come into this category. The patients, themselves, are invariable pleased when they finally stop and there is no doubt they are the better for it, even though the problem of coping with attacks of anxiety without the drugs remains.

What follows is a first hand account of benzodiazepine withdrawal provided by a female patient of the Clinical Psychopharmacology Unit at Newcastle University.

'I am 39 years old, married with two children aged 18 years and 14 years. The younger child was a very active baby, and when he was 18 months old I mentioned to the doctor that he was sleeping very little and though he did not seem tired in any way, I certainly was! After a course of vitamins I still felt worn out and this was when I was first prescribed Valium.

This was 1971; I was then 27 years old. I remember instantly feeling a lot better – all the irritability and tiredness seemed to disappear and I became a lot more relaxed and content. The next three years seemed to fly over; the eldest child began school, my husband gained promotion, and we bought a new house. Any problems which cropped up during this time could always be wiped out just by taking a Valium. Life was pretty good! Moving house also meant changing doctor and this doctor was not very keen on repeating the monthly prescription on which I had come to depend. 'You must cut them down,' she said, 'three years is far too long.' I agreed wholeheartedly, 'Why not,' I thought, 'I don't need them now.' The youngest was at school and slept soundly – in fact had done for a long time. I started reducing the tablets and can honestly say I felt no ill effects.

During this time my life hit an emotional crisis but this time, unlike in the past, I did not have the pills to cover it up. In January 1975 I suffered a miscarriage and after this, together with the conflict in my personal life, I visited the doctor in tears. She immediately put me back on Valium, this time increasing the dosage. Although the world was not as rosy as it was before, at least it was bearable. I did not realise then that this was the beginning of a new road to despair, mental and physical pain, and nearly complete disaster.

My problems did not go away like in the early days on the pills – they seemed greater. I started to become withdrawn, insecure, and confused and suffered bouts of depression together with uncontrollable outbursts of rage. My digestive system seemed to be affected and this resulted in many visits to the hospital for the necessary tests. Some days were worse than others – sleep was no longer a welcome relief; I would lie awake in the middle of the night soaking in perspiration and feeling very ill. When sleep did come it was full of vivid dreams. The traumatic experiences in my life did not stop either, in fact they seemed greater than ever. One day I could cope no longer and the doctor recommended a top psychiatrist. This seemed the most logical solution at the time, so I agreed. It was diagnosed as endogenous depression and acute anxiety. During the following months I was prescribed many different forms of antidepressants, hypnotics, and tranquillisers to take with the Valium. None of these had any lasting good effects, in fact I gradually became worse instead of better. The relationship between our GP and myself broke down, making it necessary to change doctors. I became very paranoid and believed it was me against the world. During this time I contracted chickenpox quite badly which unfortunately caused a longstanding eye complaint to flare up. This was the start of the blackest period of my life, and by this time I felt as though I was bordering on insanity. During one particular bad spell my husband dragged me to the psychiatric inpatients, and here I saw a young doctor who told me it was not the pills I needed but psychotherapy. The pills were only covering up the mental turmoil.

The next year involved extensive analysis and although at times this was mentally distressing, it seemed to help. During the weekly sessions it was suggested I drop my dose of Valium so I quickly agreed; at first it was easy – a bit jumpy when I dropped 1 mg – but then things became much worse. My confidence began to wane dramatically – I could not go out or be left on my own. My husband finally had to give up his job, as I spent most of the time begging him to come home as I was frightened. I started to feel very ill, and even going to the shops was a mammoth task. My doctor advised me not to drop the Valium any more (I was down from 15 mg to 4 mg) as I was suffering from chronic anxiety and needed some form of sedation. What both of us did not realise was that I was in tranquilliser withdrawal.

The following year was hell for me and my family. I developed into a mental and physical wreck – suicidal thoughts were never very far away.

In July this year I begged the doctor to help me – I could not go on any more like this – it was like a 'living death'. He suggested another form of tranquilliser and took the remaining Valium away – I thought I had gone mad. In sheer desperation I remembered a newspaper article about a group of people who suffered from tranquilliser side effects and withdrawal. I made a phone call, which was the most important call of my life: I was on the verge of madness and could they help?

That was nine weeks ago and during that time I have not touched a tablet. This brought on a series of symptoms that I had experienced only mildly before. Noises jarred every fibre in my body and my eyes seemed to shun the light of day. I shook from head to foot and enormous panic attacks would sweep through my body, leaving me exhausted and totally afraid. Complete fatigue took over the feeling of tiredness and sleep no longer came with the night. Many times I thought it would be best to die.

I am lucky to have found somewhere where sufferers can be encouraged and supported through withdrawal. I have found many new friends, who, like me, were caught up in the web of addiction. Also I have the good fortune to have a very caring and warm doctor to help me through this withdrawal. It has not been easy – it has been one of the hardest jobs of my life and it is not finished yet. In the early days I began to think I had gone mad, but gradually a new world is emerging. A world that is not covered over with pills. It can be a very frightening place until my mind becomes adjusted to its colours, noises, and pictures once more.

Someone once wrote "Tranquillisers are the anaesthetic of the emotions"; this is true. When used properly, they are a 'must' in medicine, but used over the long term they poison the body and destroy the mind. One day doctors will realise the extent of the tranquilliser withdrawal syndrome but until then it is going to be a hard battle, but in the end, we sincerely hope, worth it.' [18]

(2) Dependence on benzodiazepines among drug users
This appears to be becoming increasingly common and much higher doses are taken than those found in the average patient taking prescribed benzodiazepines. Sudden cessation of such drug use can precipitate withdrawal convulsions and psychotic features are common at high doses.
Detoxification of the drugtaker should be aimed at preventing epileptic fits and should not be prolonged. If benzodiazepines are to be used, a withdrawal regime using diazepam is to be preferred because

of the long half-life of its active metabolite, N-desmethyldiazepam. A regime similar to that used for alcohol withdrawals may be helpful: Diazepam 10 mg qds. (3 days); 10 mg tds (3 days); 5 mg tds (2 days); 5 mg bd (2 days). Alternatively, a phenobarbitone withdrawal regime along the lines of that already described can be used (diazepam 15 mg = 30 mg phenobarbitone).

Psychedelic drugs and cannabis

Because the drug treatment centres are mainly geared to the problems of opioid misuse, the general practitioner may find himself asked to advise on a patient taking LSD or other hallucinogens. For example he may be asked what to do about the flashbacks in a person who perhaps has taken LSD for some weeks or even months. The family doctor is less likely to have to treat cannaboid misuse as few cannabis users regard their habit as medically remediable or even serious, but they could present with an apparent cannabis psychosis. In this case psychiatric referral is necessary both for diagnosis of the real cause and for treatment, having taken the precaution of obtaining a urine sample for a drug screen prior to referral.

Since these two classes of drugs do not produce a physical abstinence syndrome, there is no equivalent of methadone detoxification. The GP may however be called to help at the time of an unpleasant or frightening psychedelic trip. This is best treated by calm and persistent reassurance. Talking down is often better done by family or supportive friends who are well known to the user. Only if talking down fails should medication be used – either diazepam 10 mg or 25 mg chlordiazepozide orally. If the patient is quite uncontrollable, and not yet admitted to hospital, haloperidol 2-4 mg intramuscularly may be given. Transfer to hospital, however, can be threatening to the patient and should be used only as a last resort.

Flashbacks

Treatment of these may be necessary if the disturbance is confined to the actual period of altered perception. Various medications have been tried, such as chlorpromazine, nicotinic acid and sedatives. Flashbacks tend to follow periods of stress or general anxiety, so psychotherapy which takes account of this is helpful. Although only occurring as a result of LSD or other psychedelic drug use they may be precipitated by the use of cannabis, so the cannabis user should be urged to abstain entirely. Talking the person down is again the main treatment, preferably by someone known to the patient.

If the experience sets off further psychotic consequences, psychiatric referral is essential.

Volatile substances

In the management of volatile substance misuse a great deal depends on whether the sniffing is experimental or persistent over several years with attendant psychosocial problems. If the former, not much treatment may be needed and the craze will probably pass. If the latter, management may be complicated, protracted and not always successful.

The usual approach to a doctor is by worried parents who have just discovered their youngster is sniffing solvents and may be horrified or terrified about implications and dangers. They may feel it is a step on the road to hard drugs. Rarely does the glue sniffer approach the doctor unless there is a well established specialist clinic with easy access, as in Newcastle-upon-Tyne. Some of the observations in this section are based on Dr Denis O'Connor's work in Newcastle [19] and other aspects are drawn from *Sniffing Solvents*, a popular book by Eve Merrill, a social worker [20].

Some knowledge of the volatile substances used and their effects is needed to give the right sort of advice or reassurance to parents and to the teenager. One also needs to discover whether the solvent use is merely for fun and to satisfy curiosity; to share experiences with friends; to help cope with emotions about teenage life; to escape from problems or to maintain compulsively an intoxicated state.

The doctor is advised therefore to see parents or other supporters first, with or without the patient, then the patient alone, and then perhaps both together. He needs to consider:

Assessment
The history, types of substances used (plus other drugs and alcohol) and the reasons for use and circumstances.

Talking to the patient alone
The solvent user is likely to have faced much recrimination or protest from parents or others in authority, and apart from the young and

early experimenter who may be successfully frightened off sniffing by a stern talk, a sympathetic approach is more likely to bring cooperation. Again, one is looking for the extent of and reasons for use. Warning the user about the dangers needs to be carefully done if one is to be believed, as sometimes an attractive feature of sniffing (or drug use in general) is the risk involved. Since few sniffers will want to stop immediately, one must ensure they know how to avoid certain situations, such as sniffing alone, or using certain products.

Medical examination

The youngster may be tired, languid or dull with poor coordination, rhinitis, red eyes, confusion or poor concentration. He/she may have a cough and wake up each day with headaches or nausea. Taking blood for urea and electrolytes, LFTS, and a full blood count and routine urine testing may be useful not because they will usually show any pathology, but, in most cases, they will reassure parents that no serious physical damage has been done.

For casual and recent solvent use there is no need to refer. Support to the family and factual information to the youngster may be sufficient.

Long-term or serious misuse generally springs from a series of underlying disturbances, family maladjustment or deprivation, school and social failure. Dr O'Connor's book states, regarding these more serious cases (regular sniffing for up to four days a week three times a day):

> 'Fundamentally, though, VSA (volatile solvent abuse) remains a psychological problem. These noxious chemical vapours offer individuals a measure of emotional discharge and fulfilment which it is felt cannot be obtained in any other way. Effective treatments for the individual will have to provide the means whereby disabling emotional states for the young person such as frustration, depression, overexcitement, can be acted out in reality rather than internalised in fantasy. VSA seems to be in many ways a less threatening and less risky substitute for normal living.
>
> The antidote lies in encouraging children and adolescents to learn how to live happily and fully through their own experiences. This task is beyond the treatment capabilities of the individual therapist alone. It is a long-term management task which lies more within the province of the parents and teachers responsible for the child's development. Psychological approaches to the treatment of VSA have this in common: they seek to provide, albeit very often in a crisis situation, a substitute form of loving care and attention

imbued with sensible discipline and guidance. The effectiveness of the treatment is conditional upon the degree to which the sniffer perceives sniffing as a habit he would like to stop and experiences the caring relationship as a healing process sufficiently strong to enable him to change his behaviour. It would seem therefore that the most effective approach to treatment of VSA is a multidisciplinary one. The ideal is for all the main child caring services, including the Police Community Services, to work as a team to make caring support for the young person and his family effective enough to overcome VSA practices in favour of health-promoting activities which will keep the adolescent in touch with the real life of the community to which he belongs.' [19]

Psychological approaches vary with individual users but cover the following person-centred approach, behaviour therapy and hypnotherapy.

A short questionnaire at the outset adapted from Alcoholics Anonymous helps the counsellor to understand the individual's reasons for sniffing, and how best to help him:

- Do you sniff because you have problems?
- When you are alone?
- When you get mad?
- Are you skiving off work or school?
- Do you suffer loss of memory due to sniffing?
- Do you get really high even when you don't want to?
- Do you feel big to be able to sniff and get high?
- Do you get low marks at school?
- Do you ever try to sniff less or stop and fail?
- Do you sniff a lot quickly because you are craving for it?
- Do you tell lies about how much you sniff?

If no other help is available for sniffers, or families, one can give them the telephone number of Release, (01-377 5905 or 24-hour emergency, 01-603 8654) or the National Campaign against Solvent Abuse (01-274 7700 ext. 22/01-733 7330 (24-hour helpline)).

On the national scale, Dr Dorothy Black (senior medical officer at the DHSS) has written:

'Studies in Avon and elsewhere have shown that locally established groups involving the relevant professions (social service and youth workers, the police, medical, nursing and educational services) can act not only in identifying the local prevalence of the condition, but also to establish a focus of expertise, using the already existing skills of these bodies. Wider dissemination of the known facts about solvent misuse has already been initiated by many of these multidisciplinary groups, and by individual social service and local education authorities. Relevant publications are available from national voluntary organisations in the education, social work, and drug dependence fields. The involvement of parents is of paramount importance ...

Response should accordingly be local and multi-professional, and should be aimed predominantly at providing adolescents with access to alternative rewarding activities, improving health education within schools and in the community generally, and identifying the minority of children for whom solvent sniffing may have become the inappropriate response to other more severe problems, and who will require specialist social work or psychiatric intervention.' [21]

Emergency treatment of unconscious or similar cases
If many cases are seen, these instructions could be photocopied, and handed to those concerned with solvent sniffers, including other children.

(1) Don't panic or run away.
(2) Remove solvent and bag. Loosen tight clothing. If indoors, open windows.
(3) If person is breathing put him on his side in the recovery position (ask a teacher or first aider to show you this) to prevent inhalation of vomit and make sure the airway is clear. Cover and keep warm. If breathing is shallow, send for ambulance. If not breathing, carry out artificial respiration. Stay until ambulance or doctor comes.
(4) When recovering give nothing to eat or drink. Inform parent or other authorities.
(5) If a child recovers before the ambulance arrives, hospital treatment may not be needed, but a check-up may be a useful warning to the child.

Treatment if 'high' or intoxicated

(1) Remove solvent and ensure access to fresh air.
(2) Tell him to breathe deeply, slowly. If he starts to overbreathe or tingle, get him to breathe into a paper bag or cupped hands.
(3) Give nothing by mouth. Stay till fully conscious.
(4) If available, pass on to a responsible adult who will inform parents, etc. The community police will also be able to advise. Check whether local shopkeepers are allowing children who they

know or suspect might be misusing it, to get glue. If so, the shopkeeper is breaking the law.

Summary
The Newcastle advice may be summed up as follows:

(1) Talk to the solvent sniffer without demands or threats.
(2) Mobilise the family for support or solving the background problems.
(3) Get specialist advice, in more persistent or emotionally disturbed cases.
(4) Meanwhile make sure sniffers understand simple safety rules. Never sniff alone. Don't use plastic bags over the head, but rather a small potato crisps bags. Don't use solvents other than glue – some can be instantly fatal. Don't sniff in dangerous places such as high buildings, on cliffs or on river banks.

Chapter 7

Long-term Care

Introduction

As family doctors we need to keep in mind the longer view of rehabilitation from the very first contact with a drug user and introduce it either during the argument for not giving an immediate prescription and/or later as the relationship develops. However, a straightforward progression from the first contact with a doctor or drug worker to becoming drug-free is not all that common. Drug users may have several attempts before breaking out of the cycle of failure. The GP must not therefore be too discouraged by his own failure or that of others. A doctor has a valuable role to play in keeping in touch over the years and stimulating fresh efforts to come off drugs.

Few of us can do the job on our own and we must therefore look at the range of facilities available to help us. General practitioners should have received the first edition of the SCODA Directory *Where to Get Help*, a comprehensive listing of facilities by region. Copies of the second edition may be obtained from SCODA or ISDD (see Appendix B). The accompanying manual to the DHSS video *'Working with Drug Users* has a section devoted to drug facilities also compiled by SCODA. Readers will also find a selected listing of facilities in Appendix B. This is not intended to be comprehensive, but an indication of the main centres of advice and treatment in each region. They can all be contacted for further information about local facilities.

Where to refer

The varieties of services may be very briefly summarised under the following headings:

(1) *Hospitals*

There are about 40 NHS drug dependency units and a larger number of general psychiatric hospitals who have a psychiatrist with a special interest in drug problems. Drug users here may have to take their turn with general psychiatric patients and may only be admitted as and when a bed is available. Most hospitals with outpatient facilities offer a short or long-term reducing prescription of opioid drugs to achieve abstinence. Nearly all operate a strict catchment area and many require referral via a general practitioner. Some NHS authorities have established advice and counselling centres, and are training CPNs (Community Psychiatric Nurses) to work specifically with drug-dependent people in the community. These services form a valuable support for all patients. Outside London in particular, Community Drug Teams and GPs have been working together to provide home detoxification for users.

(2) Day projects

These are non-residential projects offering help to drug users living independently in the community. Often these projects will also advise and support former drug users or the families and friends of drug users. These predominantly social work or youth work projects may offer:

- advice on practical problems such as housing, employment, legal proceedings;
- information and advice on drug problems;
- long-term counselling and support aimed at stabilising drug use, minimising harm, or achieving abstinence, in cases where more formal treatment or rehabilitation may be unsuitable or unavailable;
- daytime activities in a drug-free environment;
- assessment and referral to treatment and rehabilitation services.

These projects are often suitable referral options or sources of consultation for a wide range of problem drugtakers, including those seeking onward referral to formal treatment or rehabilitation, and those for whom the more formal options are unsuitable. Some also offer continuing support and liaison to clients entering prison or attending clinics or rehabilitation houses.

Important exceptions to this wide remit include several projects limiting their services to young people, the Parole Release Scheme for parolees, and TRANX for tranquilliser dependents.

A unique service, for those in the North West of England, is provided by the Lifeline Project in Manchester. In addition to a day centre providing support to drug users and advice to families and professionals, there is an induction programme. This offers assessment and preparation for long-term rehabilitation programmes.

It is as well for the doctor to find out something about any local projects and note down in the SCODA Directory additional details for future reference, opening times, referral names etc.

(3) Self-help groups

In many areas of Britain there are projects run entirely as self-help groups or by unpaid volunteers. Such groups often spring from parental concern and operate primarily as support groups for parents of drug users; many also offer counselling or advice to drug users. At least one (Narcotics Anonymous) is a self-help organisation for drug users themselves. More local information about the groups in your area may be obtained from SCODA. ADFAM, Narcotics Anonymous, Families Anonymous and the National Campaign against Solvent Abuse have a number of local contacts or groups and therefore operate to some extent on a national scale.

(4) Crisis intervention

An unusual project in the drugs world, is *City Roads*. This is a crisis intervention service where young drug users are taken through a maximum of three weeks detoxification. As a crisis centre, it receives new residents at any time of day or night. During the reduction regime of their drugs, users are helped, and also assessed for referral, if they wish, to long-term rehabilitation. Some clients leave before the end of the course, others may relapse after it, but there is a chance for drug users to return at a future date. Some pass through two or three times before finally 'making it to the rehabs' and becoming drug-free. It is important to note, however, that the City Roads catchment area is restricted to Greater London.

(5) Private residential clinics

All private centres make charges directly on the individual resident. In some instances, these charges may be paid through private health insurance and in a small number of cases 'assisted places' may be offered. Residents on assisted places will have their basic costs met through payment of supplementary benefit from the DHSS and local authority payments, which is the standard way costs are met at residential projects in the voluntary sector for people with drug problems. In some instances, costs may be exclusive of consultation, medical and pathology fees, although some negotiation of fees may be possible.

Treatment varies, but of about sixteen private clinics in the UK, roughly a third operate the Minnesota Method – a combination of reality therapy (group work and individual counselling) with an introduction to the philosophy of Narcotics or Alcoholics Anonymous as appropriate.

(6) Non-specialist services

Many professionals specialising in drug problems believe that non-specialists, who may already be in contact with the drug user and their family/friends are equipped to deal with less severe drug problems (especially among younger drug users) and are often more appropriate and more available than specialist agencies.

Generic workers or services that may be able to offer help to drug users and their families include:

- neighbourhood youth workers, who can advise youngsters and help them find fulfilling activities that don't involve drugs. These can be contacted through local authority education departments.
- youth counselling services, which offer advice and longer term counselling to young people (approx. 16-25) and their families. Contact the National Association of Young People's Counselling and Advisory Services (NAYPCAS), 17-23 Albion Street, Leicester LE1 6GD, for the address of your nearest service(s).
- Citizen's Advice Bureaux, which may be a useful source of information on local volunteer or self-help projects.
- child guidance clinics, which see schoolchildren with behavioural problems or problems at school. They have access to psychiatric support and may be able to see young people (and their parents) with drug-related behavioural or emotional problems. Referral is usually through the school or GP.
- Family Network Service branches around the country, which offer a telephone 'listening' advice or counselling service to families, young people or older individuals, as well as sometimes running more specialised services. If required, telephone calls may be followed up by a personal interview. For a list of local branches,

write to the National Children's Home, 85 Highbury Park, London N5 1UD.
- the Samaritans, who aim to help the suicidal and despairing by making trained counsellors available, usually 24 hours a day by phone, and in person during the day and evening at local 'drop-in' centres. They may be able to offer befriending, advice and longer term support to drug users and their families unable or unwilling to attend specialist services. Look in the telephone directory for your nearest branch.

The nature of rehabilitation

Much of the discussion on rehabilitation applies to heroin users, but is also relevant to other types of drug misuse.

In the drug treatment world, ideas about rehab can be as conflicting as theories about detox, so the family doctor would do well to discuss what is suitable with those experienced in the field. We may not have to arrange for rehabilitation ourselves, but it is an advantage to know the options. The subject is fully discussed in the DHSS video *Working with Drug Users*, and in the City Roads *Drug Resource Pack*, available from ISDD at £47 and £3.45 respectively.

So what is rehabilitation? City Roads provides the best definition: 'Any process by which the client can be returned to as normal a life as possible within the community'. Because in the UK there are only about 500 beds for the whole country and most of them in the South East, the majority of drug users coming off drugs need to have rehabilitation at home, with community support. The minority are those who prove suitable for a stay of a year or more at a rehab house but not all of these can get a place or the financial support from the social services to go there.

(1) Residential rehabilitation

At some stage your drug user or their family are going to say: 'What are these rehabs like, doctor?'.

At some rehabs (but by no means all) residents would be a long way out in the country, so they can't easily get back to the drug scene. They would be in a large mansion or country house with up to 30 or so other drug-free users, and initially they won't be allowed outside the grounds. There's a programme of things to do all through the day, helping in the garden or in the workshop, cooking and cleaning, times for leisure, music or TV so there isn't much time to sit and dream about drugs. A *general house* like the Cranstoun Project in Surrey offers support and counselling. A *concept house* like Alpha House in Southampton or the Ley Community in Oxford, is run mostly by the clients who all start at the bottom rung of the ladder doing the chores. Others may boss a resident around or shout, or challenge another's way of thinking in encounter groups but if the client can stick it, he or she begins to move up the hierarchy. This is aimed to help residents to start feeling again – heroin has been like a shell, a protection from emotions – so if a client starts to get angry or worried about the future, or starts to like people, this is all part of the return to a normal life.

In most centres, all drugs are prohibited and in some places no cigarettes are allowed. At the start residents will be searched and have their luggage checked to make sure no drugs creep into the house, and mail and visitors will be restricted. It may sound like prison but it's not. However, the concept houses tend to have the largest communities within rehabilitation and some people have problems being in an 'institutionalised' setting with a number of others. For those who can't take the toughest places, they may choose a *Christian-based house* like Yeldall Manor near Reading, where they are still fairly strict but not quite so hard as the concept houses. The nature of Christian-based houses varies, but their common factor is an emphasis on the importance of a resident's acceptance of Jesus in the healing process. Other houses like the Coke Hole Trust have Christian staff, but there is a less intensive compulsory Christian teaching program. No Christian houses expect one to embrace Christianity as a condition of entry. But some drug users want it the tough way – they know they need really strong medicine to stay off drugs and the ones who stay to the end of the course usually do stay off.

Quite a few people do leave either soon after they join or halfway through. If a resident is only out on the street for 24 hours, the other clients in the house may agree with the staff to let that person in again. However, if this chance is lost, most rehabs will give a user another one later on.

General houses vary in their philosophical approach, but in all cases group and individual support is provided. Residents are encouraged to take a positive part in determining their therapy. Examples include Bridge in Bradford, the Cranstoun Project in Surrey and St. Mary's House in Hove, East Sussex.

Finance
There is the question, 'How shall I pay for all this?'. The doctor must tell either parents or drug users that they have to get in touch with

social services to get a grant. If they press hard, and are lucky, social services may be able to fix it with the DHSS who may pay board and lodging to the rehab and give the person a little bit of pocket money which can go a long way when they don't have drugs to buy.

Selection

Who is suitable to go to rehab? *Not* the following:

(1) therapeutic addicts – people who have been started on an addictive drug for a medical purpose, like DF118 for pain or Valium for anxiety;
(2) drug users with families, jobs or mortgages to look after;
(3) recent or mild drug users;
(4) people over 35 (with exceptions recently).

More suitable candidates include:

(1) the under-35, unemployed or homeless drug users with no support;
(2) the long-term, heavy users who need a lot of help sorting out problems away from their drug-using environment;
(3) those who have tried coming off in a home setting and failed;
(4) those sent by the court who may not be well-motivated or may even be unwilling to come off drugs;
(5) those who are drug-free for at least 24 or 48 hours and are motivated at that time to stay off drugs;
(6) those who have been to rehab before and not completed the course.

Full details of facilities, catchment areas, conditions of entry, financial assistance etc. can be obtained from SCODA.

(2) Rehabilitation in the community

The scarcity of residential houses and the conditions of suitability mean that the majority of users will not be able to go away for rehabilitation. Yet, once they have finished detoxification, with or without methadone, they desperately need skilled assistance to stay off drugs and establish a new lifestyle.

Fortunately, it is not the doctors who have to organise everything. They should be linking up with some kind of back-up support or a community drug team if one has been formed in the area. Others will be doing most of the hard work both from the statutory and voluntary side. For instance, a probation officer who asks us if we will undertake a detox course for his client will continue to see him weekly, possibly arrange accommodation and a job.

In less well-served areas, doctors may have to arrange residential rehabilitation themselves or form their own support team for users living locally.

One must harness the friends or family or look for any sort of specialised or generic worker available and encourage their training. Parents' groups may form, the local psychiatrist may agree to start seeing problem drug users and train one of his CPNs. The GP himself might send a health visitor for training, and select only those few patients who appear well motivated, with family or other support. The doctor may find himself working with parents in his own practice to assist young heroin smokers to come off, with simple advice and encouragement. Other patients in the practice may be upset but many will learn to understand.

Therapy possibilities

Within the context of rehabilitation the following types of therapy have been used.

Family therapy

Where family tensions over drug use are perhaps perpetuating the situation family therapy can be one answer. As practised from centres, it is not widely available and psychotherapists generally are not keen on taking on cases while drug use is still active. Rehabilitation needs to take place and the whole family needs to be desirous of such therapy before it can be successful.

The sort of dysfunctions dealt with are lack of communication, poor organisation, inability to make decisions and solve problems, and over-closeness or too much distance in relationships. Parental disharmony and cross-generation tensions may be indications for such treatment.

The techniques, using family 'trees' and 'circle' diagrams, talking and listening to one another, are varied, with a common aim of getting the family to solve its own problems. The therapist then merely acts as a catalyst.

Dr Lask's article in the *British Medical Journal* [1] urges those in paediatric and general practice to learn the techniques and apply them in their own settings. Solving the former drug user's family tensions is a big step forward in avoiding future trouble.

Cognitive therapy

This is an attempt to help the patient recognise and alter maladaptive thought patterns.

The cognitive therapist sets out to alter some of the cognitive processes, like perception, memory and controllability in order to correct counter-productive styles of thinking. The emphasis is on coping with disabling symptoms such as misperception and misinterpretation rather than eliminating them altogether.

Inappropriate beliefs and expectations can influence alcoholics and drug users, so techniques of altering these and stopping negative thoughts are sought and found. Abstinence violation is one concept being applied when a user has become abstinent, and improving 'self-efficacy'. One relapse violates this abstinence and the drug user or alcoholic then has to tackle this violation before the old phrase 'once an addict, always an addict' becomes a self-fulfilling prophecy.

> 'There is little doubt that an increasing number of workers in the field are using cognitive methods whether in the context of individual or group work as an integral part of their treatment program. This is in contrast to insight-based psychotherapeutic approaches which seem to have waned in popularity over recent years' [2].

Behaviour therapy

Raistrick and Davidson in their textbook say of this subject: 'Craving is regarded as a classically conditioned response (Wikler, 1973) as it can be linked with previously neutral stimuli and a number of behavioural treatments have been developed accordingly'. Aversion therapy has been used less of late but the process of 'extinction' for a craving has met with more success. In this, a conditioned stimulus is presented but the usual behaviour resisted; an example being to enter a public house, where the therapist urges you not to have a drink. This 'cue exposure' is thought to play a part in the use of opioid antagonists, where craving can be attenuated by repeated 'non-euphoriant' injections.

Operant conditioning is also used, but lately 'self-control' or 'self-management' has become more popular. The subject identifies the clues which influence drugtaking behaviour, boredom, the type of company, withdrawal symptoms, etc., and then the consequences that occur. Coping strategies are developed, such as relaxation or assertion training which appear to be more successful than previous treatments.

Goal-setting for the drugtaker

There are many things that a drug user must face up to and tackle on the way to recovery. Dr Chang, in her booklet *Coping with Drug Misuse in General Practice*, has characterised these things as short-, mid- and long-term goals.

Planning goals

Short-term goals

- Harm reduction
- Better health
- Confrontation of personal problems without recourse to drugs
- Solving some of the physical problems, such as housing, relationships, etc.
- Reduction of chaos in life
- Realisation of need for personal change
- Truthfulness

Mid-term goals

- Improvement in self-esteem
- More truthfulness
- General consolidation
- Self-assessment regarding progress
- Improvement in relationships
- Future plans for employment
- Increased insight into personal problems

Long-term goal

- A drug-free life

Restoration of health
Better health means starting to look after oneself with good food, regular sleep and exercise. Drugtakers have been used to lying in bed, sleeping off the effects of the drug until withdrawal forces them to look for more drugs.

Responsibility
For all their recent life drugtakers may have avoided responsibilities, to their family, to themselves and to society. Now they must be willing to

change and face their responsibilities without blotting them out in a chemical haze.

Reality
Again, for years the real person may have been hidden behind the mask of the junkie. He or she have been kidding themselves and conning others in an unreal world of false optimism and broken promises. Feelings of anger, love and concern, and guilt have been suppressed. This all has to be rediscovered in sometimes painful contact with friends, drug workers, authorities, even police, and others living in the 'real' world.

Reorganisation
This means learning or relearning accepted standards of behaviour down to even elementary social customs ('sorry', 'thank you' in some cases), punctuality, discipline, not letting the doctor and others down or doing things they don't like. Drugtakers must transfer their skills in acquiring and spending large sums of money illegally. Earning an honest living may be dull and boring after the thrills of 'scoring' but employment, where it can be found, can be a new and satisfying experience. The low self-image drug users have, will be overcome as they gain confidence, so if jobs are not available, taking part in voluntary work or creative activities is important. At a rehab, these aspects are catered for, but at home one may have to point them out to family, friends or workers as goals to be achieved, sooner or later.

Recovery
'Losing' a drug problem or even the comfort of the needle, has been compared to losing a spouse or a parent. Intense grief, loneliness and loss of purpose follow. Recovery follows the usual pattern of anger ('why me?') and denial ('drugs are not *so* bad'), bargaining ('I'll settle for less, I'll stay off heroin but not cannabis or alcohol'). There is a stage of depression as the full implications of life without a crutch, the bleakness of an existence without heroin hits the drug user. A doctor-addict speaking on a TV programme said he hadn't experienced the world without a mood-altering chemical for 12 to 15 years. Finally, there is a stage of acceptance and the need to change. A doctor's experience in helping bereaved people to cope will give him insight and skill in discussing this.

Recovery from fear and worry is another aspect to remember. For years, possibly, the chronic drug user has feared pain, feared withdrawals and pushed away misery with the help of the drug. Now he or she must learn to accept suffering as a part of life. Perseverance in the face of setbacks is something different from the frenzied hunt for drugs.

Realisation
This is the realisation that one must go through a stage of dependence on other people before emerging into independence and self-sufficiency – the realisation that people still care about you, even after being rejected by society and even scorned by other drug users, and the realisation that you care about them too. Planning the next few days or looking ahead opens up new horizons. One can experience with other 'normal' people the anticipation of a brighter future, ambitions and plans for a job or family. The doctor can find satisfaction as well as relief in being able to share in this recovery.

Rehabilitation, therefore, is a highly complicated process, but after ploughing through all these aspects, the family doctor new to the field need not feel discouraged. He is not personally responsible that all these aspects are covered, and may in fact be only a small link in the chain that helps a drug user into recovery. One fact is inescapable – that for the drugtaker and those who help him, life is full of surprises – sometimes pleasant but often with setbacks and disappointments. Planned goals may often be very limited and in a few chronic cases, the goal of complete abstinence may not be achievable. Truthfulness may also be hard to achieve, but if, after deceiving the doctor for some time, the drug user does admit the deception, and frankly admits failure, some ground has been gained. Progress may be seen as people begin to feel better about themselves.

Chronic drug abuse

One of the criticisms levelled at the DHSS *Guidelines on Good Clinical Treatment of Drug Misuse* is that they fail to deal with the problem of chronic drug misuse. Since drug addiction from one point of view tends to be a relapsing condition, there should be some areas in which the general practitioner comes into the picture.

The problem of the stable or long-term drug user is recognised on page 5 of the *Guidelines*. The heading describes drug users as a heterogenous group. They include:

'Stable drug users who are psychologically and/or physically dependent on opioids or other drugs which may initially have been prescribed to treat physical disorders. They rarely have associated problems and may require continued medication for the underlying organic condition. Within this small group of 'therapeutic' addicts, however, is a minority whose main need has become their desire for drugs. Symptoms may be complained of which are no longer present. Identification, assessment, and treatment of these patients may be difficult. They may also have additional social and legal problems.'

Some long-term drug users may have initially obtained controlled drugs for the treatment of their addiction or may have always obtained their supply from illicit sources. They may nevertheless have maintained stability in their social and working lives, but may present with anticipated or current legal problems.

The only separate advice given for these small but important groups of drug users is:

'We consider that a doctor should not undertake to treat drug misusers by long-term prescription of opioids unless in consultation and conjunction with a specialist in a drug treatment clinic or elsewhere who has experience of this approach.'

This would equally apply to the care of a stimulant user or a person unable to come off benzodiazepines. The working group which produced the *Guidelines* recognised that to take on, possibly for life, the care and continued drug supply of a stable user is an enormous commitment in the context of general practice, and is beset with pitfalls for the inexperienced.

The historical background to this brief piece of guidance (and the reason for its negativity) lies mainly in the experience of the Drug Dependency Units set up in the 1960s, principally in London. At the outset, heroin was issued on a daily maintenance basis, without reduction to notified users for injection, a system which often led to a 'junkie' subculture centred round the clinics. It also put enormous strains on the staff and the programme was eventually switched to one of methadone maintenance. Finally, in the last five to ten years the majority of long-term drug users were told they must come off drugs altogether. They were offered longer- or shorter-reducing courses of methadone and then discharged. Some users managed to stay off drugs, some went onto the black market for supplies and others applied to private or independent doctors in London to continue their maintenance. Some of these doctors were not concerned with the ultimate welfare of the drug user and tended to overprescribe, risking a leakage of drugs on to the illicit scene.

Other private practitioners and GPs, the responsible majority, tried to control the users' drug use. They had to guard against misuse and the selling of prescriptions to pay for private treatment and tried to look to the patients' well-being. Two of these doctors served on the DHSS working group which produced the *Guidelines*.

The move away from maintenance prescribing, however, led to a long controversy between the DDUs and the independent doctors. The problem of how to look after stable, 'therapeutic' or other 'respectable' wage-earning drug users with families who fail to come off or wish to stay on drugs, still remains. Outside London, in the rest of the British Isles the few private practitioners available who are willing to go on prescribing indefinitely tend to be those who are either so sympathetic that they see drug users' immediate needs as paramount, or those who perhaps under pressure prescribe whatever is asked for indefinitely. Occasionally such doctors are brought before Tribunals for unwise overprescribing and failing to look into the relevant aspects of drug use which are now outlined in the DHSS *Guidelines*. However, as mentioned previously, AIDS has added a new dimension to the debate about prescribing not just in terms of 'to prescribe or not' but also in relation to long-term maintenance, and more flexible prescribing is apparent in many DDUs across the country.

So what should the GP do about long-term stable drug users who seek his help? The local clinic may say it has no longer any policy for maintaining, or there is perhaps no nearby clinic or private doctor. A family doctor may:

(1) Agree to look after the medical needs of the drug user and his family (if any) while telling him he cannot give him a legal supply of drugs indefinitely. The supply must then come from wherever it has been obtained up till now. This overall medical care means that the doctor can be in touch with various agencies and supporting friends when crises occur and have a relationship with his patient so that if ever the user decides to come off, he is there to help.

(2) Agree to an indefinite drug supply (with the qualification that if circumstances change or the doctor cannot manage it any more he should be free to withdraw and this should be written into the contract). The *Guidelines* do not actually forbid this, and so long as special care is exercised, we do not think that the Home Office would object. The *Guidelines* do give a very important reminder that consultation with a clinic or someone who has specialised in maintenance is advisable. There are pitfalls in diagnosing the situation, in deciding the level of drugs supplied, in avoiding tablets or injectables and ensuring no drug reaches the black market. There is a place for support from the

family or others, for advice and testing for AIDS or hepatitis. If one is in a group practice, the rest of the partners should be in agreement, there should be cover for holidays etc. and there may have to be an understood contract with the user or a procedure for crises or alterations in dosage. A single practitioner – while free to do what he wishes – is more vulnerable to pressure and to misjudgement unless he has good back-up elsewhere. The course of drug use, like that of true love, rarely runs smoothly and if an average length of drug use in someone's life is fifteen and a half years, a stable drug user may not require the cooperation of a doctor for more than a few years.

On the indications for methadone maintenance in America, *Drug Abuse for the Primary Care Physician* notes:

> 'Methadone maintenance is indicated for heroin-dependent persons who are not strongly motivated to achieve immediate abstinence. While maintenance therapy does not offer the prospect of full social rehabilitation, it does reduce illicit drug use and associated criminal activity, facilitate employment and increase self-esteem, often with attendant improvements in family and community functioning. Thus, methadone maintenance can provide help to a large number of persons who otherwise might return to full-scale criminal activity and illicit drug use.' [3]

Chapter 8

Women and Drugs, Pregnancy and Child Care

Introduction

Women attend their general practitioners more frequently than men but this finding only partly accounts for the fact that they are more likely than men to receive a prescription for tranquillisers. Twice as many adult females than males at each age level receive tranquillisers from their GP and women also continue on these drugs longer than men [1]. Attitionally, women who are retired, unemployed, or not in the labour force are the highest consumers of psychotropic drugs [2].

There is disagreement as to the reasons why such prescribing is at a greater level for women. Do women suffer more mental illness than men, or is it that the male-dominated medical profession attach this label more readily to women? In one study [3] Horwitz concluded that women accept the self-label of psychiatric illness more readily than men and he later found men to have less awareness of both emotional disorders and physical symptoms [4]. He attributed these findings to the expected role of women in society: that of nurse to children and elderly relatives, which he considered made them more sensitive to the emotional needs of others. Other authors have concluded that the true level of psychiatric disorder among women in the community is about twice that of men [5].

These interpretations are open to the criticism that they are the result of bias in the observer. Certainly a marked degree of bias is sometimes openly encountered in the medical profession. Writing in *Woman* magazine (April 1978) one consultant stated: 'the whole developmental period of youngsters in terms of the two sexes is still vastly different ... boys tend to be more adventurous, more outgoing, more experimental, by virtue of their manhood ... a girl tends to be less of a wanderer, or seeker after other experiences, because child-bearing is such a fundamental experience.'

Modern medicine has been accused of incorporating 'stereotypes of women as emotional, sensitive, introverted and physically and psychologically weak, with interpretations of Freud attributing these deficiencies to biological factors ...' [6]. The question as to what extent prescribing by doctors is influenced by their own preconceptions requires further exploration. There is no doubt that there are great variations in prescribing patterns by GPs, not only of tranquillisers but also other drugs of dependence such as the more powerful analgesics.

Women who misuse illicit drugs meet more social disapproval than their male counterparts. As one author put it [6]: 'The illicit user attracts additional moral disapproval for selfish pleasure-seeking and an assumption that she is rootless, rejecting 'normal' family life. These images are drawn from a view of woman's major role as centrally responsible for the 'private' side of life – housework, childcare, emotional support and family servicing, the value of these being sentimental rather than economic, and crucially dependent on responsible self-supervision. The illegal addict is seen as first rejecting and then being rendered incapable of performing these functions effectively by a lifestyle which is initially willfully perverse and then, inescapably pathetic. The dependent housewife is seen as an unfortunate individual unable to cope with the stresses of her family responsibilities without drug support.'

Perhaps because of society's prejudices women may be more likely to conceal their drug use. In the Wirral, women drug users are said to be 'more likely than men to remain in the hidden sector. They are less likely to commit crime and ... when they are "busted" by the police, particularly for dealing with a male partner, the woman is often not arrested, with her boyfriend or cohabitee "taking the rap" instead, particularly if the couple have children' [7]. They are, therefore, less likely to appear in front of the courts on a drugs or drugs-related charge.

Women are known to be less likely than men to use specialist alcohol services [8] and primary health care professionals may too easily fail to identify alcohol as a problem in female patients [9]. However, the question as to whether women are more or less likely to seek help for a drug problem remains unclear in the UK. Various surveys have shown wide variations in male to female ratios in different populations and the relationship of these variations amongst those who attend the treatment services to gender use in local catchment populations has still to be elucidated. In spite of apparent wide local variations of the use of treatment services by women, notifications to the Home Office of drug users who have attended doctors throughout the UK have consistently shown a figure of approximately 29% to be women.

There is some evidence too that women present for treatment at a later stage than men. Commonly amongst those attending DDUs there is an initial peak of attendance 2 years after commencing regular drug use for men, but 3 years for women.

There are practical problems surrounding the care of young children which may be a deterrent to help-seeking. In a survey of facilities for women misusing drugs and alcohol conducted in 1984, DAWN (Drugs Alcohol Women Nationally) found that in reality only one in five agencies made any particular effort to help mothers with drug/alcohol problems [10]. Subsequent to this a number of rehabilitation centres throughout the country have set up mother and baby units. Many day centres, street agencies and DDUs have also taken steps to be more accommodating to women who are looking after young children. In Stevenage a scheme has been set up whereby volunteers come into the house for three weeks and take over the running of the household, doing the cooking, cleaning, taking the children to school, etc. while the mother is undergoing detoxification with the help of her GP.

In spite of such advances, it appears that one real deterrent which prevents women drugtakers reaching out for help has been the worry that, if they present for treatment, their children will be taken into care. If this is indeed the case then the potential health risks to both mother and child are considerable. It may be that the family doctor who is known and trusted is in a better position than other agencies to help women with such fears. Certainly a higher proportion of women drug users do attend their GPs than attend the DDUs [11] and GPs may attend women drugtakers for other problems such as contraception, gynaecological disorders and pregnancy which may act as a ticket to allow them to talk about their other more difficult problem – their drug use.

Contraception

Women who are regular opioid users taking $\frac{1}{4}$ gram of street heroin per day or more (or the opioid equivalent of this) often have amenorrhoea for several months or even years. It is not unusual for such women to assume that they are infertile and not to worry about using any method of contraception. Although there is no doubt that their fertility is lowered, breakthrough ovulation may occur at times, together with an unwanted pregnancy. In addition to this, opioid suppression of LH and FSH usually stops the moment the drug is withdrawn and women who undergo opioid detoxification should be warned that they will probably start having their periods again and that their fertility will increase considerably. Not only do their chances of conceiving rise, but so too does their libido, further increasing the possibility of pregnancy. It is therefore important to give contraceptive advice to all women who are using drugs, particularly those who are undergoing opioid detoxification.

Drug dependence is a relapsing condition and however well-motivated a person is, if drugs have been used for a protracted period of time, relapse is very likely to occur. Therefore those who lead very disorganised lifestyles when taking drugs are best discouraged from taking the contraceptive pill as they are unlikely to take it regularly. A better solution might be an injectable long-acting progestogen or the IUCD.

Some women taking drugs regularly become prostitutes as a means of raising sufficient funds to buy their drugs. Such women commonly have a history of pelvic inflammatory disease and in these cases the IUCD should be avoided. It is common practice these days for prostitutes to ensure that their male customers are wearing the sheath but this is more in order to reduce the risk of contracting HIV infection than to prevent them getting pregnant, and women drug users appear to be less likely to take this precaution than regular prostitutes.

It must not be overlooked that women drug users who have been involved in prostitution are also at high risk of developing carcinoma of the cervix, now that a clear association has been established between this condition and the sexually transmitted human papilloma wart virus. Women in this group should have regular cervical smears, preferably on a yearly basis. It may be convenient to combine this with a routine contraceptive check.

Barbiturate takers, as a result of induced enzyme activity in the hepatic P450 cytochrome system, metabolise the contraceptive pill at an increased rate and low-dose pills are liable to be ineffective. If the pill is to be prescribed, one containing 50 rather than 30 micrograms of oestrogen is preferable. However, since barbiturate users tend to lead chaotic lifestyles, oral contraception may be best avoided altogether.

Pre-conception counselling

Whatever his or her personal feelings about the matter, no professional is able to prevent a currently active drugtaker from attempting to conceive. However, those patients who admit their intentions do present an ideal opportunity for pre-conception counselling and may be receptive to ideas of changing to a drug-free existence.

Pre-conception counselling should include information about the possible harmful effects of drugs on the fetus, including the fetal alcohol syndrome and the effects of smoking in pregnancy. After pre-test counselling including a full explanation of the implications of a positive result, testing for HIV antibodies can be arranged if the woman consents and further post-test counselling should be organised for all who have a positive test. An enquiry into dietary habits will often reveal gross inadequacies and vitamin supplements are likely to be beneficial. A cervical smear should be taken.

Pre-conception counselling should include a tactful exploration of the reasons for wishing to conceive. It is not unknown for some women to think that having a baby will make them change their lifestyle and to use conception as a means of overcoming their own personal difficulties. Although there may be more than a grain of truth in this argument, a stable drug-free state needs to be achieved prior to conception if they are to avoid potentially damaging the prospective child.

Similar reasons for wishing to conceive may be apparent in women who are problem drinkers. Any woman with a history of heavy drinking who wishes to conceive should be given vitamin B compound forte tablets BPC and folic acid 5 mg daily. There is evidence that neural tube defects can be prevented by giving vitamin supplements prior to conception [12].

Pregnancy

Over the last few years an increasing number of women drug users have attended their GPs for confirmation of pregnancy. This reflects the rise in drug use in women of child-bearing age. For reasons already discussed many such women disguise their drug use if they are pregnant, or if they are known drug users, they may not attend until late in their pregnancy.

Sometimes there are additional reasons for this such as the worry that they will have to stop using drugs straight away, that there will be disapproval by the medical staff (which there often is), that they will make an inadequate mother, that they will not be allowed to keep the child, or pressure will be applied for them to have a termination. Others attend late because their lives have become chaotic through drug use. When the drugtaker does finally attend for antenatal care, the pregnancy can be regarded as being at risk. For pregnant women drug users in general, irrespective of the drug or drugs taken during pregnancy:

(1) *there is an increased risk of having a low birth-weight baby*. In one study of drug use in pregnancy, 29% of babies weighed less than 2,500 g at birth compared to 11% of controls [13]. Post-mortem evidence

suggests that growth retardation is due to a reduced cell number with all organs affected [14], and although intra-uterine growth retardation has been demonstrated to improve with good antenatal care from 26% below normal to 20% in one series [15] the main cause for this, which is probably multifactorial, is outside the control of the obstetrician.
(2) *there is an increased risk of perinatal mortality,* mainly in association with low birth-weight babies.
(3) *there is an increased likelihood of other complications to the pregnancy* resulting from malnutrition and anaemia, venereal disease, hepatitis B, HIV and other infections, drug-related psychiatric disorder, fits of hopelessness and depression, and maternal rejection of the baby. These complications may be compounded by a difficult social situation. The pregnant drug user may be isolated and lack support from cohabitee, family or friends. She may not be aware of the amount of professional social support that is available to her locally or she may be frightened of accepting it. She then misses out on the practical and financial help she could get and suffers further.
(4) *the incidence of congenital abnormalities lies between 2.7% and 3.2%*, which is the high normal range.
(5) *multiple pregnancy and multiple ovulation appear to be common* [16].

The effects of individual drugs of misuse on pregnancy and the fetus

Evidence has been accumulating for some time about the effects of individual drugs in pregnancy and a resumé of present-day knowledge is cited below. The effects of smoking and alcohol are also included for convenience. It is not always known whether a particular drug increases the incidence of abortion in the first trimester as it is not always certain, when a period is late, whether a gestation sac was present or not. Research indicates that some drugs such as cocaine might increase the risk of early miscarriage. However, where the situation is not clear, other drugs should be viewed with particular suspicion if, like heroin, they interfere with placental functioning at a later stage in pregnancy.

Smoking

There is no evidence that congenital malformations are increased by cigarette smoking. However, in heavy smokers, the placenta may develop specific histopathological changes. There is broadening of the basement membrane, intimal damage within the placental vessels and the villi have an increased collagen content. Such changes are characteristic of uterine underperfusion, and indeed decreased intervillous blood flow has been shown to be caused by cigarette smoking. In the light of this, it is not surprising to find that smoking in pregnancy is also associated with low birth-weight babies (less than 2,500 g) and pre-term deliveries (before 37 weeks).

Smoking has been known for a long time to worsen perinatal mortality figures. A study of 150,000 births by the British Perinatal Mortality Survey in 1958 showed clearly that perinatal mortality was greater when the mother had smoked during pregnancy. Both stillbirths and neonatal deaths were 28% higher in smokers. This increased perinatal mortality could be totally accounted for by prematurity and intra-uterine growth retardation.

Cigarette smoking has also been shown to reduce fetal breathing movements *in utero*, and this appears to be a direct physiological effect of nicotine rather than carboxyhaemoglobin. In addition there is a slight increase in the risk of antepartum haemorrhage but the incidence of pre-eclamptic toxaemia is reduced. This latter beneficial effect may possibly be a result of thiocyanate production which is known to produce hypotension.

Although it is far better to stop smoking before conception occurs, stopping or even cutting down on cigarette consumption during pregnancy will help. Davis *et al*. [18] showed that if smoking is stopped for only 48 hours there is an 8% rise in available oxygen from maternal blood.

Alcohol

On theoretical grounds, no drug should be taken in pregnancy unless absolutely necessary and, as a result, the Health Education Authority recommended that alcohol should be completely avoided during pregnancy. There is no evidence that occasional social drinking is harmful to the fetus, (although alcohol crosses the placenta barrier freely), but large amounts of alcohol taken during pregnancy are known to damage the developing baby. The drinking level where there is known to be a definite risk is in the region of four units daily (one unit = half a pint of ordinary beer, one single measure of spirits, or one glass of wine/sherry). At this level, there is some degree of intrauterine growth retardation and minor abnormalities are observable in

10% of babies born. When daily consumption is twice this level there is a 20% chance of damaging the fetus.

Although alcohol was noted to increase perinatal mortality and morbidity during the English gin epidemic of 1720-1750, a definite syndrome linked with excessive alcohol consumption during pregnancy was not generally recognised until 1973 when Smith and his colleagues coined the term 'fetal alcohol syndrome'. There are four features typifying this syndrome:

- antenatal growth retardation
- a characteristic facial appearance
- neurological defects
- a tendency to other major abnormalities

At least two of these need to be present to make a diagnosis, one of which must be the abnormal facial appearance, typical of the syndrome. The facial features comprise the presence of short palpebral fissures either alone or in combination with multiple dysmorphic facial features including epicanthic folds, a broad, low nasal bridge together with a broad flat midface, a short upturned nose, short philtrum and facial hirsutism. In addition, there may be ear abnormalities, small nails, abnormal palmar creases, large haemangiomata (purple birthmarks) and limited joint movement.

The antenatal growth retardation is usually associated with short stature in later life. In the eight cases described by Jones et al. [18], none of the children reached normal height or weight for their age, even though some had been admitted for investigation of failure to thrive and one had been fostered. In addition to their small size, they all had microcephaly.

The most serious neurological defect is mental deficiency, but abnormal neurological behaviour, not unlike the neonatal opioid withdrawal syndrome may be observed following delivery. There is irritability, insomnia, increased yawning and sneezing and increased head preference to the left [19].

Most of the major congenital abnormalities associated with the fetal alcohol syndrome are cardiac in origin, and include ventricular and atrial septal defects and patent ductus arteriosus. Of the eight cases originally described by Jones et al., five had abnormalities of this type. There is evidence that vitamin and dietary deficiencies, as found in some heavy drinkers, may cause congenital abnormalities to occur.

Postmortem studies of babies that have been exposed to excessive alcohol use while *in utero* have shown structural abnormalities within the CNS. In one series, four brains had similar abnormalities, caused by a failure of neuronal and glial migrations.

There is some evidence that it is acetaldehyde, an alcohol metabolite, rather than alcohol itself, which is responsible for the fetal alcohol syndrome. A case has been recorded where an alcoholic woman on disulfiram (antabuse) had consumed minimal amounts of alcohol during her pregnancy but gave birth to a baby with the fetal alcohol syndrome. Disulfiram works by blocking the oxidation of acetaldehyde causing this metabolite to build up to extremely high levels. In experiments with lymphocyte and fibroblast cell cultures, acetaldehyde has been shown to cause cell death and chromosomal aberrations, findings that did not occur with high levels of ethanol.

Solvents and other volatile hydrocarbons

All of these substances cross to the placenta as they are strongly lipophilic and there is a theoretical risk of teratogenic effects if they have been misused in pregnancy. However, to date there are no relevant reports recorded in the literature.

Opioids

There is no evidence that opioid use in pregnancy causes congenital malformations. In the first trimester it may increase the risk of miscarriage although there is, as yet, no conclusive evidence of this. In the third trimester, however, there is evidence that heroin causes episodes of acute placental insufficiency leading to episodic intrauterine fetal distress and sometimes stillbirth. The stillbirth rate is increased, although overall increase in perinatal mortality is mainly attributable to neonatal deaths. Rementaria and Nuang [20] found a stillbirth rate of 65–70 per 1,000 births in 1973 in pregnant heroin users. They also showed that if such women were maintained on methadone throughout their pregnancy, the stillbirth rate fell to normal levels although the perinatal death rate increased by a factor of three.

Any opioid drug used repeatedly in pregnancy is liable to cause physical dependence not only in the mother but also in the fetus and neonate. In these circumstances it is best if possible to substitute oral methadone during pregnancy because its long duration of action makes it less likely that mother and fetus will experience intermittent physical withdrawal effects. It is probably better to use methadone linctus (2 mg/5 ml) than methadone mixture (5 mg/5 ml), as the latter compound contains a small amount of chloroform which could, in theory, have a detrimental effect on the fetus.

Opioid withdrawals during pregnancy have been shown to increase catecholamine levels within the amniotic fluid [21]. In addition, withdrawal effects can cause uterine irritability and, in some patients, premature labour [22].

Several studies have shown that opioid use is linked with intrauterine growth retardation in about one-third of cases, and this figure remains unchanged in those who have received methadone maintenance throughout their pregnancy. For this reason, and the fact that opioid withdrawals can be life-threatening to the newborn baby, it is preferable in most cases slowly to reduce the opioid at a rate that will not harm the fetus.

Barbiturates

All barbiturates cross the placenta and attain higher levels in fetal tissues than maternal tissues, because of poor fetal elimination of these substances [23, 24].

A prospective study of 9,000 pregnancies by the Royal College of General Practitioners [25] showed a marginal increase in congenital malformations when therapeutic doses of barbiturates had been taken. For mothers on anticonvulsants of all types, there is a two- to four-fold increase in malformations. Barbiturates appear to be less teratogenic than other anticonvulsants.

Large doses of barbiturates in pregnancy may lead to more serious consequences. A syndrome resembling the fetal hydantoin syndrome has been reported in association with massive phenobarbitone dosage in pregnancy. There are dysmorphic facial features, digital hypoplasia and growth retardation [26].

Cocaine

There is some evidence that cocaine, when taken in the first trimester, may be teratogenic to the fetus, although as yet the evidence is not conclusive. There has been one report of capillary angiomata in two of eight children born to cocaine addicts. There is, however, firmer evidence that cocaine use in early pregnancy significantly increases the rate of spontaneous abortions [27].

Cocaine causes placental vasoconstriction and transient hypertension and tachycardia secondary to increased levels of circulating catecholamines. There have been several reports of abruptio placentae and premature labour in cocaine users. Some papers have reported instances of such events immediately following an intravenous injection of cocaine. Intra-uterine growth retardation does not seem to be a general feature of cocaine use *per se*, but babies may be small for dates due to the appetite suppressant action of the drug.

Amphetamines

There is a link between amphetamine taking in pregnancy and congenital abnormalities. Milkovich and Van der Berg [28] found an excess of oral cleft defects. Cases of biliary atresia have been described, and two cases of microcephaly in association with mental retardation and motor dysfunction, when mothers had been taking methamphetamine during their pregnancies. A retrospective study of babies born with congenital heart defects has shown a relationship with amphetamine use in pregnancy. Like cocaine, premature labour may also be induced by amphetamine use, and babies may be small for dates.

Benzodiazepines

All benzodiazepines should be considered potentially teratogenic. Three studies have shown a relationship between benzodiazepine ingestion in the first trimester and oral cleft malformations. However, although all benzodiazepines are suspect, there are several drugs belonging to this group (including chlordiazepoxide, medazepam, lorazepam, oxazepam, temazepam, chlorazepate, clonazepam and clobazem) where there have been no reports of harmful effects to the fetus when these were taken in pregnancy. Chlordiazepoxide is probably the safest of all the benzodiazepines to take in this respect. In a retrospective study [29] of 50,282 pregnancies, 257 took this drug in the first trimester, 590 in the remainder, and 107 throughout. There was no difference in the percentage of malformations and perinatal mortality from the control group.

When diazepam is taken in pregnancy, it achieves higher levels in cord plasma than in maternal plasma [30] and tissue levels of the drug remain high, particularly in the gastrointestinal tract, liver and CNS because the young fetus is unable to metabolise diazepam to any appreciable extent [31]. Pre-term and term babies, however, have a limited capacity to metabolise this drug and its active metabolites following delivery. Furthermore, diazepam and its active metabolites may persist for one to two weeks following delivery, causing respiratory depression, hypotonia, poor feeding and impaired thermogenesis in the neonate.

Cannabis

There is no evidence at the time of writing that cannabis is teratogenic in humans, although some reports have indicated an increased likelihood of psychiatric disturbance in the mother.

LSD

The picture here is confusing and shows some conflicting evidence. In a review of the literature, Long felt that there was no firm evidence of teratogenesis by LSD in humans [32]. In spite of this, one study found a 10% incidence of major congenital abnormalities, the majority being neural tube defects, and 50% of all cases had minor chromosomal abnormalities at birth, although these were no longer detectable at three to six months [33]. Long did, however, note five cases of limb deficiencies and urged caution.

Management of the pregnant drugtaker

At first consultation a full history and examination should take place. The history should include details of smoking, drinking, past and current drug use, whether or not the patient injects, the sharing of injection equipment, and any history suggestive of hepatitis. It is also important to know details of the drug user's social situation and whether there is support from relatives or cohabitees who are non-users. A urine sample should be sent for analysis for drugs at this first consultation and consideration should be given as to whether further samples should be sent at later stages in the pregnancy. Early booking is helpful and later the GP should ensure that the hospital has arranged for a blood test to screen for hepatitis B, as this may have implications for the neonate. Screening for hepatitis B is now routine in some hospital obstetric departments, but this is by no means universal.

Although these points apply to all pregnant drug users, subsequent management will vary according to which drug or drugs are being taken.

Women and Drugs, Pregnancy and Child Care   263

Management of the pregnant opioid drugtaker

The opioid drugtaker sometimes misses the fact that she is pregnant, mistakenly thinking that her amenorrhoea is due to drug use. When she does find out she may attempt to stop taking her drugs abruptly, thinking that they will harm the fetus. In fact the reverse is true; sudden cessation of opioid use may be life-threatening to the fetus. In view of this, *it is correct practice for any doctor confirming pregnancy in an opioid user to prescribe a temporary maintenance dose of methadone linctus immediately, without waiting for the results of urine analysis for drugs.* Counselling can then be undertaken and a decision made as to whether the pregnancy will be continued or terminated. During this period it is helpful to know the result of the patient's HIV test if consent is given for this to be done, and appropriate pre- and post-test counselling should be given.

If the test for HIV antibodies is negative and/or the patient wishes to continue the pregnancy, early referral to an obstetrician is indicated. A decision will then need to be made by the obstetrician as to whether the opioid-dependent user should be admitted to an antenatal ward and a slow inpatient detoxification undertaken whilst monitoring placental and fetal functioning, whether she can be slowly detoxified as an outpatient, or whether she should be maintained on a steady dose of methadone. Some high-dose, long-term opioid users may be best treated with methadone maintenance as the risk of relapse is so high and this may be life-threatening to the fetus. These risks have to be balanced against the risk to the neonate of the opioid withdrawal syndrome, if the mother is maintained on a stable dose of methadone throughout her pregnancy.

Inpatient and outpatient opioid detoxification are best conducted during the second trimester as this minimises the risk of abortion and premature labour, although in practice it is not always possible to do this. Methadone is the drug of choice because its long duration of action gives a plateau effect on blood levels, minimising the risk of interdose withdrawals. It is best given in the form of methadone linctus (2 mg/5 mls) and although it may be given as a single daily dosage to an outpatient, on an inpatient basis where more ideal conditions may prevail it is preferable to split the dose and give it twice daily.

Inpatient detoxification is usually anticipated to last for about 12 weeks. The advantages of inpatient care are (a) the methadone dosage can be titrated against withdrawal symptoms, (b) fetal and placental function can be monitored, and (c) detoxification is more likely to be successful with less chance of additional illicit drugs being used on top of the prescription. Inpatient care is particularly suitable for those whose social situation is unstable.

For those users who have good support at home, outpatient detoxification is the treatment of choice. Compliance as an outpatient is likely to be better with a single daily dose rather than a split dose of methadone elixir. Reduction should again be slow with dosages being reduced at a rate no greater than 5 mg methadone per week, even at the early stages of detoxification where there is normally greater flexibility for dose reduction. Again, complete detoxification would normally be expected to occur within a period of 12 weeks.

For those with a history of regular opioid use extending over several years, methadone maintenance may be the treatment of choice. Partial detoxification followed by maintenance on a low fixed dose of methadone, say 15 mg daily, has limited effects on the fetus and may be an ideal compromise solution. Some women who present too late for full detoxification may also fit into this category.

The management of pregnancy in other drug users

Amphetamines and cocaine should be stopped at once. Substitute withdrawal is not appropriate and is potentially harmful to the fetus. Concurrence with the advice to stop should be confirmed at a later stage by urinalysis.

Volatile substance misuse and the taking of psychedelic drugs should also, where possible, be stopped. Advice to do this is more likely to be adhered to as dependence on these substances does not occur to any significant extent. However, cessation of their use cannot be confirmed by urine testing as this is not possible in ordinary hospital laboratories.

Barbiturate withdrawal in pregnancy should be dealt with on an inpatient basis in order to prevent fitting. Phenobarbitone elixir is a useful tool for a smooth withdrawal programme because of its long duration of action. In contrast to opioid dependence in pregnancy, there is no need to prolong the withdrawal phase of barbiturates because the patient is pregnant, and chemical detoxification can usually be completed within eight days. A method for doing this is described elsewhere in this book. It is useful to extend the inpatient stay for, say, another two weeks beyond completion of detoxification, if immediate relapse is to be avoided.

Benzodiazepines, when these have been taken in ordinary therapeutic doses, should be withdrawn on an outpatient basis and this is usually achievable over a 4-week period. However, when they are taken in large amounts (e.g. 60 mg diazepam or more/day) inpatient withdrawal to prevent fitting is appropriate. A detoxification timescale of up to 1–2 weeks using diazepam syrup t.d.s. is helpful during the first and second trimesters. But in the third trimester it is better to use phenobarbitone elixir because of the danger to the neonate of benzodiazepines (15 mg diazepam may be regarded as being roughly equivalent to 30 mg phenobarbitone).

The management of labour

As we have seen, drug use in the third trimester can lead to an obstetric emergency with abruptio placentae or impending intrauterine death from placental insufficiency. Such cases may require urgent delivery by Caesarean section if the baby is to survive. Other drug use in late pregnancy may induce premature labour. This applies particularly to the use of amphetamines or cocaine.

If a woman goes into labour while she is still taking opioids, barbiturates, cocaine or amphetamines, the fetus is at high risk of developing distress. Under these circumstances, it is important that admission is arranged to a hospital labour ward at an early stage, so that the labour may be closely monitored and also so that special care facilities will be available for the newborn child if required.

As a general principle, for all known drug users in labour, if analgesia is necessary, this is best done on a regional basis, with local or epidural anaesthesia.

Sometimes a woman will have concealed her drug use during pregnancy, the problem being recognised for the first time during labour. Any drug user who goes into opioid withdrawals during labour should be treated by a small dose of an opioid by injection. Fetal distress is sometimes dramatically improved by this. Generally speaking the wellbeing of both mother and child is maintained by prescribing a dose of drug to the mother that is sufficient to prevent withdrawal symptoms, but does not produce intoxication in the mother or respiratory depression in the neonate.

Both methadone and pethidine have an advantage over most other opioids of not affecting uterine contractility and it is, therefore, helpful to use one of these two drugs. A dose of less than 10 mg of methadone is unlikely to cause depression of the fetal respiratory centre. However, if depression of respiration does occur in the neonate this is likely to be particularly long-lasting if methadone has been given. A better approach may be to give small aliquots of pethidine through an intravenous line, titrating the dose against maternal symptoms and monitoring the fetus. *In the event of opioid overdose in pregnancy or labour,* naloxone (Narcan) must not be given as this will precipitate abrupt withdrawal symptoms in both fetus and mother.

Depression of the respiratory centre in the newborn by opioid drugs taken by a dependent mother just prior to delivery can cause a difficult management problem. *Naloxone (Neonatal Narcan) should never be given, except as an absolutely last resort, in this situation, as it is likely to precipitate immediate severe life-threatening withdrawals and convulsions in the neonate.* The preferred treatment is intubation and ventilation under the supervision of a skilled paediatrician until the drug-induced depression of spontaneous respiration no longer occurs. In cases where there is immaturity of neonatal hepatic enzyme systems needed to metabolise the drug, it may be several hours or sometimes days before this happens.

Breast feeding

Most drugs of misuse do not pass into the breast milk to affect the neonate. Some drugs are present in breast milk in such small amounts that they have no observable effects on the baby. Opioids fall into this last category. The quantities ingested are so small that they are very unlikely to affect the baby and will not prevent the onset of the neonatal opioid withdrawal syndrome.

There is some variation amongst the benzodiazepines. Diazepam passes into the milk and may cause sedation in the neonate. Chlordiazepoxide and nitrazepam also go into the breast milk, but in such small quantities that the baby remains unaffected.

If the mother takes a high dose of barbiturates while she is still breast feeding the drug is excreted in the breast milk in sufficient quantity to cause drowsiness in the neonate.

Any mother who is HIV positive, or who is untested but considered to be at high risk of HIV infection, should be advised not to breast feed.

The neonate

Whenever possible, a paediatrician should be present at the birth of any baby whose mother has been misusing drugs in pregnancy, as the newborn baby is likely to be distressed and may have breathing difficulties.

Opioids and the neonate

In this country, heroin is the most common drug of misuse likely to affect the fetus. In 1985, one Thames Health Regional Authority reported the birth of 60 heroin-addicted babies. Most of these were breathing normally at birth but some had respiratory depression with respiratory and metabolic acidosis at birth as a result of maternal opioid use. The management of this condition and the importance of avoiding the use of naloxone (Neonatal Narcan) in the neonate has already been described.

Although most babies of opioid-dependent women are normal at birth, after 24–72 hours (longer with methadone) they will start developing the neonatal opioid withdrawal syndrome, in up to 90% of cases. They become restless and irritable, with a shrill cry and a squirming that excoriates knees, toes and face. There is muscular hypertonia with occasional brief periods of hypotonia. Persistent high-pitched crying and constant sucking and chewing of the fingers which cannot be relieved by swaddling and comforting are frequent features. The neonatal head circumference is reduced in comparison with controls [34] and babies are often small and of a low birth weight. Reflexes are exaggerated and sleep is difficult. Such babies feed poorly and diarrhoea is common. Their colour changes. In severe withdrawals neonatal death can be caused by convulsions. In less severe cases and at a later stage, autonomic symptoms such as yawning, sneezing, nasal stuffiness and sweating occur. Owing to immaturity of hepatic enzyme systems, in approximately 10% of babies, the opioid withdrawal syndrome does not appear until anything up to the thirty-sixth day following delivery. If this is recognised it can be effectively treated; if left untreated, there is a chance that it may be fatal. The greatest danger is when the withdrawal syndrome remains unrecognised. This is, of course, most likely to occur when drug misuse is not detected in the mother and when mother and baby have returned home from the hospital. Experience has shown that the neonatal opioid withdrawal syndrome is liable to occur when the mother has been taking 20 mg methadone a day or more, or its equivalent, or if she has been using a mixture of opioid drugs plus alcohol.

Barbiturates and the neonate

If a high dose of barbiturates has been taken in the six-hour period before delivery this causes a less responsive baby with poor sucking ability and weight gain. For mothers who are dependent on barbiturates at the time of delivery, a neonatal barbiturate abstinence syndrome has been described. The clinical features of this are: restlessness, irritability, tremors, hyperreflexia, shrill cry, sleep disturbance, hyperphagia and vomiting [35]. Convulsions may occur.

Barbiturates may also deplete serum folate and cause hypoprothrombinaemia in the neonate, although this will respond to vitamin K. In addition, these drugs can cause a platelet deficiency, further increasing the risk of neonatal haemorrhage.

Cocaine and amphetamines and the neonate

Cocaine use in late pregnancy can lead to marked behavioural disturbances in the neonate. There is shrill crying, irritability with increased tremulousness and startle responses, and there is commonly repeated sneezing. Neonatal gestational age, birth weight, length, and head circumference are not affected by cocaine use [27]. A similar neonatal deprivation syndrome has also been described in association with maternal amphetamine use [36].

Benzodiazepines and the neonate

Neither chlordiazepoxide nor diazepam when taken in normal therapeutic doses during labour affect fetal pH or Apgar score. However, a single dose of 30 mg diazepam or more, given in the 15 hours preceding delivery can cause respiratory depression, hypotonia, poor feeding and impaired thermogenesis in the neonate.

A neonatal benzodiazepine withdrawal syndrome has also been described and is typified by tremors, irritability, hyperactivity, hypertonicity, tachypnoea and frantic sucking. As the fetus develops much higher tissue levels of the drug than the mother, this withdrawal syndrome is of greater severity than might otherwise have been anticipated from the dosage taken by the mother.

Treatment of the neonatal withdrawal syndromes

As can be seen there are many similarities between the different neonatal withdrawal syndromes. These similarities have in fact been so great that many paediatricians treat them all in the same way, believing in a single non-specific neonatal withdrawal syndrome, irrespective of the type of drug used by the mother. Traditionally chlorpromazine in a dose of 1 mg/kg/4-hourly by mouth, reducing over a period of 3-6 weeks, has been regarded as the treatment of choice for any neonate that is withdrawing, but chloral hydrate, phenobarbitone, diazepam, methadone, and paregoric have all been used at times.

Recent research, however, lends support to the suggestion that there is not one but several neonatal withdrawal syndromes. Studies at the Beth Israel Medical Centre in New York [37] have shown that, although it is not so good in other respects, paregoric is superior to phenobarbitone in the prevention of seizures in the neonate withdrawing from opioids. This indicates that there are separate withdrawal syndromes for opioids and barbiturates at a biochemical level and some authorities feel that the most logical and probably the best approach is, therefore, to prescribe a scaled down drug withdrawal programme similar to that which might be prescribed for an adult. This principle would not, however, be acceptable for the neonatal cocaine and amphetamine withdrawal syndrome. In the authors' view the following can be recommended as treatments for the different neonatal withdrawal syndromes:

The neonatal opioid withdrawal syndrome

Paregoric (camphorated tincture of opium) should be given at an initial dose of 4–6 drops every 4 hours increasing by 2 drops per dose if symptoms persist. In some babies this induces vomiting. Intramuscular morphine sulphate in a dose of 0.06–0.1 mg per kg is said to be less likely to cause emesis and is sometimes used for initial stabilisation. Oral methadone at a dose of 0.1–0.5 mg/kg/day is often used instead of paregoric. During the first 24 hours the dose is titrated by giving small increments every 2 hours until symptoms subside. Once stabilisation is achieved a single daily dose can be given allowing for smooth detoxification.

Treatment of the neonatal amphetamine and cocaine withdrawal syndrome

The neonatal amphetamine and cocaine withdrawal syndrome is probably best treated by chlorpromazine in the dosage already stated.

Treatment of the neonatal barbiturate, alcohol, and benzodiazepine withdrawal syndrome

The neonatal withdrawal syndromes from each of these three CNS depressant drugs are probably identical. For treatment purposes it is best to use sodium phenobarbitone elixir in a total daily dose of 5 mg/

kg. This dose should be divided by three and given 8-hourly. Blood levels should be monitored. Diazepam in a total daily dose of 3–6 mg/kg is recommended by some authorities for the neonatal benzodiazepine withdrawal syndrome. Again this dose is divided by three and given every 8 hours. This regime works well if the baby's liver enzyme system is mature. However, when this is not the case, accumulation of the drug will occur with potentially fatal results. Phenobarbitone, on the other hand, acts as an enzyme inducer in the neonatal liver and speeds up the maturation of hepatic enzyme systems as well as acting in its own right to counteract CNS depressant drug withdrawal effects.

For all neonates who are withdrawing

It is traditional practice for all newborn babies who are withdrawing to be swaddled, cuddled and laid on their stomach in a darkened room to reduce external stimulation to an already irritable nervous system. In fact, there is very little that can be done to comfort them and this can be very distressing for their mothers, who should be advised not to try to feed them every time they frantically suck their fists and continue the shrill cry.

Other neonatal problems

Poor bonding

The failure of withdrawing babies to respond to maternal comforting can start an ongoing process of maternal rejection [38] by someone who is already experiencing guilt about her drug use. Negative emotions may be compounded in the mother to produce a feeling that she is unable to love the baby or plan for its future. Drug-using mothers need understanding and persistent encouragement if effective bonding is to be achieved to lay the foundations for a good mother-child relationship. Where a baby's withdrawals, prematurity, or other neonatal problems enforce separation of mother and child, hospital staff should try to mitigate the anguish of separation.

Good bonding is even more important if the mother and baby, instead of going to a supportive husband or family, are returning to inadequate housing shared with drug users, a violent husband, life as a single parent, or other social difficulties which may be associated with previous drug use in the mother. Sympathetic and persistent care from the family doctor, midwife, health visitor and social or street worker can help to conquer the formidable obstacles in a deprived baby's development.

The transmission of hepatitis B and HIV

Children born to high risk hepatitis B carriers should be treated by a mixture of passive and active immunisation. This gives good antibody levels and reduces the carrier state in these infants by 90%. It is sometimes said that the children of low risk (anti HBe positive) carriers do not require prophylaxis. Twelve per cent of these women transmit the virus and it is very rare for the infected neonate to become a carrier. However, as there is still a degree of risk, albeit small, it is wise to give combined active/passive immunisation to all neonates whose mothers carry the hepatitis B virus.

Transplacental transmission of HIV from a seropositive mother may occur in up to 50% of cases. Whether or not the virus has crossed the placenta is difficult to determine in the neonate because the mother's antibodies also cross over into the baby's circulation, so that a positive test in the neonate merely reflects seropositivity in the mother. If AIDS develops, the time-span from diagnosis to death is on average 9 months faster than that in the adult.

Care Orders

The GP will also be involved in the thorny question of taking the baby into care, if this arises. In Britain, as in the USA, the seventies saw an emphasis on the parents' rights so that it was hard to get a child into care if the drug-using parents could not cope. Then a series of tragic cases hit the headlines in which social work departments were blamed when an abused child finally died. In the eighties the pendulum has swung over in favour of the rights of the fetus and child. As a result drug-using parents are tending to act defensively, concealing problems because of fears that they will lose their children to the State.

The American 'State Child Abuse Programs' insist that harm and danger to the fetus and newborn child must be reported. Drug misuse is specifically included within this category of harm and danger and if a physician fails to report drug misuse in pregnancy he can be held to be responsible for later child abuse.

A recent case in Britain has created apprehension in many drug-using parents, and those caring for drug users. The case began in 1985 when the child of a 30-year-old mother from Reading was put into care at birth because it had become addicted to methadone *in utero*. The mother fought the case all the way to the House of Lords, but on 4 December 1986 her appeal against the magistrate's care order was lost. Lord Brandon was reported as saying that in the present case, the juvenile court had had ample material on which to find that on 23 April 1985, when the child was still in hospital, 'her proper development had been avoidably prevented, and her health had been avoidably impaired'. The situation could have been avoided if the mother had not persisted in taking excessive doses of narcotic drugs throughout her pregnancy.

He saw no reason either why the court should not look back at the time before the child had been born, but Lord Goff made it clear that the *law does not imply that if a woman refuses to stop indulging in potentially dangerous activities during pregnancy, such as taking drugs, smoking or drinking, she risks having her child taken away by the local authority*. Even sports, vigorous intercourse or failing to attend antenatal appointments could all constitute dangers to the child, so if other social services take advantage of this judgement to press for custody, they are indeed opening the Pandora's box so frequently mentioned in comments about this case.

With all this in mind, the family doctor and other workers must work even harder for the mother's cooperation in pregnancy, and should try to be involved in decisions about the welfare and custody of the child, not leaving it entirely to social workers and lawyers.

Medically, it is reckoned that the mother and child should be seen by the doctor or paramedical staff once a week for the first three months at least. If parents fail to cooperate in this, lack of care must be suspected. Authorities on postnatal care in drug dependence differ as to the suitability of a family who continue to use drugs while bringing up a child. As it is, a third to over half of drug users' children do end up for some period in care through neglect or abuse, although there are a number of parents who, while unable to overcome their drug use completely, do fiercely work to ensure that their children will not suffer as a result. When the children reach school age, any faltering in health, behaviour or punctuality which would be accepted in normal families, is automatically suspected of being due to drug misuse in these parents. A recent case of a 15-year-old girl being put in care when she confided to a teacher that her mother was a drug user is also alarming. This case was pressed home despite the family doctor's opinion that the woman was a good mother to her child.

Intervention must therefore be regarded with great care, and a balanced medical viewpoint must be brought into situations where emotion, prejudice and lack of awareness may appear in case conferences about placements. As one authority put it [39] 'The future of the child must be assumed to lie in the hands of the parents, and the aim of treatment must be to enable them to undertake this responsibility'.

Chapter 9

Drugs, the Family and the GP

On discovering the problem

The initial response of parents and other close family members is almost always described as shock.

Parents in particular, feel guilt, bewilderment, and a sense of stigma. This may be followed by a period of grief or mourning for the loss of the child, and often tied in with this are fears of imminent physical death of their child. Feelings of bewilderment may be increased if, as is usually the case, parents feel unable to give direction to their children, who probably know far more about drugs than they do. Sometimes, parents feel that they themselves are destroying their own children.

Strategies adopted by concerned non-users

Coercion to seek help

Most concerned non-users will attempt to coerce a friend who is using regularly to seek help. With family and intimate friends such coercion may take extreme forms: threats, blackmail, temper tantrums, verbal abuse, physical violence and other types of bad behaviour appear to be common – perhaps as an expression of intense frustration as much as manipulative devices. The drugtaker may continue to use drugs just to win the interpersonal battle or possibly give in to such onslaughts and seek help in order to please the person concerned, but if he or she does not really want to stop, then complete cessation of drug use is unlikely. It can, however, be constructive to open doors to someone who has been coerced in this way so that when they are more ready in themselves to accept help, they will know where to go. Most users who allow themselves to be coerced into seeking help are fairly ambivalent in their attitudes but it is not beyond the bounds of possibility that for a few, treatment will be successful. Taking a broader view, most people who seek help are at least to some degree ambivalent about their drug use and have several goes at getting straight before they finally manage it.

Interfering with the consequences of drug misuse

Alternatively, those involved may try to protect the user from the consequences of drugtaking: money may be given to buy drugs in order to prevent stealing or other criminal activity (an Amsterdam father was granted tax relief for this); sometimes non-using parents or spouses will buy the drugs themselves if the user is too ill with withdrawals to go out; employers may be telephoned to say that the drugtaker is too ill to go to work through influenza; friends and acquaintances may be similarly lied to; doctors may be approached by relatives requesting a day's prescription to stop drug withdrawals.

It is perfectly understandable that most parents could not sit back and do nothing – the urge to act is overpowering and it must be said that these strategies can be effective. However, anything that prevents the consequences of drug misuse will also reduce the user's motivation to stop; drugtaking rather than the drugtaker will be supported and the user will carry on for longer before he or she is motivated to stop.

A persistent drugtaker in the family

Families Anonymous, a self-help group for the families and close friends of drugtakers, describes the whole family of a persistent drugtaker as becoming sick. Relationships within such a family become strained and distorted, and no family member will remain unharmed, least of all the drugtaker himself who may become the scapegoat of all the family's ills and the safety valve for family distress.

Max Glatt's description [1] of the children of alcoholics could be equally applied when one parent is a drugtaker:

'Children are torn in their loyalties between father and mother and are continually called upon to make fresh readjustments in an atmosphere characterised by continual quarrels, emotional upheavals, mutual recrimination, threats of separation with temporary reconciliations, the emergence of hope from time to time, only to be followed by sad disappointments ... children may feel depressed and neglected and the vicious circle described by Bowlby may be set in motion – today's deprived neglected children may grow up into tomorrow's psychopathic, neglectful, unstable parents who are again unable to provide a normal home life for their children.'

Sources of help for the family

Apart from the GP and other generic workers such as social workers, other sources of help that can be considered are:

(a) Family therapy

Although this is a facility that is not widely available, it is interesting to note that there is some evidence of a decrease in drug misuse when family therapy is instituted even when the misuse itself is not treated. In family therapy, psychopathology is viewed as an impairment in communications between two or more family members, rather than a condition affecting a single person. For the family to be helped constructively, individual roles need to be examined in a non-blaming way.

(b) Families Anonymous (FA)

Just as Al-Anon and Al-Ateen are sister organisations of Alcoholics Anonymous and are for the families, close friends and teenage children of problem drinkers, so Families Anonymous is the sister association of Narcotics Anonymous. All of these organisations are self-help groups which are run along similar lines and have branches throughout the country. (Interestingly, further self-help groups based on the same 12 steps have recently started up. These include groups for the adult children of alcoholics and others for people with anorexia nervosa, and for those suffering from anxiety.)

The families and close friends of drug users share many common problems; the drugtaker's anger against himself is projected onto them. Their money and possessions may be stolen in order to buy drugs, there is often a social stigma against them; the drugtaker may at times become violent towards them, and unlike professional carers, they have to live with the problem 24 hours a day, seven days a week. They may need as much if not more help than the drug user. Their support and help may be invaluable provided that it is support for the drugtaker rather than his or her habit.

The FA approach of controlling yourself rather than the user and giving tough love (not accepting unacceptable behaviour but showing that you really do care) may set the framework for the recovery of the user and they recommend that it is not advisable to make a threat when it is not intended to be kept.

(c) Other non-statutory groups

However, the FA approach is not suitable for all situations and over the last few years, a number of voluntary organisations have been launched to help and support the parents and families of drug users.

These organisations have quickly built up expertise on drugs and local networks of help and many offer groups where parents can meet and share mutual problems. Staff in these organisations will offer practical help, where possible, such as attending court with a parent, giving appropriate information about individual drugs, or facilitating professional help for a family member who is taking drugs. Some are national organisations, such as OPUS, ADFAM and the National Campaign Against Solvent Abuse. ADFAM in particular has taken over from FA in many areas as the main national body providing family support. Others are a local response to meet the needs of parents in particular.

GP help to family and friends

We have dealt with the reactions of the family to a drug user and possible sources of help. Here we look at what the GP can do when people come to the surgery.

As family doctors, we may have dealings on two levels with the families or supporting friends of drug users:

(1) those who come for advice;
(2) those whose cooperation we need to help drug users we are dealing with.

In both cases we should look at the special needs of those who are in this situation. People think that their own doctor should know all about drugs or they are told in government and other literature to seek the advice of a GP. What happens when they do? In a BBC programme where one of the authors was the only medical person in a very large group, the presenter asked the assembled parents, drug users and others, if they thought that, on the whole, GPs were helpful in this. The answer was a resounding 'No' from the whole audience and this is borne out by the following section from *Coping with a Nightmare*, a book published by ISDD [2] in which families tell in their own words, their emotional and practical experiences of having a long-term drug user in the family.

For some parents, turning to their GP is the obvious first source of help in dealing with something that may seem like a physical illness. Indeed, GPs may be an important point of contact for referral to any treatment facilities available within the National Health Service.

However, while some parents do find their GPs helpful – 'We had a super GP...' – very many do not seem particularly happy with the responses they have had from their doctors:

> 'So I went to my doctor and I might as well have talked to the wall really, he really did not want to know. I tried to get a doctor to talk to.'

Another mother wanted a doctor to visit her daughter when she was in a bad way:

> 'I wanted someone to (come and) see her like I was seeing her, and that doctor made me feel that small. He really went to town on me, that I ought to be ashamed of myself for even thinking anything's up with her. He just didn't know.'

Other parents feel that doctors do their best but are not in a good position to be able to help:

> 'They try and listen, the doctors, but they don't know anything about it, that's the problem. I'm not saying they're not willing to help, they can't help because they don't know what they're dealing with. Half the local GPs are frightened because they've been ripped off so many times by the users which is understandable.'

> 'She'd asked for more help from the doctor, and she went. But really I think it was because she knew it would probably be a ticket to more drugs that she could swap or sell for things she wanted, and that's what it turned out to be.'

There may also be a tendency for GPs to offer the parents tranquillisers for themselves, which some parents do not expect:

> 'I've been up to the doctor and he tried to give me tranquillisers. I said "I don't want those, that's the last thing I want. My son's got drug problems; I don't want to go on drugs." Sam was going mad because I was on tablets.'

To save repetition, let us use the word 'parents' to represent those in a supporting situation since they are probably the largest group. So...

What brings parents to the doctor?

Sometimes it is only suspicions and worries that a child who is run down and not acting as usual may be taking drugs. Sometimes it is a disastrous situation where there is no doubt; unexpected trouble with the law, stealing in the house, an overdose, seeing a family member intoxicated or perhaps violent attacks upon parents from a child who has been getting increasingly disturbed or rebellious. Parents may bring a young person to be warned off – or say that he or she refuses to come and they ask what they should do.

What are they asking of us?

We can point out to parents whose children are not obvious addicts that things may be not so bad as they imagine. A child may be only experimenting and a violent reaction could push them into more serious drug misuse. Families have had their information about drugs mainly from sensational media stories and picture a 'slippery slope' downhill from a taste of cannabis to a grisly death in the gutter. They can be reassured that this rarely occurs. On the other hand, a youngster may be taking drugs regularly, confident that he or she can handle it and be able to give them up when they wish.

What information do they need?

The more families know about drugs, their effects and how to handle things, the more hope there is. Apart from what the doctor tells them, the parents would do as well to meet or discuss matters with those who are experienced drugs workers, or in self-help groups. It is useful to give them the address of ISDD and suggest they write for the book list and point out booklets like *Drugs: What Every Parent Should Know*, and *Drug Abuse Briefing*. Doctors should continue to keep a stock of the DHSS leaflets including *Drug Misuse, A Basic Briefing* to hand out. If they learn more about the subject they should not only be less worried, but can discuss matters with the youngster more confidently. The parents may have sought desperately for help and be angry or despairing that they have found none for their child, so information about facilities, however few, brings some relief. GPs themselves are advised to read *Coping with a Nightmare*. It gives valuable insights into the reactions of families and how they tried to cope. While not an advice book as such, it becomes clear that a number of options for coping are available which can be put to distressed families whom the GP might have to deal with. Which one(s) they try, if any, will depend on individual circumstances.

Appendix A

GP Training and Self-awareness

On the subject of drug misuse, doctors have long been saying that they receive no real training as medical students and that postgraduate training is also conspicuous by its absence. Even the teaching films of the pharmaceutical industry have avoided the subject until only very recently, preferring the safe and overcrowded waters of arthritis therapy and hypertension to the cold, stormy seas of drug misuse. Now, like the alcohol and tobacco industries, they are being forced to take up the challenge.

Some GPs use the lack of training as a reason for turning their back on the subject. Others feel helpless in the face of drug problems. There is no need for either reaction because there is a wealth of material and means by which we can teach ourselves how to cope with the needs of drug users. We can do much to help the teaching situation by writing to the medical educational boards and the Royal Colleges and pressing for local and national seminars for GPs.

In the meantime, here are some of the sources of self-teaching we can use:

(1) Pamphlets and books from ISDD and SCODA (for addresses see Appendix B). Some ISDD materials are free; you can keep a stock of these to hand out or perhaps hand out the ISDD publications list to drug users and their families and friends, worried parents and so on.

(2) DHSS and Home Office literature (much of which is also available from ISDD).

(3) The DHSS *Guidelines* and the introductory chapter in the *British National Formulary*. These are both on the lines of Highway Codes rather than instruction manuals, but we need to be familiar with them, even if they only emphasise one aspect of drug treatment. In November 1988 the Royal College of GPs will be producing an important information folder for GPs on substance misuse entitled *'Alcohol and Drug Use – Everybody's Concern'*.

(4) Collecting articles from the medical and lay press. The medical articles are often both instructive and up-to-date. While both

the national and local press tend to concentrate on the more sensational aspects of the subject, they can alert us to new developments in the field.
(5) Collecting literature from voluntary groups and centres.
(6) Recording TV programmes on drug use and AIDS. (This appears to be permissible under copyright law as long as the programme is to be viewed for private purposes only and in your own home.)
(7) Studying the relevant video material, in particular the DHSS video *Working with Drug Users* (see Appendix C for further details) and British Medical TV series Nos. 25 and 26 on drug misuse.
(8) Attending study days and multidisciplinary training such as the courses held at St. George's Hospital in London.
(9) Discussions with experienced workers.
(10) Visiting any local drug facilities. By arrangement with the workers you might be able to speak with some of the clients while keeping a low profile if you did not want to take on any drug-using patients at the time.
(11) Trying to familiarise yourself with the local drug scene. Some general idea of what is going on in your locality can be gauged from talking to your local chemist, the officers at the drugs squad or even your own teenage children, as well as, of course, any drug-using patients you may see. The police themselves are very considerate about not pressing doctors for information about their drug-using patients, but perhaps surprising to drug users, the police as well as those working in casualty departments, probation and social services may ask a doctor's advice about treatment facilities.
(12) Talking to, if not necessarily treating, drug users in the practice. Temporary residents who are only seeking a legal supply of drugs are not people to be avoided. If you cannot persuade them to return and consider coming off drugs, you may learn from the argument something to help the next drug user or at least help you to remain unruffled!
(13) Examining your own attitudes to drug misusers as compared to your other patients. Your own philosophy and sense of priorities are very important in a field of work which can be both demanding and at times disappointing. Your beliefs, attitudes and prejudices will probably be strained to the limit, although temperament is not necessarily a hindrance. Those doctors who deal with drug users learn to become extremely firm, irrespective of their normal style with other patients.

Appendix B

Sources of Advice and Information

Apart from national agencies which can give advice and information there are now local services and self-help and support groups in many areas of the country.

A full listing of advice, counselling and information agencies, broken down by county, can be found in a national directory called *Drug Problems: Where To Get Help*, published by SCODA (address below) price £3.95.

This directory covers England, Scotland, Wales and Northern Ireland, but there is also a special directory for Scotland produced by the Scottish Health Education Group (address below).

It is not possible to reproduce the contents of both directories here. The list below is aimed at giving readers a lead-in to the services available and those organisations and projects listed will be able to direct readers to more appropriate or local help.

England

National organisations

Publications and information
ISDD (Institute for the Study of Drug Dependence)
1, Hatton Place
London EC1N 8ND
(01-430 1991)

Advice and information about services
SCODA (Standing Conference on Drug Abuse)
1, Hatton Place
London EC1N 8ND
(01-430 2341)

Telephone advice about drug effects, accidental ingestion of substances and overdoses
National Poisons Information Service
01-635 9193 (24-hour cover)

Self-help and support organisations for relatives and friends
ADFAM (Aid for Addicts and Family)
Adfam National Office
99/101, Old Brompton Road
London SW7 3LE
(01-581 4163)

Families Anonymous
5-7, Parsons Green
London SW6 4UL
(01-731 8060: Helpline)

OPUS (Organisation for Parents Under Stress)
106, Godstone Road
Whyteleafe
Surrey CR3 OEB
(01-645 0469)
(Nottingham 0602-470551: 24-hour crisis line)

Self-help groups for drug users
Narcotics Anonymous
PO Box 246
c/o 47, Milman Street
London SW10
(01-351 6794/6066: 24-hour answerphone)
Also a contact point for NA branches throughout the UK

Legal advice and information
Release
169, Commercial Street
London E1 6BW
(01-603 8654: 24-hour emergency service)

Regional contacts
North East England
North East Council on Addictions (NECA)
1, Mosley Street
Newcastle-upon-Tyne NE1 1YE
(0632-327878 and 320797: 24-hour answerphone)

The Bridge Project
Equity Chambers
40, Piccadilly
Bradford BD1 3NN
(0274-723863)

North West England
Drug and Alcohol Advisory Centre
Croft House
Wigton Road
Carlisle CA3 2EP
(0228-49605)

Lifeline Project
Joddrell Street
Manchester M3 3HE
(061-832 6353: 24-hour answerphone)

Merseyside
Mersey Regional Drug Training and Information Centre
10, Maryland Street
Liverpool L1 9BX
(051-709 3511: 24-hour answerphone)

Midlands
Drugline
Dale House
New Meeting Street
Birmingham 4
(021-632 6363: 24-hour answerphone)

East Anglia
Bridge Project
154, Mill Road
Cambridge
(0223-214604/214614: 24-hour answerphone)

London and the South East
Blenheim Project
7, Thorpe Close
London W10 5XL
(01-960 5599: 24-hour answerphone)

Community Drug Project
30, Manor Place
London SE17 3BB
(01-703 0559)

Hungerford Drug Project
First Floor
26, Craven Street
London WC2
01-930 4688: 24-hour answerphone)

DAIS (Drugs Advice and Information Service)
38, West Street
Brighton
(0273-21000: 24-hour service)

South West England
BADAS (Bath Area Drugs Advisory Service)
James Street West
Bath BA1 2BX
(0225-69479)

Scotland

National organisations

Information/co-ordination services
Scottish Drugs Forum
266, Clyde Street
Glasgow G1 4JH
(041-221 1175)

Scottish Health Education Group
Woodburn House
Canaan Lane
Edinburgh EH10 4SG
(031-447 8044)

Regional contacts

Lothian
Addictions Resource Unit
19, Jarvey Street

Bathgate
West Lothian
(0506-633801)

Gateway Exchange
2-4, Abbeymount
Edinburgh EH8 8EJ
(0341-661 0982)

Muirhouse/Pilton Drugs Project
Department of Social Work
34, Muirhouse Crescent
Edinburgh EH4 4QL
(031-343 1991)

Strathclyde
Information and Resource Unit on Addiction
82, West Regent Street
Glasgow G2 2QF
(041-332 0062)

Castlemilk Drug Project
9-11, Ballantay Quadrant
Castlemilk
Glasgow G45 0DY
(041-634 0711)

Calderhead Addiction Unit
The Cottage
Kirk Road
Shotts
Lanarkshire
(0501-23539)

Wales

National organisations

SWAPA Counselling Network (South Wales Association for the Prevention of Addiction)
111, Cowbridge Road East
Cardiff CF1 9AC
(0222-383313: 24-hour service)

Regional contacts

Clwyd
Clwyd Drugs Prevention Service
21b, Chester Road West
Shotton
(Deeside 0244-817798: 24-hour answerphone)

West Glamorgan
Sand (Swansea Advice on Narcotics and Drugs)
St Phillip's Community Centre
Bathurst Road
Swansea
(0792-472002)

Northern Ireland

Londonderry
Northlands – Alcohol and Drug Abuse Advice Centre
68, Northland Road
Derry
(0504-263011)

Appendix C

Resource List

The following items are all available from the Institute for the Study of Drug Dependence (ISDD). Prices include postage and packing and a full catalogue detailing all ISDD's services is available free on request. Doctors are also recommended to contact the Standing Conference on Drug Abuse (SCODA) for their list of publications including referral guides to rehab and detox facilities, regional lists of drug treatment services and fieldwork reports.

Booklets, leaflets

Drug Abuse briefing: a guide to the effects of drugs and the social and legal facts about their non-medical use in Britain. ISDD, 1988. 24 pages, £1.50. (Strongly recommended.)

Drugs: What Every Parent Should Know. ISDD, 1985. 32 pages, £1.15.

The Addiction Experience by Stanton Peele. Hazelden, 1980. 32 pages, £1.75.

Recreation or Desperation: a practical guide to assessing drug problems by Rowdy Yates. Lifeline Project, 1982. 4 pages, 40p.

How to Help: a practical guide for the friends and relatives of drug users. Blenheim Project, 1982. 20 pages, 95p.

How to Stop: a do-it-yourself guide to opiate withdrawal. Blenheim Project, 1982. 20 pages, 95p.

The Misuse of Drugs Act Explained. ISDD, 1986. 6 pages, 45p.

Women and Drug Use: an unfeminine dependency. ISDD, 1980. 4 pages, 40p.

Sniffing for Pleasure : guidance notes on counselling young solvent users by Rowdy Yates. Lifeline Project, 1982. 4 pages, 40p.

Books

Street Drugs by Andrew Tyler. New English Library, 1986. 342 pages, £4.40.
This reference work on the current legal and illegal drug scene in Britain allocates one chapter per drug, the author detailing effects and consequences, prevalence, patterns and methods of use, social and political history.

What Everyone Should Know About Drugs by Kenneth Leech. Sheldon Press, 1983. 94 pages, £3.30.
Widely held beliefs about drugs and their effects are discussed with advice to parents on talking to their children about drugtaking.

Drugs in Perspective by Martin Plant. Hodder and Stoughton, 1987. 176 pages, £6.50.
An overview reflecting current research on the misuse of drugs both legal and illegal.

Treatment and Rehabilitation. Report of the Advisory Council on the Misuse of Drugs. HMSO, 1982. 146 pages, £4.40.
A report from the government's advisory body reviewing the history of treatment and the present pattern of services, culminating in a far-reaching set of recommendations for change.

Living with Drugs by Michael Gossop. Wildwood House, 1987. 242 pages. £6.50.

Coping with a Nightmare: Family feelings about long-term drug use by Nick Dorn et al. ISDD, 1987. 72 pages, £2.50.
Families tell in their own words what their emotional and practical responses were to having a long-term drug user in the family.

Not available from ISDD
Coping with Drug Misuse in General Practice: A personal view by Dr Jackie Chang.
This introductory booklet to the subject is being distributed to all GPs by Abbot Laboratories.

Guidelines of Good Clinical Practice in the Treatment of Drug Misuse. DHSS, 1984.
All GPs should have received a free copy. Those who didn't or wish for a replacement copy should write to DHSS Store, Government Buildings, Honeypot Lane, Stanmore, Middx HA7 1AY enclosing a cheque for £1 made payable to the DHSS.

Videos

Working with Drug Users. Optic Nerve Ltd/DHSS, 1986.
Video training pack to use with those who come into contact with drug users in their everyday work. Materials include 2¾ hour modular video and full back-up materials for tutor and course participants. This video can be hired from CFL Vision, Chalfont Grove, Narcot Lane, Gerrards Cross, Bucks. The cost is £10 which is deducted from the retail price of £47 should you then decide to buy the film. The £10 entitles you to the training pack which you can keep whether or not you buy the film.

On the face of it this DHSS training video is an absorbing 2¾ hour panorama across the range of dependence management. When one has a little, or only local experience of one or two drug problems it gives one a wide view, from London to Scotland and from experimental drug use in a youth club to the burnt-out old junkie almost past redemption. One sees how both doctors and lay workers, parents and drug teams deal with an astonishing variety of dependence situations using actual drugtakers. The medical interviews are models of careful, sympathetic but firm discussion with drug users. The video gives a clear and comprehensive view of drug treatment, and it will either intrigue you in the subject or put you off for life.

The training pack with it has unfortunately to be purchased for £10, even if one is borrowing the video for a few days free on one's own. As a partnership or group expense the large handbook is good value, but even for the single GP it is worthwhile. The handbook not only explains and teaches in the different modules of the video but gives a section on assessment and a section on nationwide facilities. The module explanations are more geared to group discussion and multidisciplinary teaching, than to study by a single doctor, but are still helpful. If one is trying to train or introduce one or two staff, or other team workers to the subject, the course and the video are excellent materials to choose. From the drug facilities point of view, the video presents the ideal situation, a 10-day waiting list to see the clinic instead of 6–12 weeks; highly experienced workers instead of raw volunteers. Where a GP is working 'out in the sticks' or in a desert of facilities the picture is something to aim at – a target to present to health and local authorities, or voluntary workers in one's area. Even on a national scale, if financial pressures continue and the central government-supported projects under the three-year plan are not taken over by the NHS and local councils, facilities in many areas will be hard pressed. Doctors with other team members will need to adapt the principles and practical advice of the training video to their own situation.

Merck Ltd. have produced a 20-minute video specially designed for doctors by selecting extracts and editing a shortened version of the DHSS tape. This will be shown by their representatives to groups of doctors but you can write to the company about seeing it on your own.

Understanding Problem Drug Use. Manchester: North West Regional Drug Training Unit, 1986.

A video training pack which sets out to put drug use into perspective and tries to show that the skills already possessed by generic workers are vital to the success of dealing with drug-related problems. The video can be hired from the Training Unit at Kenyon Ward, Prestwich Hospital, Bury New Road, Manchester M25 7BL. The cost is £7.

Abbot Laboratories have produced a video for GPs which can be viewed free of charge by contacting the company on 0795-663371 or writing to their office at Queensborough, Kent ME11 5EL.

A list of videos available in this country can be obtained from ISDD, price 20 pence.

Appendix D

Drugs Controlled under the Misuse of Drugs Regulations

Explanatory notes on the schedules

Schedule 1

The Misuse of Drugs Regulations divide controlled drugs into five schedules. Drugs in schedule 1 are the most stringently controlled. These drugs (such as LSD and cannabis) are not authorised for medical use and can only be supplied, possessed or administered in accordance with a Home Office licence. Such licences are issued only for research or other special purposes. Outside these rare exceptions there are no circumstances in which possessing, supplying, producing, etc., these drugs is permitted. Doctors cannot prescribe them nor pharmacists dispense them. This is the closest British law comes to absolute prohibition.

Schedule 5

At the other end of the scale is schedule 5, listing preparations of drugs considered to pose minimal risk of abuse. Some of these dilute, small-dose, non-injectable preparations are allowed to be sold over-the-counter at a pharmacy without a prescription, and all may be possessed by anyone with impunity. But once bought they cannot legally be supplied to another person, a restriction that is probably ignored more often than it is enforced. Among these schedule 5 preparations are some well-known cough medicines, anti-diarrhoea agents and mild painkillers.

Schedules 2, 3 and 4

Between the extremes of schedules 1 and 5 are schedules 2, 3 and 4, including the vast majority of controlled drugs. These drugs are available for medical use, but can only be supplied or administered in accordance with a prescription or other authority. Here we find heroin, a drug that can still legally be prescribed by any doctor to any patient for the treatment of physical disease or injury.

It is illegal to possess drugs in schedules 2 and 3 without a prescription or other authority; but so long as they are in the form of a medicinal product, the benzodiazepine tranquillisers in schedule 4 *can* legally be possessed, even *without* a prescription. So it is an offence for Mr X to give (i.e. 'supply') Ms Y some of the diazepam his doctor prescribed him, but Ms Y would be in the clear as she merely possessed the drug.

Schedule 1

1. The following substances and products, namely:
    (a) Bufotenine
    Cannabinol
    Cannabinol derivatives
    Cannabis and cannabis resin
    Coca leaf
    Concentrate of poppy-straw
    Eticyclidine
    Lysergamide
    Lysergide and other N-alkyl derivatives of lysergamide
    Mescaline
    Psilocin
    Raw opium
    Rolicyclidine
    Tenocyclidine
    4-Bromo-2, 5-dimethoxy-α-methylphenethylamine
    N,N-Diethyltryptamine
    N,N-Dimethyltryptamine
    2,5-Dimethoxy-α, 4-dimethylphenethylamine
    (b) any compound (not being a compound for the time being specified in sub-paragraph (a) above) structurally derived from tryptamine or from a ring-hydroxy tryptamine by substitution at the nitrogen atom of the sidechain with one or more alkyl substituents but no other substituent;
    (c) any compound (not being methoxyphenamine or a compound for the time being specified in sub-paragraph (a) above) structurally derived from phenethylamine, an N-alkylphenethylamine, α-methylphenethylamine, an N-alkyl-α-methylphenethylamine, α ethylphenethylamine, or

an N-alkyl-α-ethylphenethylamine by substitution in the ring to any extent with alkyl, alkoxy, alkylenedioxy or halide substituents, whether or not further substituted in the ring by one or more other univalent substituents.
2. Any stereoisomeric form of a substance specified in paragraph 1.
3. Any ester or ether of a substance specified in paragraph 1 or 2.
4. Any salt of a substance specified in any of paragraphs 1 to 3.
5. Any preparation or other product containing a substance or product specified in any of paragraphs 1 to 4, not being a preparation specified in Schedule 5.

Schedule 2

1. The following substances and products, namely:
Acetorphine
Alfentanil
Allylprodine
Alphacetylmethadol
Alphameprodine
Alphamethadol
Alphaprodine
Anileridine
Benzethidine
Benzylmorphine
   (3-Benzylmorphine)
Betacetylmethadol
Betameprodine
Betamethadol
Betaprodine
Bezitramide
Clonitazene
Cocaine
Desomorphine
Dextromoramide
Diamorphine
Diampromide
Diethylthiambutene
Difenoxin
Dihydrocodeinone
   O-carboxymethyloxime
Dihydromorphine
Dimenoxadole
Dimepheptanol
Dimethylthiambutene

Dioxaphetyl butyrate
Diphenoxylate
Dipipanone
Drotebanol
Ecgonine, and any derivative of ecgonine which is convertible to ecgonine or to cocaine
Ethylmethylthiambutene
Etonitazene
Etorphine
Etoxeridine
Fentanyl
Furethidine
Glutethimide
Hydrocodone
Hydromorphinol
Hydromorphone
Hydroxypethidine
Isomethadone
Ketobemidone
Lefetamine
Levomethorphan
Levomoramide
Levophenacylmorphan
Levorphanol
Medicinal opium
Metazocine
Methadone
Methadyl acetate
Methyldesorphine
Methyldihydromorphine (6-methyldihydromorphine)
Metopon
Morpheridine
Morphine
Morphine methobromide, morphine N-oxide and other pentavalent nitrogen morphine derivatives
Myrophine
Nicomorphine
Noracymethadol
Norlevorphanol
Normethadone
Normorphine
Norpipanone
Oxycodone
Oxymorphone

Pethidine
Phenadoxone
Phenampromide
Phenazocine
Phencyclidine
Phenomorphan
Phenoperidine
Piminodine
Piritramide
Proheptazine
Properidine
Racemethorphan
Racemoramide
Racemorphan
Sufentanil
Thebacon
Thebaine
Tilidate
Trimeperidine
4-Cyano-2-dimethylamino-4,
 4-diphenylbutane
4-Cyano-1-methyl-4-
 phenylpiperidine
1-Methyl-4-phenylpiperidine-
 4-carboxylic acid
2-Methyl-3-morpholino-1, 1-
 diphenylpropanecarboxylic acid
4-Phenylpiperidine-4-carboxylic
 acid ethyl ester

2. Any stereoisomeric form of a substance specified in paragraph 1 not being dextromethorphan or dextrorphan.
3. Any ester or ether of a substance specified in paragraph 1 or 2, not being a substance specified in paragraph 6.
4. Any salt of a substance specified in any of paragraphs 1 to 3.
5. Any preparation or other product containing a substance or product specified in any of paragraphs 1 to 4, not being a preparation specified in Schedule 5.
6. The following substances and products, namely:

Acetyldihydrocodeine
Amphetamine
Codeine
Dextropropoxyphene
Dihydrocodeine
Ethylmorphine
 (3-ethylmorphine)

Mecloqualone
Methaqualone
Methylamphetamine
Methylphenidate
Nicocodine
Nicodicodine
 (6-nicotinoyldihydrocodeine)
Norcodeine
Phenmetrazine
Pholcodine
Propiram

7. Any steroeoisomeric form of a substance specified in paragraph 6.
8. Any salt of a substance specified in paragraph 6 or 7.
9. Any preparation or other product containing a substance or product specified in any of paragraphs 6 to 8, not being a preparation specified in Schedule 5.

Schedule 3

1. The following substances, namely:

    (a) Benzphetamine
    Chlorphentermine
    Diethylpropion
    Ethchlorvynol
    Ethinamate
    Mazindol
    Mephentermine
    Meprobamate
    Methylphenobarbitone
    Methyprylone
    Pentazocine
    Phendimetrazine
    Phentermine
    Pipradrol

    (b) any 5,5 disubstituted barbituric acid.

2. Any stereoisomeric form of a substance specified in paragraph 1.
3. Any salt of a substance specified in paragraph 1 or 2.
4. Any preparation or other product containing a substance specified in any of paragraphs 1 to 3, not being a preparation specified in Schedule 5.

Schedule 4

Controlled drugs excepted from the prohibition on importation, exportation and, when in the form of a medicinal product, possession and subject to the requirements of Regulations 22, 23, 25 and 26

1. The following substances and products, namely:

    Alprazolam
    Bromazepam
    Camazepam
    Chlordiazepoxide
    Clobazam
    Clonazepam
    Clorazepic acid
    Clotiazepam
    Cloxazolam
    Delorazepam
    Diazepam
    Estazolam
    Ethyl loflazepate
    Fludiazepam
    Flunitrazepam
    Flurazepam
    Halazepam
    Haloxazolam
    Ketazolam
    Loprazolam
    Lorazepam
    Lormetazepam
    Medazepam
    Nimetazepam
    Nitrazepam
    Nordazepam
    Oxazepam
    Oxazolam
    Pinazepam
    Prazepam
    Temazepam
    Tetrazepam
    Triazolam

2. Any stereoisomeric form of a substance specified in paragraph 1.
3. Any salt of a substance specified in paragraph 1 or 2.
4. Any preparation or other product containing a substance or product specified in any of paragraphs 1 to 3, not being a preparation specified in Schedule 5.

Schedule 5

Controlled Drugs excepted from the prohibition on importation, exportation and possession and subject to the requirements of Regulations 24 and 25

1. (1) Any preparation of one or more of the substances to which this paragraph applies, not being a preparation designed for administration by injection, when compounded with one or more other active or inert ingredients and containing a total of not more than 100 milligrammes of the substance or substances (calculated as base) per dosage unit or with a total concentration of not more than 2.5 per cent (calculated as base) in undivided preparations.
    (2) The substances to which this paragraph applies are acetyldihydrocodeine, codeine, dihydrocodeine, ethylmorphine, nicocodine, nicodicodine (6-nicotinoyldihy-drocodeine), nor-codeine, pholcodine and their respective salts.
2. Any preparation of cocaine containing not more than 0.1 per cent of cocaine calculated as cocaine base, being a preparation compounded with one or more other active or inert ingredients in such a way that the cocaine cannot be recovered by readily applicable means or in a yield which would constitute a risk to health.
3. Any preparation of medicinal opium or of morphine containing (in either case) not more than 0.2 per cent of morphine calculated as anhydrous morphine base, being a preparation compounded with one or more other active or inert ingredients in such a way that the opium or, as the case may be, the morphine, cannot be recovered by readily applicable means or in a yield which would constitute a risk to health.
4. Any preparation of dextropropoxyphene, being a preparation designed for oral administration, containing not more than 135 milligrammes of dextropropoxyphene (calculated as base) per dosage unit or with a total concentration of not more than 2.5 per cent (calculated as base) in undivided preparations.
5. Any preparation of difenoxin containing, per dosage unit, not more than 0.5 milligrammes of difenoxin and a quantity of atropine sulphate equivalent to at least 5 per cent of the dose of difenoxin.
6. Any preparation of diphenoxylate containing, per dosage unit, not more than 2.5 milligrammes of diphenoxylate calculated as base, and a quantity of atropine sulphate equivalent to at least 1 per cent of the dose of diphenoxylate.
7. Any preparation of propiram containing, per dosage unit, not

more than 100 milligrammes of propiram calculated as base and compounded with at least the same amount (by weight) of methylcellulose.

8. Any powder of ipecacuanha and opium comprising –

   10 per cent opium, in powder,
   10 per cent ipecacuanha root, in powder, well mixed with
   80 per cent of any other powdered ingredient containing no controlled drug.

9. Any mixture containing one or more of the preparations specified in paragraphs 1 to 8, being a mixture of which none of the other ingredients is a controlled drug.

Appendix E

A Note About Drug Slang

In our first edition we gave a moderately comprehensive list of the words and phrases used by street addicts mainly in the London area, when they discussed drugs. The heyday of such jargon was the sixties, as the colourful subculture of drug users and the alternative society swung from Haight-Ashbury in San Francisco to Piccadilly and the cities of Europe and Asia. With the enormous explosion in drug use, and the abandonment of secrecy a more matter-of-fact language has emerged varying widely in the newly penetrated regions of the UK. It is no longer necessary to talk to 'junkies' in their own jargon except in a limited way, and one can at the beginning ask a patient what he or she means by a particular phrase without losing face, or looking a fool.

Some of the more common words and phrases used in most areas are as follows:

Heroin still has several synonyms – 'smack', 'junk', 'skag' or is referred to in bags or sizes. (The colour may be helpful also, and ask about its purity.) *Physeptone* may be 'phy' or 'amps' or 'linctus'. *Diconal* – 'dike'. *Palfium* – 'peach palf' is much prized. *Dihydrocodeine* – will probably remain 'DF's'.

Stimulants. Now that 'Rit' (Ritalin) is no longer prescribed, 'speed' (amphetamine sulphate) or 'sulfate' or 'whizz' remains the main product, with 'coke' for cocaine.

Sedatives tend to be known by derivatives (barbs, mogies etc.) or just as 'sleepers' and 'downers'.

Psychedelics and cannabis are described more in their various forms – 'dots' (microdots of LSD) 'acid' (a tab of LSD) and 'acapulco', 'mexican' or 'lebanese gold' for cannabis. With 'blow', 'grass', 'dope' and 'pot' for marijuana. 'Joint' remains common for a cannabis cigarette and a 'roach' for the cardboard support of such a rolled cigarette.

People. Descriptions probably vary in different areas, but a 'barb freak' or 'speed freak' explain themselves and a derogatory word like 'junkie' for the gutter-type street addict. The police still have their colourful names (the 'Bill', 'Fuzz', 'Pigs') and you may still be 'busted' (arrested) and put in the 'nick' or 'slammer' (gaol).

Drugtaking. It is important to recognise some of these phrases like 'gear' or 'works' for the equipment used in injecting. 'Scoring' means getting drugs illegally and 'fixing', 'shooting' or 'jacking up' the actual injection. 'Chasing the dragon' (inhaling heroin vapour) probably has other phrases in different areas. 'Skin popping' and 'joypopping' refer to subcutaneous injection. 'Track marks' are the injection lines in the veins and 'bread' is the money needed to buy drugs. 'Coming down' or 'freaking out' and 'crashing out' mean withdrawals. 'Cold turkey' still means the involuntary withdrawal. 'Hooked' (addicted) is now in normal language as are many other former phrases.

Appendix F

Advice for People who are HIV Antibody Positive

by Charles Farthing (MRCP, St Stephen's Hospital (1986)

Individuals who have a positive HIV antibody test have at some stage been infected with HIV (The Human Immunodeficiency Virus – formerly known as HTLV-III/LAV). This virus has recently been discovered to be the cause of AIDS but it is not known what percentage of infected individuals will go on to develop AIDS. To date only a minority have done so.

Most infected individuals however do appear to be carriers of HIV and to remain infectious. The presence of antibodies in the blood does not mean, as it does with some other infections, that the virus has left the body and the individual is immune.

The commonest way HIV causes illness in an individual, if it is going to do so, is by lowering the body's resistance to infectious disease i.e. damaging the body's 'immune system'. It does this by infecting a certain subset of one of the types of white blood cell. All white blood cells are concerned with defence against infection (i.e. they are part of the body's immune system) but it is a certain subset of the lymphocytes that HIV infects. Lymphocytes are particularly concerned with defence against viral, fungal and parasitic infection and some types of tumour. The particular subset of the lymphocyte population that gets infected is the 'T helper lymphocytes' – sometimes referred to as the 'OKT 4 positive lymphocytes'. These T helper cells are an important component of the immune system and if their function is reduced or their numbers significantly depleted by HIV, defects in cell-mediated immunity develop which may result in the development of major or minor opportunistic infections or tumours.

Individuals who have been infected with HIV can be divided into four general groups:

1. Well with no signs of infection or immunosuppression. Such individuals could be called asymptomatic carriers.
2. Well with glandular swellings (lymphadenopathy) in armpits, neck etc. Such individuals are said to have persistent generalised lymphadenopathy (PGL).

3. Less than well with fatigue, often night sweats, and often a low T Helper lymphocyte subset count. Such individuals have minor infections such as shingles or oral thrush which indicate a degree of immunosuppression. These individuals have been classified as having AIDS related complex (ARC).
4. Individuals who meet the Centre for Disease Control's (CDC) criteria for the acquired immune deficiency syndrome (AIDS). To meet this definition the individual must have Kaposi's sarcoma or have had a life-threatening opportunistic infection such as pneumocystis pneumonia or toxoplasmosis. Such individuals nearly always have a low T helper lymphocyte count.

Although one can only state with certainty that individuals in category three and four are immunocompromised it is often true that those in categories one and two are also immunocompromised to some degree. The T helper lymphocyte count whilst a useful guide to immune status only measures the number of OKT4 positive cells and not their function and thus should not be relied upon too heavily. Anyone who is HIV antibody positive should therefore regard himself as possibly immunocompromised and take note of the following health guidelines.

Report early

If you are immunocompromised and you develop an infection it is best to report early to the physician who cares for your HIV disease for assessment and for an antibiotic if necessary. This is standard advice given to any group of immunocompromised patients, e.g. kidney transplant recipients, as infections may develop more quickly and be more severe in any immunocompromised individual. Having said this however, an individual immunocompromised from HIV infection is not at risk of dying from the common cold and minor infections are more common than major ones. Identifying that you have an infection is usually not difficult, but signs of infection do very much depend on the site of that infection – cough and breathlessness usually means a chest infection, diarrhoea a bowel infection, a rash possibly a skin infection, etc. Infection is often accompanied of fever. An increased swelling of your lymph glands usually does not mean an acute infection. It is usual for glands to swell intermittently in individuals with PGL, particularly if you get over-tired, and you should not be alarmed by this – if anything it may be reassuring in as much as it indicates activity in the immune system. Rest if your glands swell. If any particular gland is persistently enlarging however, show it to your doctor.

Rest

Fatigue is the commonest symptom experienced by individuals with HIV infection. The fatigue may come and go with patients feeling quite well for variable periods of time and then experiencing periods of severe fatigue with loss of energy, loss of ambition and drowsiness. It is often difficult to separate true fatigue from the lassitude that accompanies depression, which is occasioned by the fear engendered by the knowledge that one has been exposed to HIV. The fatigue should be acknowledged and patients should rest as much as possible. We recommend at least 8 hours of sleep each night and short naps during those periods when the fatigue is profound. If fatigue is so severe that you have difficulty in completing a day's work, a week or two of sick leave with ample rest is certainly appropriate.

This recommendation may require a major change in your social life. If you are accustomed to going out at the weekend, staying up late, spending time with friends at a bar, or dancing until the early hours of the morning these behaviour patterns need to be recognised and altered. You should attempt to see friends for small dinners or evenings in the theatre or cinema. You should decide which hour each night you will be in bed, and your friends must be made aware that your health is the most important thing in your life, and that you are going to stick to your schedule of getting to bed by 10 or 11 each evening. Of paramount importance is that you should listen to your body and if you feel that you should rest, that should be the course of action that you follow.

Exercise

Regular exercise is desirable but to overdo it is tiring and unwise. If you attend a gym it is probably best to continue but not to necessarily step up your programme – exercise to keep fit but not to exhaustion. If you have not been in the habit of exercising you should begin slowly – perhaps with regular walking or swimming. We advise against competitive sports because in the heat of competition an individual may push himself harder than he should.

Diet

A balanced diet with a reasonable calorie and fibre content is recommended. Potatoes and rice are good sources of carbohydrate. Beans, cheese and meat are high in protein. Vegetables and fruit are high in fibre. You may consider adding bran to your diet for further fibre. There is no need to go on any 'special' diet however.

Vitamins

If your diet is adequate in greens and fruit, vitamin supplementation is usually unnecessary. Some signs of HIV infection however may mimic Vitamin C and zinc deficiency so occasionally we recommend to some patients that they take Vitamin C or zinc tablets.

Drugs

Alcohol in moderation (2 drinks per day) does not appear to have any adverse effect. The most common opportunistic infection experienced by people with HIV is however pneumocystic pneumonia – a chest infection. Smoking cigarettes will irritate your lungs, and theoretically could increase your chance of pneumocystis infection. Patients are urged to stop smoking cigarettes. Other recreational drugs are probably also unwise – especially stimulant drugs (cocaine, speed, poppers) as they give a false sense of 'energy' which when used leaves the body exhausted. Moderation is probably the key word.

Sex

Individuals infected with HIV are capable of transmitting this agent to their sexual partners before they develop any symptoms whatsoever. Indeed they may be more infectious before they are symptomatic than after their T helper cells are depleted.

Exactly which sexual activities transmit the virus and which do not is unknown. However surveys of gay men who restrict themselves to only certain practices give us an indication of relative risk.

Men who are only passive in anal intercourse are much more likely than others to be HIV antibody positive. Men who restrict themselves exclusively to active anal intercourse or oral sex are far less likely to be HIV antibody positive. It is impossible to prove however that any particular sexual practice is safe and there are now many HIV antibody positive patients who insist they have never had passive anal intercourse.

What therefore are the guidelines on sexual practice for HIV antibody positive patients? Different doctors will give different advice but we feel it is important to remember that if, as an HIV antibody positive individual, you have unprotected vaginal or anal intercourse with an individual who is HIV antibody negative or whose status is unknown, you are very likely to transmit the AIDS virus.

Remember also that a condom whilst probably a reasonable protection if it remains intact, can break easily with anal intercourse and if it does is no protection at all. It would seem wise therefore to cease altogether active anal (or vaginal) intercourse with partners who are HIV antibody negative or who do not know their status.

What of other sexual practices with HIV antibody negative individuals? The only way to be absolutely certain of not transmitting infection is to have entirely non-mucous membrane contact or 'dry' sex. However as mentioned above oral sex appears to be low risk. Passive anal sex on the part of the HIV antibody positive individual with the negative partner wearing a condom continuously is also probably low risk.

Kissing must be very low risk, if a risk at all, as nearly all cases of HIV infection have had actual intercourse or received blood and one would expect many unexplained cases if kissing alone could transmit the virus. However live virus has been isolated from semen and saliva and therefore considerable saliva exchange or any semen exchange could theoretically transmit the virus.

What about sex with other HIV antibody positive individuals? Here medical opinion is again divided. Arguments against having sex with other patients are that you may pick up another strain of HIV worse than your own or you may pick up another infection such as syphilis which may further damage the immune system or trigger dormant HIV infection. Another worry is that sperm in the rectum if absorbed into the blood may itself be immunosuppressive. These worries whilst logical are theoretical. It would seem wise however if you do intend having anal sex with other HIV antibody positive individuals to use condoms. If you intend using condoms buy a generous supply of a tough brand, such as 'Prophyltex – red stripe' and use plenty of water-based lubricant to prevent tearing from friction. Do not use saliva or oil based lubricants. Saliva may contain the virus, and oils dissolve the latex of condoms causing them to split. We recommend using Duragel (which contains nonoxinol 9 – a spermicidal agent which destroys HIV) or KY.

Ultimately the decision of whom to have sex with and what practices to indulge in is of course a personal one. Restricting anal sex only to an already regular partner or to have partners whom you know to be positive, using condoms, and having only 'safer', or entirely safe dry sex with antibody negative individuals is what most antibody positive individuals decide. Obviously it is vital not to transmit this infection to those who are not already infected or to do anything that would further impair your own immunity.

Social activities

It is now common knowledge that an HIV antibody positive individual is not an infective risk to others in an ordinary social or family setting. The only advice we would give is that an HIV antibody positive individual should not share a toothbrush or razor blade with others as these objects allow the possibility of blood contact. Sharing glasses and knives and forks is probably not a good practice for anyone to indulge in but is very unlikely to transmit HIV if it occurred accidentally. Dishes should be washed in hot soapy water but no other special precaution is necessary. Soiled linen only requires to be laundered in a hot wash. Blood or other body fluid spills should be mopped up using household bleach as an anti-virus disinfectant (one in ten dilution). On surfaces that may be damaged by bleach hot soapy water will suffice.

There is no reason for an HIV antibody positive individual to avoid social contact for the protection of his own health. We know of no situation where immunocompromised people have suddenly developed pneumocystis or other opportunistic infections from being exposed to individuals suffering from these diseases. It would appear that nearly all of us already carry many opportunistic organisms such as Pneumocystis Carinii and Cytomegalovirus (CMV). What determines whether we become ill from them or not is the state of our immune system and not whether we are re-exposed to these agents.

Blood/organ donation

No HIV antibody positive individual should carry an organ donor card or donate blood to the blood transfusion service. This in fact applies to all gay men and intravenous drug users whether HIV antibody positive or not.

Vaccinations

Although they have not yet proved to be harmful, HIV antibody positive individuals should probably not receive live vaccines such as those for polio or yellow fever. All inactivated (dead) vaccines such as Hep B Vac and 'flu Vaccine' must be safe however. If you are going to travel specify NO LIVE VACCINES.

Treatment

Nearly all the opportunistic infections acquired secondary to immunosuppression are treatable, but there is a greater chance of success if treatment is commenced early.

There are also various treatments available for the underlying immunosuppression itself. Such treatments are of two kinds: 'Immunostimulant' drugs which to date have shown only slight if any benefit, and 'antiviral' anti-HIV drugs, also called 'reverse transcriptase inhibitors' which are very new and in the early phases of assessment. We do not yet know if they will prove to be a control or cure of AIDS but we are hopeful. It is possible you may be asked to partake in the assessment of these drugs. If you are it is very important that you understand fully the possible risks and benefits and not be frightened to ask questions.

Alternative therapies

As there is at present no known cure for HIV infection and AIDS we are often asked about the benefits of alternative therapies offered by homeopathy, herbal medicine etc. Just as there is as yet no good scientific evidence that conventional medicine can reverse AIDS neither is there any evidence that any other therapies work either. Alternative therapies are often quite harmless however and may possibly be of some benefit. If you are contemplating them ask for full information, discuss them with your doctor, and do not put your trust in literature that is not from a reliable scientific source. Be especially sceptical if a large amount of money is being charged for any alternative therapy.

Support agencies

You are not alone. There are thousands of HIV antibody positive people in the United Kingdom. If you feel lonely or in need of more information the Terrence Higgins Trust or the Body Positive Group are two helpful organisations you can turn to. The Trust provides buddy support and assistance for patients who are unwell and also runs counselling groups where antibody positive individuals can meet to learn more about HIV disease and to talk to others with the same problem. The Trust can be contacted via the helpline (01-833 2971) any night between 7 and 10 pm. The Body Positive Group run a disco every other Tuesday at the Market Tavern (corner of Nine Elms and Wandsworth Road, SW8) as well as other social activities. Both organisations are largely voluntary. They may be able to help you and later you may be able to help them.

Who should know?

With so much misunderstanding about HIV disease around we recommend that someone who is HIV antibody positive tells as few people as possible the result of his test. It may of course help to discuss the problem with one or two trusted friends; however if there is no one you feel you can fully trust then it may be best to talk only to people at your hospital, the Terrence Higgins Trust or the Body Positive Group. Do not tell your employer – he does not need to know and however understanding he may appear we have known many employers to turn nasty. We are often asked if patients should tell their general practitioners their result. An argument against telling your GP is that he would have to include this information in any medical report you may require. However if you are consulting your GP while unwell with unexplained symptoms then you must tell him as it might be vital to your medical care, but if you are currently quite well then there is probably no need to make a special point of telling your GP. You should inform your dentist or any doctor who is going to perform a surgical procedure. Also you should inform a tattooist, acupuncturist or ear piercer that your blood may be infectious.

The future

A question often asked by HIV antibody positive individuals is 'am I going to get AIDS?'. No one can answer this question for any one individual. Hopefully the majority of HIV antibody positive individuals will never become unwell let alone develop AIDS. Amongst those who are unwell with AIDS related complex a question often asked is 'does having ARC mean that I shall definitely develop AIDS?' Again no one can answer this question for any one individual either. Some patients unwell with ARC improve greatly on changing their lifestyle and taking better care of themselves – many have lived several years without developing AIDS and look less like doing so now than they did when we first saw them. Finally, patients with AIDS often ask 'how long have I got to live?' No one can accurately predict how long anyone will live. AIDS can move quickly but it can be a very slow disease. Many patients with AIDS in this country are alive and well and in full-time occupation some years after diagnosis.

Take care of yourself. Think positively. Do not transmit this infection to others. Soon there may be a successful treatement for this new disease.

References

Chapter One

1. Inglis, B. (1975) *The Forbidden Game: A Social History of Drugs.* London: Hodder & Stoughton.
2. Picardie, J. & Wade, D. (1985) *Heroin: Chasing the Dragon.* Harmondsworth, Middx: Penguin.
3. *Report of the Departmental Committee on Morphine and Heroin Addiction.* (1926) London: HMSO.
4. UK Interdepartmental Committee on Drug Addiction. (1961) *Report.* [chaired by Sir Russell Brain]. London: HMSO.
5. UK Interdepartmental Committee on Drug Addiction. (1965) *Second Report.* [chaired by Sir Russell Brain]. London: HMSO.
6. Strang, J. (1984) Abstinence or abundance – what goal? *Brit. Med. J.* **289**, p.604.
7. UK Department of Health and Social Security. (1982) *Treatment and Rehabilitation: Report of the Advisory Council on the Misuse of Drugs (ACMD): Central Funding Initiative.* London: DHSS.
8. UK. Department of Health and Social Security, Medical Working Group on Drug Dependence. (1984) *Guidelines on Good Clinical Practice in the Treatment of Drug Misuse.* London: DHSS.
9. Wiepart, G.D., Bewley, T.H. & d'Orban, P.T. (1978) Outcomes for 575 British opiate addicts entering treatment between 1968 and 1975. *UN Bull. Narcotics* **30** (1), 21–32.
10. Oppenheimer, E., Stimson, G.V. & Thorley, A. (1979) Seven year follow-up of heroin addicts: abstinence and continued use compared. *Brit. Med. J.* **2**, 627–630.
11. Blumberg, H.H. (1976) British users of opiate-type drugs: a follow-up study. *Brit. J. Addict* **71** (1), 65–77.
12. Mott, J. (1978) A long-term follow-up of male non-therapeutic opiate users and their criminal histories. In: *Problems of Drug Abuse in Britain.* (ed. D.J. West). Cambridge: University of Cambridge Institute of Criminology, 80–84.
13. UK Home Office. (1984) *Prevention. Report of the Advisory Council on the Misuse of Drugs.* London: HMSO.
14. *AIDS and Drug Misuse: First Report of the Advisory Council on the Misuse of Drugs.* London: HMSO. (In Press).

15 UK House of Commons Social Services Committee. (1985) *Misuse of Drugs with Special Reference to the Treatment and Rehabilitation of Misusers of Hard Drugs*. Fourth report of the Social Services Committee session 1984-1985. Together with proceedings and minutes of evidence. London: HMSO.
16 Home Office. (1985) *Tackling Drug Misuse*. London: HMSO.
17 Home Office. (1986) *Tackling Drug Misuse*. 2nd edn. London: HMSO.
18 Strang, J.S. (1985) Treatment of drug dependence – the role of the satellite clinic. *Health Trends* **17**, (1) 17-18.
19 Bennett, T. & Wright, R. (1986) Opioid users' attitudes towards and use of NHS Clinics, general practitioners and private doctors. *Brit. J. Addict* **81**, 757-763.
20 Robertson, J.R. (1985) Drug users in contact with general practice. *Brit. Med. J.* **290**, 34-35.
21 Parker, H. & Chadwick, C. (1987) *Unattractive Alternatives. Dilemmas for Drugs Services in Wirral*. The Fifth Report of the Misuse of Drugs Research Project for the Wirral Drug Abuse Committee and the Wirral District Drug Dependency Problem Team. Sub-Dept of Social Work Studies, University of Liverpool.
22 Kosten, T.R., Jalali, B., Hogan, I. *et al.* (1983) Family denial as a Prognostic Factor in Opiate Addict Treatment Outcome. *J. Nerv. Ment. Dis.* **171**, (10) 611-616.
23 Gossop, M., Green, L., Phillips, G. *et al.* (1987) What happens to opiate addicts immediately after treatment: a prospective follow up study. *Brit. Med. J.* **294**, 1377-1380.
24 Glanz, A. & Taylor, C. (1986) Findings of a national survey of the role of general practitioners in the treatment of opiate misuse. [3 parts]. *Brit. Med. J.* **293**, 427-430.
25 Glanz, A. & Taylor, C. (1986) Findings of a national survey of the role of general practitioners in the treatment of opiate misuse. [3 parts]. *Brit. Med. J.* **293**, 486-488.
26 Robertson, J.R. & Bucknell, A.B.V. (1985) Heroin users: notification to the Home Office Addicts Index by general practitioners. *Brit. Med. J.* **291**, 111-113.
27 Strang, J. & Shah, A. (1985) Notification of addicts and the medical practitioners – an evaluation of the system. *Brit. J. Psychiat.* August, (L,C,S), **147**, 195-198.
28 Glanz, A. & Taylor, C. (1986) Findings of a national survey of the role of general practitioners in the treatment of opiate misuse. [3 parts]. *Brit. Med. J.* **293**, 543-545.
29 Anderson, P. (1985) Managing alcohol problems in general practice. *Brit. Med. J.* **290**, 1873-5.
30 *WHO Mental Health report on the First Session of the Alcoholism Subcommittee*. (1951) WHO Technical Report series, (42).
31 *WHO Expert Committee on Drugs Liable to Produce Addiction. Third Report*. 1952 WHO Technical Report Series (57).

32 WHO Expert Committee on Addiction-producing drugs. Seventh report. 1957 *UN Bull. Narcotics* **9** (1), 45–47.
33 Eddy, N.B., Halbach, H., Isbell, H. *et al.* (1965) Drug dependence: its significance and characteristics. *Bull. WHO* **32**, 721–733.
34 Young, J. (1971) *The Drugtakers: the Social Meaning of Drug Use*, p.95. London: MacGibbon and Kee.
35 Wikler, A. (1973) Dynamics of drug dependence: implications of a conditioning theory for research and treatment. In: *Opiate Addiction: Origins and Treatment*. 7–21 (eds. Fischer, S. Freedman, A.M.) Washington, D.C.: Winston.
36 Kales, A, Scharf, M.B. & Kales, J.D. (1978) Rebound insomnia: a new clinical syndrome. *Science* **201**, 1039–1041.
37 Edwards, G., Arif, A. & Hodgson, R. (1982) Nomenclature and classification of drug-related and alcohol-related problems – a WHO Memorandum. *Brit. J. Addict* **77**, (1), 3–20.
38 Sutherlands, G., Edwards, G., Taylor, C. *et al.* (1986) The measurement of opiate dependence. *Brit. J. Addict* **81**, (4), 485–494.
39 Edwards, G., Gross, M.M., Keller, M. *et al.* (1977) *Alcohol-related Disabilities*. WHO offset publication **32** (Geneva WHO).
40 WHO Expert Committee on Drug Dependence (1969) **407**, WHO Technical Report Series.
41 Hughes, P.H., Senoy, E.C. & Parker, R. (1972) The medical management of a heroin epidemic. *Arch. Gen. Psychiat.* **27**, (11), 585–591.
42 Parker, H., Bakx, K. & Newcombe, R. (1986) *Drug Misuse in Wirral. A Study of Eighteen Hundred Problem Drug Users Known to Official Agencies*. The first report of the Wirral Misuse of Drugs Research Project. Liverpool: The University.
43 Brill, H. (1977) Introductory thoughts regarding treatment and rehabilitation. In: *Rehabilitation Aspects of Drug Dependence*, 1–9. (ed. A. Schecter). Cleveland, Ohio: CRC Press.
44 Lukoff, I.F. & Kleinman, P.H. (1979) The addict life cycle and problems in treatment evaluation. In: *Rehabilitation Aspects of Drug Dependence*, 163–175. (ed. A. Schecter) Cleveland, Ohio: CRC Press.
45 Guardian. September 23rd 1986.
46 Guardian. January 4th 1984.
47 Henman, A., Lewis, R. & Malyon, T. (1985) *Big Deal: the Politics of the Illicit Drugs Business*. London: Pluto.
48 UK Home Office. (1987) *Statistics of the Misuse of Drugs in the United Kingdom*, 1986. London: HMSO.
49 Tippell, S. (1986) *The Parole Release Scheme and Sisters Avenue: 1984/86 Monitoring Report*. London: PRS.
50 Scott, R.T.A. (1986) Medical aspects of drug misuse during one year in a rehabilitation unit. *J. Roy. Coll. Gen. Pract.* **36**, (292), 514–516.
51 Mott, J. & Taylor, M. (1974) *Delinquency Amongst Opiate Users: a Home Office Research Unit Report*. London: HMSO. vi, 31 pp. (Home Office Research Studies 23).
52 Ball, J.C., Rosen, L., Flueck, J.A. *et al.* (1981) The criminality of heroin

addicts: when addicted and when off opiates. *In: The Drug-crime Connection*, 39–65. (ed J.A. Inciardi). Beverly Hills, Calif: Sage.
53 Commissioner of Police for the Metropolis. (1983) *Speech to the Pharmaceutical Society of Great Britain*. New Scotland Yard press release.
54 Chief Constable of the Lothian and Borders Police. (1984) *Report in the Times newspaper*, 19th April.
55 Goldstein, P.J. (1981) Getting over: economic alternatives to predatory crime among street drug users. *In: The Drugs-crime Connection*, 67–84. (ed. J.A. Inciardi) Beverly Hills, Calif: Sage.
56 Johnson, B.D. (1977) How much heroin maintenance (containment) in Britain? *Int. J. Addict* **12** (2–3), 361–398.
57 Dupont, R.L. (1972) Heroin addiction treatment and crime reduction. *Amer. J. Psychiat.* **128**, 856–860.
58 Schut, J., Steer, R.A. & Gonzalez, F.H. (1975) Types of arrests recorded for methadone maintenance patients before, during and after treatment. *Brit. J. Addict* **70**, (1), 89–93.
59 Trebach, A.S. (1982) *The Heroin Solution*. New Haven: Yale University Press.
60 Ditton, J. & Speirits, K. (1981) *The Rapid Increase of Heroin Addiction in Glasgow in 1981*. Glasgow: Glasgow University.
61 Bennett, T. & Wright, R. (1986) The impact of prescribing on the crimes of opioid users. *Brit. J. Addict* **81**, (2), 265–273.
62 Stimson, G.V. & Ogborne, A.C. (1970) Survey of addicts prescribed heroin at London clinics. *Lancet* May 30, **2**, 1163–1166.
63 Idänpään-Heikkila, J. & Khan, I. (eds) (1982) *Public Health Problems and Psychotropic Substances*, p.85. Helsinki: the Government of Finland.
64 WHO (1981) *The Influence of Alcohol and Drugs on Driving*. Report of a WHO ad hoc Technical Group. Copenhagen: WHO Regional office for Europe. (EURO Reports and Studies No. 38).
65 Dembo, R. & Shern, D. (1982) Relative deviance and the process (es) of drug involvement among inner-city youths. *Int. J. Addict* **17** (8) 1373–1399.
66 Donoghoe, M., Dorn, N., James, C. et al. (1987) How families and communities respond to heroin. *In: A Land Fit for Heroin*. (eds. N. Dorn, N. South). Basingstoke: Macmillan Education Ltd.
67 Laing, R. & Esterson, A. (1964) *Sanity, Madness and the Family*. Harmondsworth: Penguin.
68 Vogt, I. (1980) Mother-child interaction and patterns of drug consumption. *In: Aspects of Alcohol and Drug Dependence*. (eds J.S. Madden, R. Walker & W.H. Kenyon). London: Pitman Medical.
69 Edwards, G. (1982) *The Treatment of Drinking Problems – a Guide for the Helping Professions*. Bath: Grant McIntyre.
70 Lavenhar, M.A. & Sheffet, A. (1973) Recent trends in non-medical use of drugs reported by students in two suburban New Jersey communities. *Prev. Med.* **2**, (4), 490–509.
71 Blum, R.H. et al. (1969) *Students and Drugs. Drugs II: College and High School Observations*. San Francisco, Ca.: Jossey-Bass Inc.

72   Rosenberg, C.M. (1971) Sons of alcoholic fathers. *Brit. J. Psychiat.* **118** 469–470.
73   Hoffmann, F.G. (1983) *A Handbook of Drug and Alcohol Abuse: the Bio-medical Aspects.* 2nd ed. Oxford: Oxford University Press.
74   Raistrick, D. & Davidson, R. (1985) *Alcoholism and Drug Addiction.* Edinburgh: Churchill Livingston.
75   Hafen, B.Q. & Peterson, B. (1978) *Medicines and Drugs: Problems and Risks, Use and Abuse.* 2nd ed. Philadelphia: Lea and Febiger.
76   Rotter, J. (1966) Generalised expectancies for internal *vs* external control of reinforcement. *Psych. Monogr.* **80**, (60).
77   Wallston, B.S. & Wallston, K.A. (1978) Locus of control and health: a review of the literature. *Hlth Ed. Monogr.* **6**, 107–117.
78   Young, J. (1971) *The Drugtakers: the Social Meaning of Drug Use.* London: MacGibbon and Kee.
79. Plant, M.A. (1987) *Drugs in Perspective* (Revised edition). London: Hodder and Stoughton.
80   Murray, R.M. (1980) An epidemiological and clinical study of alcoholism in the medical profession. In: *Aspects of Alcohol and Drug Dependence.* (eds J.S. Madden, R. Walker and W.H. Kenyon) London: Pitman Medical.
81   Bale, R.N. (1986) *The Sick Doctor.* p.1027 Update, 1-12-86.
82   Louria, D. (1977) The epidemiology of drug abuse and drug abuse rehabilitation. In: *Drug Dependence: Current Problems and Issues,* 105–118. (ed M.M. Glatt). Lancaster: MTP Press.
83   Plant, M. (1975) *Drugtakers in an English Town.* London: Tavistock.
84   Dembo, R., Schmeidler, J., Burgos, W. (1980) Life-style and drug involvement among youths in an inner city junior high school. *Int. J. Addict.* **15**, (2) 171–188.

Chapter Two

Volatile substance misuse

1   Ramsay, A.W. (1982) Solvent abuse: an educational perspective. *Human Toxicology,* **1**, (3), 265–270.
2   Gay, M., Mellor, R. & Stanley, S. (1982) Drug abuse monitoring: a survey of solvent abuse in the county of Avon. *Human Toxicology:* **1**, (3), 257–263.
3   Francis, J., Murray, V.S.G., Ruprah, M. *et al.* (1982) Suspected solvent abuse in cases referred to the Poisons Unit, Guy's Hospital, July 1980–June 1981. *Human Toxicology* **1**, (3) 271–280.
4   King, M.D., Day, R.E., Oliver, J.S. *et al.* (1981) Solvent encephalopathy. *Brit. Med. J.* **283**, (6292), 663–665.
5   Anderson, H.R., Dick, B., Macnair, R.S. *et al.* (1982) An investigation of 140 deaths associated with volatile substance abuse in the United Kingdom (1971–1981). *Human Toxicology* **1**, (3), 207–221.
6   Anderson, H.R., Bloor, K., Manair, R.S. *et al.* (1986) Recent trends in

mortality associated with abuse of volatile substances in the UK. Brit. Med. J. **293**, (6560), 1472-1473.
7   Bass, M. (1970) Sudden sniffing death. *J. Amer. Med. Ass.* **212**, (12), 2075-2079.
8   Watson, J.M. (1978) Clinical and laboratory investigations in 132 cases of solvent abuse. *Med. Sci. Law* **18**, (1), 40-43.
9   Institute for the Study of Drug Dependence, Library and Information service. (1980) *Teaching about a Volatile Situation: Suggested Health Education Strategies for Minimising Casualties Associated with Solvent Sniffing.* London: ISDD, 1979. New edition 1980.
10 Fornazzari, L., Wilkinson, D.A., Kapur, B.M. *et al.* (1983) Cerebellar, cortical and functional impairment in toluene abusers. *Acta Neurol. Scand.* June, **67** (6), 319-329.
11 King, M.D., Day, R.E., Oliver, J.S. *et al.* (1982) Neurological sequelae of toluene abuse. *Human Toxicology* **1**, (3), 281-287.
12 Ron, M.A. (1983) The alcoholic brain: CT scan and psychological findings. *Psych. Med. Monogr.* (suppl) **3**. Cambridge: Cambridge University Press.
13 Zur, J. (1983) *The Cognitive and Affective Sequelae of Chronic Solvent Abusee.* M. Phil, London University.
14 Devathasen, G. Low, D., Teoh, P.C. *et al.* (1984) Complications of chronic glue (toluene) abuse in adolescents. *Aust. NZ. J. Med.*: February, **14**, (1), 39-43.
15 Taylor, G.J. & Harris, W.S. (1970) Cardiac toxicity of aerosol propellants. *JAMA* **214**, 81-85.
16 Powars, D. (1965) Aplastic anemia secondary to glue-sniffing. *N. Eng. J. Med.* **273**, (13), 700-702.
17 Sharp, C.W. & Brehm, M.L. (eds) (1977) *Review of Inhalants: Euphoria to Dysfunction.* Rockville, Md: NIDA. NIDA Research Monograph 15.
18 Young, R.S.K., Grzyb, S.E. & Crismon, L. (1977) 'Recurrent Cerebral Disfunction related to Chronic Gasoline Sniffing in an Adolescent Girl: Lead Poisoning from Leaded Gasoline as an Attendant Complication.' *In: Clinical Pediatrics* **16**, p.706.
19 Recknagel, R.O. (1967) *Pharmacological Review*, **19**, p.145.

Cannabis

20 Mott, J. (1985) Self-reported cannabis use in Great Britain in 1981. *Brit. J. Addict* **80**, (1), 37-43.
21 Atha, M. & Blanchard, S. (1985) Cannabis use in Great Britain. *In: Big Deal: The Politics of the Illicit Drug Business.* 103-107. (eds A. Henman, R. Lewis & T. Malyon). London: Pluto Press.
22 Wagstaff, A. & Maynard, A. (1986) The consumption of illicit drugs in the UK. *Brit. J. Addict* **81**, (5), 691-696.
23 Smart, R.G. (1983) The epidemiology of cannabis use and its health consequences in western countries. *In: Cannabis and Health Hazards:*

Proceedings of an ARF/WHO Scientific Meeting on Adverse Health and Behavioral Consequences of Cannabis Use, 30 March–3 April 1981, 723-761. (eds K.O. Fehr & O.H. Kalent). Toronto: ARF.

24 Isbell, H., Gorodetzsky, C.W., Jasinski, D. et al. (1967) Effects of Δ9-trans-tetrahydrocannabinol in man. *Psychopharmacologia* **11**, 184-188.

25 Jaffe, J.H. (1980) Drug addiction and drug abuse. In: *The Pharmacological Basis of Therapeutics*, 535-584. (eds L.S. Goodman & A. Gilman). 6th edn. New York: MacMillan.

26 Turner, P. (1982) Kinetic and metabolic information on cannabis and related compounds in man. In: *UK Advisory Council on the Misuse of Drugs. Report of the Expert Group on the effects of cannabis use*. London: Home office.

27 Ashton, C.H. (1987) Cannabis: dangers and possible uses. *Brit. Med. J.* **294** (6565), 141-142.

28 Calder, I.M. & Ramsey, J. (1987) A survey of cannabis use in offshore rig workers. *Brit. J. Addict* **82**, (2), 159-161.

29 Chopra, G.S. & Smith, J.W. (1974) Pyschotic reactions following cannabis use in East Indians. *Arch. Gen. Psychiat.* **30**, (1) 24-27.

30 Carney, M.W.P., Bacelle, L. & Robinson, B. (1984) Psychosis after cannabis abuse. *Brit. Med. J.* **288**, (6423), p.1047.

31 Thacore, V.R. & Shukla, S.R.P. (1976) Cannabis psychosis and paranoid schizophrenia. *Arch. Gen. Psychiat.* **33**, (111), 383-386.

32 Rottanburg, D., Robins, A.H., Ben-Arie, O. et al. (1982) Cannabis-associated psychosis with hypomanic features. *Lancet* **2**, (8312), 1364-1366.

33 Knudsen, P. & Vilmar, T. (1984) Cannabis and neuroleptic agents in schizophrenia. *Acta Psychiat. Scand*, **69**, (2), 162-174.

Opioids

34 Hartnoll, R., Lewis, R., Mitcheson, M. et al. (1985) Estimating the prevalence of opioid dependence. *Lancet* **1**, (8422), 203-5.

35 Hartnoll, R. & Lewis, R. (1984) *The Illicit Heroin Market in Britain: Towards a Preliminary Estimate of National Demand.* Mimeo (University College Hospital, Drug Indicators Project) 1984.

36 Ditton, J. & Speirits, K. (1981) *The Rapid Increase of Heroin Addiction in Glasgow in 1981.* Glasgow: Glasgow University.

37 Wagstaff, A. & Maynard, A. (1986) The consumption of illicit drugs in the UK. *Brit. J. Addict* **81**, (5), 691-696.

38 Henderson, G. & McFadzean, I. (1985) Opioids – a review of recent developments. *Chemistry in Britain* 1094-1097.

39 Research on mental illness and addictive disorders: progress and prospects – supplement to the *Am. J. of Psychiat.* 1985, **142** (7), 8-41.

40 Jaffe, J.H. & Martin, W.R. (1980) Opioid analgesics and antagonists. In: *The Pharmacological Basis of Therapeutics.* 6th edn, (eds L.S. Goodman & A. Gilman), p.522. New York: Macmillan Publ Co.

Barbiturates

41 Madden, J.S. (1984) *A Guide to Alcohol and Drug Dependence.* 2nd edn Bristol: John Wright.
42 Bennett, J.R. (1976) *Barbiturate Abuse.* (Letter to all GPs). London: Campaign on the Use and Restriction of Barbiturates (CURB).
43 Oswald, I. & Priest, A.G. (1965) Five weeks to escape the sleeping-pill habit. *Brit. Med. J.* **2**, 1093–1099.

Benzodiazepines

44 Parish, P.A. (1971) The prescribing of psychotropic drugs in general practice. *J. Roy. Coll. G.P.* **30**, 603–6.
45 Marks, J. (1985) The benzodiazepines – for good or evil. *Neuropsychobiology* **10**, (2–3), 115–126.
46 Skegg, D.C.G., Doll, R. & Perry, J. (1977) Use of medicines in general practice. *Brit. Med. J.* **2**, 1561–1563.
47 Balter, M.B., Manheimer, D.I. *et al.* (1984) A cross-national comparison of anti-anxiety/sedative drug use. *Curr. Med. Res. Opin:* **8**, (suppl 4), 5–17.
48 Cooperstock, R. & Hill, J. (1982) *The Effects of Tranquillization: Benzodiazepine Use in Canada.* Toronto: Health Promotion Directorate.
49 US National Institute on Drug Abuse. (1978) *Nationwide Survey on Drug Abuse: 1977. A Nationwide study – Youth, Young Adults and Older People. Volume 1. Main Findings.* Rockville, Md: NIDA.
50 Robertson, J.R., Steed, M.E. & Bucknall, A.B.V. (1986) Letter. *J. Roy. Coll. Gen. Pract.*
51 Squires, R.F. & Braestrup, C. (1977) Benzodiazepine receptors in rat brain. *Nature* **266**, 732–734.
52 Mohler, H. & Okada, T. (1977) Benzodiazepine receptor: demonstration in the central nervous system. *Science* **198**, 849–851.
53 Covi L., Lipman, R.S., Pattison, J.H. *et al.* (1973) Length of treatment with anxiolytic sedatives and response to sudden withdrawal. *Acta Psychiat. Scan.* **49**, (1) 51–64.
54 Tyrer, P., Rutherford, D. & Huggett, T. (1981) Benzodiazepine withdrawal symptoms and Propanolol. *Lancet* **1**, (8219), 520–522.
55 Hallstrom, C. *et al.* (1981) Benzodiazepine withdrawal phenomena. *Int. Pharmacopsychiat.* **16**, (4), 235–244.
56 Hallstrom, C. & Lader, M. (1982) The incidence of benzodiazepine dependence in long-term users. *J. Psychiat. Treat. Eval.* **4**, (3), 293–296.
57 Tyrer, P., Owen, R. & Dowling, S. (1983) Gradual withdrawal of diazepam after long-term therapy. *Lancet* **1**, (8339), 1402–1406.
58 Tyrer, P. & Seivewright, N. (1984) Identification and management of benzodiazepine dependence. *Postgrad. Med. J.* **60**, (suppl. 2), 41–46.
59 Owen, R.T. & Tyrer, P. (1983) Benzodiazepine dependence: a review of the evidence. *Drugs* **25**, (4), 385–398.
60 Fontaine, R., Chouinard, G. & Annable, L. (1984) Rebound anxiety in

anxious patients after abrupt withdrawal of benzodiazepine treatment. *Amer. J. Psychiat.* **141**, (7), 848–852.
61 Murphy, S.M., Owen, R.T. & Tyrer, P.J. (1984) Withdrawal symptoms after six weeks' treatment with diazepam. *Lancet* **ii** (8416), p.1389.
62 The CRM on benzodiazepines. (1980) *Drug and Therapeutic Bulletin* **18**, 97–98.
63 Burrows, G.D. & Davies, B. (1984) Recognition and management of anxiety. *In: Antianxiety Agents*, 1–11. (eds G.D. Burrows, T.R. Norman & B. Davies). Amsterdam: Elsevier Science, BV publishers.
64 Fitzsimmons, C. (1988) 'Addicts to sue over "happy pill" misery'. *The Observer*, 14 February.
65 National Tranquilliser Advisory Council Annual Report (1985).
66 Mandelli, M., Tognoni, G. & Garrattini, S. (1978) Clinical pharmacokinetics of diazepam. *Clin. Pharmacokinet* **3**, 72–91.
67 Kales, A., Scharf, M.B., Kales, J.D. *et al.* (1979) Rebound insomnia. A potential hazard following withdrawal of certain benzodiazepines. *J. Am. Med. Ass.* **241**, 1692–1695.
68 Tyrer, P., Rutherford, D. & Huggett, T. (1981) Benzodiazepine withdrawal symptoms and propranolol. *Lancet* (i), 520–522.
69 Lader, M.H., Ron, M. & Petursson, H. (1984) Computed axial brain tomography in long-term benzodiazepine users. *Psychol. Med.* February **14**, (1), 203–206.

Amphetamines

70 Duquesne, T. & Reeves, J. (1982) *A Handbook of Psychoactive Medicines*, p.217. London: Quartet.
71 Gossop, M. (1987) *Living with Drugs*. 2nd edn. p.169. Aldershot: Wildwood House.
72 Steel, J.M. & Briggs, M. (1972) Withdrawal depression in obese patients after fenfluramine treatment. *Brit. Med. J.* July, **3**, 26–27.
73 Levin, A. (1973) Abuse of fenfluramine. *Brit. Med. J.*: 7 April **2**, p.49.
74 Home Office Statistical Bulletin, issue 28/86.
75 Connell, P.H. (1958) Amphetamine psychosis. London: Oxford University Press.
76 Snyder, S.H. (1972) Catecholamines in the brain as mediators of amphetamine psychosis. *Arch. Gen. Psychiat.* **27**, (2), 169–179.
77 Snyder, S.H. (1973) Amphetamine psychosis: a 'model' schizophrenia mediated by catecholamines. *Amer. J. Psychiat.* **130**, (1), 61–67.

Cocaine

78 Goodman, L.S. & Gilman, A. (eds) (1980) *The Pharmacological Basis of Therapeutics*. 6th edn New York: Macmillan.

79 Ellinwood, E.H. Jr. (1979) Amphetamines/anorectics. *In: Handbook on Drug Abuse*, 221-231. (eds R.L. Dupont *et al.*) Rockville, Md: NIDA.
80 Fischman, M.W., Schuster, C.R., Rosnekov, L. *et al.* (1976) Cardiovascular and subjective effects of intravenous cocaine administration in humans. *Arch. Gen. Psychiat.* **33**, (8), 983-989.
81 Matsuzaki, M. (1978) Alteration in pattern of EEG activities and convulsant effects of cocaine following chronic administration in the rhesus monkey. Electroencephalogy *Clin Neurophysiol.* **45**, 1-15.
82 Castellani, S., Ellinwood, E.H. Jr. & Kilbey, M.M. (1978) Behavioural analysis of chronic cocaine intoxication in the cat. *Biol. Psychiat.* **13**, 203-215.
83 Caldwell, J. (1976) Physiological aspects of cocaine usage. *In: Cocaine: Chemical, Biological, Clinical, Social and Treatment Aspects*, 187-199. (ed S.J. Mule). Cleveland, Oh: CRC Press.
84 Aigner, T.G. & Balster, R.L. (1978) Choice behaviour in rhesus monkeys: cocaine versus food. *Science* **201**, 534-535.

Psychedelics

85 Madden, J.S. (1984) A guide to alcohol and drug dependence 2nd edn. Bristol: John Wright.
86 Hofmann, A. (1980) *LSD my Problem Child*. New York: McGraw-Hill.
87 Johnson, C.L., Kang, S. & Green, J.P. (1975) Stereoelectronic characteristics of LSD and related hallucinogens. *In: LSD - a Total Study*, 197-244. (ed D.V.S. Sankar). Westbury, New York: PJD Publications.
88 Bennett, J.P. Jr., Snyder, S.H. (1976) Serotonin receptor binding in rat brain membranes. *Mol. Pharmacol.* **12**, 373-389.
89 Freedman, D.X. Mode of action of hallucinogenic drugs. (1981) *In: Handbook of Biological Psychiatry, Part IV. Brain Mechanisms and Abnormal Behaviour*, 858-882. (eds H.M. Van Praag, M.H. Lader, *et al*). New York: Marcel Dekker.
90 Hatrick, J.A. & Dewhurst, K. (1970) Delayed psychosis due to LSD. *Lancet* **ii**: 10 October 742-744.
91 Bowers, M.B. (1972) Acute psychosis induced by psychomimetic drug abuse. *Arch. Gen. Psychiat.* **27**, (4), 437-442.
92 McGlothin, W.H., Arnold, D.O. & Freedman, D.X. (1969) Organicity measures following repeated LSD ingestion. *Arch. Gen. Psychiat.* **21**, (6), 704-709.
93 Cooper, H.A. (1955) Hallucinogenic drugs. *Lancet* **268**, p.1078.
94 Huxley, A. (1972) *The Doors of Perception and Heaven and Hell*. London: Chatto and Windus.
95 Rawson, R.A., Tennant, F.S. & McCann, M.A. (1981) Characteristics of 68 chronic phencyclidine abusers who sought treatment. *Drug Alc. Depend.* **8**, (3), 223-227.

Miscellaneous drugs

96   Gough, S.P. & Cookson, I.B. (1984) Khat-induced schizophreniform psychosis in U.K. *Lancet* 25 February, (8374), p.455.
97   Mayberry, J., Morgan, G. & Perkin, E. (1984) Khat-induced schizophreniform psychosis in U.K. *Lancet* 25 February (8374), p.455.
98   Henshaw, D. (1986) Alcohol abuse. The Government's blurred vision over our biggest drug problem. *The Listener*, 16th October.
99   Gregg, E. & Akhter, I. (1979) Chlormethiazole Abuse. *Brit. J. Psychiat.* **134**, 627–629.
100 Pullen, G.P., Best, N.R. & Maguire, J. (1984) Anticholinergic drug abuse: a common problem? *Brit. Med. J.* **289** (6445), 612–613.
101 Banks, A. & Waller, T.A.N. (1983) Drug addiction and polydrug abuse: the role of the General Practitioner. London: ISDD.
102 Editorial. (1981) Management of alcohol withdrawal symptoms. *Brit. Med. J.* **282**, p.502.
103 Horder, J.M. (1978) Fatal chlormethiazole poisoning in chronic alcoholics. *Brit. Med. J.* **i**, 693–694.
104 Illingworth, R.N., Stewart, M.J. & Jarvie, D.R. (1979) Severe poisoning with chlormethiazole. *Brit. Med. J.* **ii**, 902–903.
105 Foster, A. (1977) Sedatives for alcoholics. *Brit. Med. J.* **i**, p.1355.
106 Stockwell, T., Bolt, E. & Hooper, J. (1986) Detoxification from alcohol at home managed by general practitioners. *Brit. Med. J.* **292**, 733–735.
107 Glatt, M.M., George, H.R. & Frisch, E.P. (1965) Controlled trial of chlormethiazole in treatment of the alcoholic withdrawal phase. *Brit. Med. J.* **ii**, 401–404.
108 Kryspin-Exner, P. & von K. Mader, R. (1971) Withdrawal delirium in chlormethiazole addiction. *Weiner Medizinische Wochenschrift* **121**, 811–812.
109 Reilly, T.M. (1976) Physiological dependence on, and symptoms of withdrawal from, chlormethiazole. *Brit. J. Psychiat.* **128**, 375–378.
110 Hession, M.A., Verma, S. & Bhakla, K.G.M. (1979) Dependence on chlormethiazole and effects of its withdrawal. *Lancet* 5th May i (8123), 952–954.
111 McGrath, S.D. (1975) A controlled trial of chlormethiazole and chlordiazepoxide in the treatment of acute withdrawal phase of alcoholism. *Brit. J. Addict.* **70**, (suppl l), 81–86.
112 Sellers, E.M., Zilm, D.H. & Degani, N.S. (1977) Comparative efficacy of propranolol and chlordiazepoxide in alcohol withdrawal. *J. Stud. Alc.* **38**, 2096–2108.
113 Weathersbee, P.S., Olsen, L.K. & Lodge, J.R. (1977) Caffeine and pregnancy: a retrospective survey. *Postgrad. Med.* September **62**, (iii), 64–72.
114 Stone, M.C. (1987) Coffee and coronary heart disease. *J. Roy. Coll. Gen. Pract.* **37**, (297), 146–147.
115 Bruce, M.S., Lader, M.H. (1986) Caffeine: clinical and experimental effects in humans. *Hum. Psychopharmacol.* **1**, 63–82.

Alcohol and its relationship to drug misuse

116 Borkenstein, R.F., Crowther, R.P. & Shumate, W.B. *et al.* (1964) The role of the drinking driver in traffic accidents. Bloominham: 1964. Department of Police Administration, Indiana University.
117 Observer & Maxwell M.A. (1959) A study of absenteeism, accidents and sickness payments in problem drinkers in one industry. *Q. J. Stud. Alc.* **20** 302-12.
118 Potter, J.F., Banaan, L.T. & Beevers, D.G. (1984) Heavy alcohol consumption and physical health problems. *Res. Adv. Alc. Drug Prob.* **8**, 149-182.
119 Thornton, J.R. (1984) Atrial fibrillation in healthy non-alcoholic people after an alcoholic binge. *Lancet* **2**, 1013-1015.
120 Idänpään-Heikkila, J. & Khan, I. (eds). *Public Health Problems and Psychotropic Substances*, p.85. Helsinki, the Government of Finland.
121 WHO (1981) *The Influence of Alcohol and Drugs on Driving*: Report of a WHO ad hoc Technical Group, Copenhagen. WHO, Regional Office for Europe. Euro Reports and Studies no 38.
122 Fischman, M.W., Schuster, C.R., Rosnekov, L., Shick, J.F.E., Krasnegor, N.A., Fennell, W. & Freedman, D.X. (1976) Cardiovascular and subjective effects of intravenous cocaine administration in humans. *Arch. Gen. Psychiat.* **33**, 983-989.
123 Morgan, M. (1982) Alcohol and Nutrition. *Brit. Med. Bull.* **38**, 21-28.
124 Harper, C.G., Krill, J.J. & Holloway, R.L. (1985) Brain shrinkage in chronic alcoholics: a pathological study. *Brit. Med. J.* **290** 501-504.
125 Morgan, M. & Pratt, O.E. (1982) Sex, alcohol and the developing foetus. *Brit. Med. Bull.* **38**, 43-52.
126 Banks, A. & Waller, T.A.N. (1983) *Drug Addiction and Polydrug Abuse: The Role of the General Practitioner.* London: ISDD.
127 Kaplan, H.S. (1974) The effects of drugs on sexuality. In: *The New Sex Therapy.* (ed. Kaplan H.S.). New York: Brunner/Mazel.
128 Kolodny, R., Masters, W. & Johnson, V. (1979) Drugs and Sex. In: *Textbook of Sexual Medicine.* (eds R. Kolodny, W. Masters & V. Johnson). First Ed. Boston: Little, Brown.
129 Gay, G.R., Newmeyer, J.A., Elion, R.A. & Weider, S. (1977-8) The sensuous hippie: Drug/sex practices in the Haight-Ashbury. *Drug Forum* **6**, (1), 27-47.
130 Jones, K.L., Smith, D.A., Ulleland, C.N. *et al.* (1973) Pattern of malformation in offspring of alcoholic mothers. *Lancet* **1**, 1267-1271.
131 Barrison, I.G., Waterson, E.J. & Murray-Lyon, I.M. (1985) Adverse effects of alcohol on pregnancy. *Brit. J. Addict.* **80**, 11-22.
132 Stoffer, S.S. (1968) A gynecologic study of drug addicts. *Am. J. Gynaecol.* **101**, 779-783.
133 Siep, M. (1976) Growth retardation, dysmorphic facies and minor malformations following massive exposure to phenobarbitone in utero. *Acta Paediat. Scand.* **65**, 617-621.

134 Milkovich, L. & Van den Berg, B.J. (1979) Effects of antenatal exposure to anorectic drugs. *Am. J. Obstet. Gynaecol.* **129**, 637–642.
135 Saxen, I. & Saxen, L. (1975) Association between maternal intake of diazepam and oral clefts. *Lancet* **ii**, p.498.
136 Chasnoff, I.J., Burns, W.J., Schnoll, S.H. & Burns, K.A. (1985) Cocaine use in pregnancy. *Nw Eng. J. Med.* **313**, (11), 666–669.
137 Rementeria, J.L. & Nuang, N.N. (1973) Narcotic withdrawal in pregnancy. Stillbirth incidence with a case report. *Am. J. Obstet. Gynaecol.* **116**, 1152–1156.
138 Jaffe J.H. (1980) Drug Addiction and Drug Abuse. *In: Pharmacological Basis of Therapeutics* (6th edn) (eds L.S. Goodman & A. Gilman). New York: MacMillan 535–584.
139 Rafaelsen, O.J., Bech, P., Christiansen, J., Christrup, H., Nyboe, J. & Rafaelsen, L. (1973) Cannabis and alcohol effects on simulated car driving. *Science* **179**, 920–923.
140 Fits, W.H., Arney, J. & Patton, A. (1973) *Self-concept Study of Alcoholic Patients.* Nashville, Tennessee: Dede Wallace Centre.
141 Robinson, J.S. (1973) *The Self-concepts of Drug Abusers.* Nashville, Tennessee: Dede Wallace Centre.
142 Keeler, M.H., Taylor, C.I. & Miller, W.C. (1979) Are all recently detoxified alcoholics depressed? *Am. J. Psychiat.* **136** (B), 586–588.
143 Bewley, T.H., Ben-Arie, O & James, I.P. (1968) Morbidity and mortality from heroin dependence. I. Survey of heroin addicts known to the Home Office. *Brit. Med. J.* 725–726.
144 Office of Health Economics (1981) *Alcohol – Reducing the Harm.* London: Office of Health Economics.
145 Jeffs, B. & Saunders, W. (1983) Minimising alcohol-related offences by enforcement of existing licensing legislation. *Brit. J. Addict.* **78**, 67–77.
146 Freeman, S.D.A. (1979) *Violence in the Home.* Hants: Saxon House, Farnborough.
147 Iversen, L. & Klausen, H. (1981) Lukningen of Nordhavns-Vaerflet. Publication 13. Institut für Social Medicin, Klobenhavns, Universitet.
148 Bailey, M.B., Haberman, P. & Alksne, (1962) Outcomes of alcoholic marriages: endurance, termination or recovery. *Q. J. Stud. Alc.* **23**, 610–623.
149 Orme, T.C. & Rimmer, J. (1981) Alcohol and Child Abuse: a Review. *J. Stud. Alc.* **42**, 273–287.
150 Chief Constable of the Lothian and Borders Police. (1984) Report in *The Times*, 19th April.
151 Creighton, S.J. NSPCC. (1987) Personal Communication.
152 Wagstaff, A. & Maynard, A. Data Note – 5. (1986) The consumption of Illicit Drugs in the UK. *Brit. J. Addict.* **81**, 691–696.
153 Carroll, J.F.X., Klein, M. & Santo, Y. (1978) Comparison of the similarities and differences in the self-concepts of male alcoholics and addicts. *J. Consult. Clin. Psychol.* **46**, iii, 575–576.
154 Wilson, I. (1980) *Drinking in England and Wales,* p.50. Office of Population Censuses and Surveys.

326 Drug Misuse

155 Green, C. & Cromwell, C. (1985) Heroin and young black people (a discussion paper). Drug indicators Project.
156 Stimmel, B., Korts, D., Cohen, M. et al. (1981) Opiate addiction and alcoholism: the feasibility of combined treatment approaches. In: Research Developments in Drug and Alcohol Use, 50–56. (eds R.B. Millman, P. Cushman & J.H. Lowinson). New York: New York Academy of Sciences.
157 Cohen, S. (1977) The Effects of Combined Alcohol-drug Abuse on Human Behaviour. A report prepared for Joint Drug–Alcohol Collaborative Project, Services Research Branch, Division of Resource Development, National Institute on Drug Abuse, Rockville, Maryland.
158 Dalton, M.S. & Duncan, D.W. (1975) Drug dependent doctors. In: Proceedings of the 31st International Congress on Alcoholism and Drug Dependence, 292–293. Lausanne: International Council on Alcohol and Addictions.
159 Glatt, M.M. (1970) Psychotherapy of drug dependence: some theoretical considerations. Brit. J. Addict. **65**, 51–62.
160 Stimmel, B. Methadone Maintenance and Alcohol Use. A report prepared for Joint Drug-Alcohol Collaborative Project, Services Research Branch, Division of Resource Development, National Institute on Drug Abuse Rockville, Maryland.
161 Ottenberg, D.J. & Rosen, A. (1971) Merging the treatment of drug addicts into an existing program for alcoholism. Q. J. Stud. Alc. **32**, 94–103.
162 Aumark, L. (1980) The effectiveness of combined vs separate treatment of alcoholics and drug addicts. In: Aspects of Alcohol and Drug Dependence. (eds J.S. Madden, R. Walker & W.H. Kenyon). Bath: Pitman Medical.
163 La Porte, D.J., McLellan, A.T. & MacGahan, J.A. (1980) Evaluation of combined treatment for alcohol and drug abusers: importance of patient compatibility. In: Aspects of Alcohol and Drug Dependence. (eds J.S. Madden, R. Walker & E.H. Kenyon). Bath: Pitman Medical.

Chapter Three

1 Bass, M. (1970) Sudden sniffing death. J. Am. Med. Ass. **212**, 2075–2079.
2 Fornazzari, L., Wilkinson, D.A., Kapur, B.M. & Carlen, P.L. (1983) Cerebellar, cortical and functional impairment in toluene abusers. Acta Neurol. Scand. **67**, 319–329.
3 Lader, M.H., Ron, M. & Peturrson, H. (1984) Psychol. Med. **14**, 203–6.
4 Bolelli, G., Lafisca, S. et al. (1979) Heroin addiction: Relationship between the plasma levels of testosterone, dihydrotestosterone, androstenedione LH, FSH, and the plasma concentration of heroin. Toxicology **15**, 15–19.
5 Tolis, G., Hickey, J. & Guyda, H. (1975) Effects of morphine on serum growth hormone, cortisol, prolactin and thyroid stimulating hormone in man. Clin. Endocrinol. Metab. **41**, 797–800.
6 Gold, M.S., Redmond, D.F. et al. (1978) Increase in serum prolactin by

exogenous and endogenous opiates: evidence for antidopamine and antipsychotic effects. *Am. J. Psychiat.* **135**, 1415-1416.
7   Lal, H.B., Drawbaugh, R., Hynes, M. & Brown, G. (1977) Enhanced prolactin inhibition following chronic treatment with haloperidol and morphine. *Life Sci.* **20**, 101-106.
8   Wallach, R.C., Jerez, E. & Blinick, G. (1969) Pregnancy and menstrual function in narcotics addicts treated with methadone. *Am. J. Obstet. Gynaecol.* **105**, 1226-1229.
9   Blatmen, S. (1973) *Methadone Effects on Pregnancy and the Newborn.* Proceedings of the Third National Conference on Methadone Treatment. Washington D.C.: U.S. GPO.
10 Cicero, T.J., Wilcox, C.E., Bell R.D. & Meyer E.R. (1976) Acute reductions in serum testosterone levels by narcotics in the male rat. Stereospecificity, blocked by naloxone and tolerance. *J. Pharmacol. Exp. Ther.* **198**, 340-346.
11 Mendelson, J.H. & Mello, N.K. (1975) Plasma testosterone levels during chronic heroin use and protracted abstinence. *Clin. Pharmacol. Ther.* **195**, 296-302.
12 Smith, D.E., Moser, C. *et al.* (1982) A clinical guide to the diagnosis and treatment of heroin-related sexual dysfunction. *J. Psych. Drugs* **14**, (1-2), 91-99.
13 Gay, G.R. & Newmeyer, J.A. *et al.* (1982) Love and Haight: the sensuous hippie revisited. Drug/sex practices in San Francisco, 1980-81. *J. Psych. Drugs* **14** (1-2), 111-123.
14 Kaplan, H.S. (1974) The effects of drugs on sexuality. In: *The New Sex Therapy.* (ed H.S. Kaplan). New York: Brunner/Mazel.
15 Dawley, H.H., Winstead, D.K. *et al.* (1979) An attitude survey of the effects of marijuana on sexual enjoyment. *J. Clin. Psychol.* **35**, 212-217.
16 Kolodny, R., Masters, W. & Johnson, V. (1979) Drugs and sex. In: *Textbook of Sexual Medicine.* 1st edn. (eds R. Kolodny, W. Masters & V. Johnson). Boston, Massachussetts: Little, Brown & Co.
17 Ungerer, J.L., Harford, R.J. *et al.* (1976) Sex/Guilt and preferences for illegal drugs among drug abusers. *J. Clin. Psychol.* **32**, 891-895.
18 Winick, C. (1981) Substances of abuse and sexual behaviour. In: *Substance Abuse: Clinical Problems and Perspectives.* (eds J.H. Lowinson & P. Ruiz). Baltimore: Williams & Wilkins.
19 Bell, D.S. & Trethowan, W.A. (1961) Amphetamine addiction and disturbed sexuality. *Arch. Gen. Psychiat.* **4**, 74-78.
20 Hall, R.C.W. *et al.* (1979) Relationship of psychiatric illness to drug use. *J. Psyche. Drugs* **11**, 337-342.
21 Waller, T.A.N., McCartney, P., Speight, L., Mainwaring-Burton, R. & Ramsey, J. Substance Misuse in an inner city practice. (In Press.)
22 Snyder, S.H. (1972) Catecholamines in the brain as mediators of amphetamine psychosis. *Arch. Gen. Psychiat.* **27**, 167-179.
23 Snyder, S.H. (1973) Amphetamine psychosis: A 'model' schizophrenia mediated by catecholamines. *Am. J. Psychiat.* **130** 61-67.
24 Hatrick, J.K. (1970) Delayed psychosis due to LSD. *Lancet* **ii**, 742-744.

25 Bowers, M.B. Jnr. (1972) Acute psychosis induced by psychotomimetic drug abuse. I. Clinical findings. II. Neurochemical findings. *Arch. Gen. Psychiat.* **27**, 437-442.
26 Brewer, C. (1985) Amphetaminea prescribing could safely be extended. *General Practitioner Newspaper*, 22nd March.
27 Caldwell, J. (1976) Physiological aspects of cocaine usage. In: *Cocaine: Chemical, Biological, Clinical, Social, and Treatment Aspects.* 187-199. (ed S.J. Mule). Cleveland, Ohio: CRC Press.
28 Gawin, F.H. & Kleber, H.D. (1984) Cocaine abuse treatment: An open pilot trial with lithium and desipramine. *Arch. Gen. Psych.* **41**, 903-909.
29 Dackis, C.A. & Marks, S.G. (1983) Opiate addiction and depression – cause or effect. Drug Alcohol Dependence **11**, 105-109.
30 Johnson, D.A.W. (1973) Treatment of depression in general practice. *Brit. Med. J.*. **2**, 18-20.
31 Tyrer, P. (1978) Drug treatment of psychiatric patients in general practice. *Brit. Med. J.* **2**, 1008-1010.
32 Johnson, D.A.W. (1983) Benzodiazepines in depression. In: *Benzodiazepines Divided. A Multidisciplinary Review.* (ed M.R. Trimble.) Chichester: John Wiley.
33 Petursson, H. & Lader, M. (1984) *Dependence on Tranquillisers.* Oxford: Oxford University Press.
34 Raistrick, D. & Davidson, R. (1985) *Alcoholism and Drug Addiction*, p.83. Edinburgh: Churchill Livingstone.
35 Harding, T. & Knight, F. (1973) Marijuana – modified mania. *Arch. Gen. Psychiat.* **29**, 635-637.
36 Abraham, H.D. (1983) Visual phenomenology of the LSD flashback. *Arch. Gen. Psychiat.* **40**, 884-889.

Hepatitis

37 Szmuness, W., Dienstag, J.L., Purcell, R.H. *et al.* (1976) Distribution of antibody to hepatitis A antigen in urban adult populations. *N. Engl. J. Med.* **295**, 755-759.
38 Gust, I.D., Lehmann, N.I., Lucas, C.R. *et al.* (1978) Studies on epidemiology of hepatitis A in Melbourne. In: *Viral Hepatitis*, 105-112. (eds G.N. Vyas, S.N. Cohen & R. Schmid) Franklin Institute Press, Philadelphia.
39 Norkrans, G., Frösner, G., Hermodsson, S. & Iwarson, S. (1979) Clinical, epidemiological and prognostic aspects of hepatitis 'Non-A, Non-B' – a comparison with hepatitis A and B. *Scand. J. Infect. Dis.* **ii**, 259-264.
40 Widell, A., Hansson, B.G., Moestrup, T.. & Nordenfelt, E. (1983) Increased Occurrence of Hepatitis A with Cyclic Outbreaks among Drug Addicts in a Swedish Community. Infection. *Eur. J. Clin. Stud. Treat. Infect.* **4**, 198-200.
41 Dietzman, D.E., Harnish, J.P., Ray, G., Alexander, F.R. & Holmes, K.K.

(1977) Hepatitis B surface antigen (HBsAg) and antibody to HBsAg: prevalence in homosexual and heterosexual men. *JAMA* **238**, 2625-2626.
42 Papaevangelou, G., Trichopoulos, D., Kremastinou, T. & Papoutsakis, G. Prevalence of hepatitis B antigen and antibody in prostitutes. *Brit. Med. J.* **ii**, 256-258.
43 Scott, R.T.A. (1986) Medical aspects of drug misuse during one year in a rehabilitation unit. *J. Roy. Coll. Gen. Pract.* **36**, 514-516.
44 Haw, S. (1985) Drug Problems in Greater Glasgow. Report of the SCODA Fieldwork Survey in Greater Glasgow Health Board.
45 Zuckerman A.J. (1983) Hepatitis Viruses. *In: Oxford Textbook of Medicine.* 5-123. (eds D.J. Weatherall, J.G.G. Ledingham & D.A. Warrell) Oxford Medical Publications.
46 Goedert, J.J. *et al.* (1987) *Abstract.* Third International Conference on AIDS. Washington. June.
47 Des Jarlais, D.C. & Freidman, S.R. (1987) HIV infection among intravenous drug users: epidemiology and risk reduction. *AIDS* **1**, 67-76.
48 Moss, A.R. (1987) AIDS and intravenous drug use: the real heterosexual epidemic. *Brit. Med. J.* **294**, 389-390.
49 Adler, M.W. (1987) Development of the epidemic. *In: ABC of AIDS.* (ed. M.W. Adler.) London: BMA.
50 Allain, J.P. (1986) Prevalence of HTLV-III/LAV antibodies in patients with haemophilia and their sexual partners in France. *N.Engl. J. Med.* **315**, 517-518.
51 Kreiss, J.U.K., Kitchen, L.W., Prince, H.E. *et al.* (1985) Antibody to human T-lymphotropic virus type 3 in wives of haemophiliacs. *Ann. Intern. Med.* **102**, 623-626.
52 France, A.J., Skidmore, C.A., Robertson, J.R. *et al.* (1988) Heterosexual spread of human immunodeficiency virus in Edinburgh. *Brit. Med. J.* **296**, 526-529.
53 Bayley, A.C. (1984) Aggressive Kaposi's sarcoma in Zambia 1983. *Lancet* **i**, 1318-1320.
54 Biggar, R.J., Melbye, M., Kestens, L. *et al.* Seroepidemiology of HTLV-III antibodies in a remote population in eastern Zaire.
55 Pilot, P., Quin, T.C., Taelman, H. *et al.* (1984) Acquired immunodeficiency syndrome in a heterosexual population in Zaire. *Lancet* **ii**, 65-69.
56 Perre, P., Rouvray, D., Lepage, P. *et al.* (1984) Acquired immunodeficiency syndrome in Rwanda. *Lancet* **ii**, 62-65.
57 Bygbjerg, I.C. (1983) AIDS in a Danish surgeon (Zaire 1976). *Lancet* **i**, p.925.
58 Vandepitte, J., Verwilghen, R. & Zachee, P. (1983) AIDS and cryptococcus (Zaire 1977). *Lancet* **i**, 925-926.
59 Hancock, G. & Carin, E. (1986) *AIDS the Deadly Epidemic.* London: Gollancz.
60 World Health Organization. (1986) *AIDS Among Drug Abusers.* Copenhagen: WHO.

61 Spira, T.J., Des Jarlais, D.C., Marmor, M. et al. (1984) Prevalence of antibody to lymphadenopathy associated virus among drug detoxification patients in New York. *N. Engl. J. Med.* **313**, 467–468.
62 Levy, N., Carlson, J.R., Hinrichs, S. et al. (1986) The prevalence of HTLV-III/LAV antibodies among intravenous drug users attending treatment programs in California: a preliminary report. *N. Engl. J. Med.* **314**, p.446.
63 Brettle, R.P., Bisset, K., Burn, S. et al. (1987) Human immunodeficiency virus and drug misuse: the Edinburgh experience. *Brit. Med. J.* **295**, 421–424.
64 Follett, E.A.C., McIntyre, A., O'Donnell, B. et al. (1986) HTLV-III antibody in drug abusers in the West of Scotland: the Edinburgh Connection. *Lancet* **1**, p.446.
65 Peutherer, J.F., Edmonds, E., Simmonds, P. et al. (1985) HTLV-111 antibody in Edinburgh drug addicts. *Lancet* **2**, p.1129.
66 Robertson, J.R., Bucknall, A.B.V., Welsby, P.D. et al. (1986) An epidemic of AIDS-related virus (HTLV-III/LAV) injection among intravenous drug abusers in a Scottish general practice. *Brit. Med. J.* **292**, 527–530.
67 World Health Organization. (1987) *Meeting on Training on AIDS for Personnel in Drug Treatment Centres: Summary Report.* Copenhagen: WHO.
68 Brettle, R.P. (1987) *Evidence to the Working Party on AIDS and Drug Misuse.* Advisory Council on the Misuse of Drugs.
69 Shillitoe et al. (1977) Changes in CMI responses to HSV in humans. *Infect. Immun.*, **18**, p.130.
70 Moharty et al. (1984) Thymus derived lymphocytes (T-cells) in patients with genital warts. *Brit. J. Ven. Dis.* **60**, p.186.
71 Levitt (1987) Immunobiology of Chlamydia. *Immunol. Today*, **8** (7), 18, p.246.
72 Musher (1975) Lymphocyte transformation in syphilis. *Infect. Immun.*, **11**, p.1261.
73 MacGregor, R.R. (1986) Alcohol and the Immune System. In: *Acquired Immune Deficiency Syndrome and Chemical Dependence.* Report of a Symposium National Institute on Alcohol Abuse and Alcoholism.
74 Cushman, P., Khurana, R. Marijuana and T lymphocyte rosettes. *Clin. Pharmaco. Therapeut.*, **19**, (3), 310–317.
75 McDonough, R.J., Madden, J.J., Rosman, H.S. et al. (1981) Opiate inhibition of sheep erythrocyte binding to T lymphocytes: reversal by naloxone and cyclid nucleotides. In: *Problems of Drug Dependence 1980*, 159–165. (ed L.S. Harris) Rockville, NIDA, **34**.
76 McDonough, R.J., Madden, J.J., Falek, A. et al. (1980) Alteration of T and null lymphocyte frequencies in the peripheral blood of human opiate addicts: in vivo evidence for opiate receptor sites on T lymphocytes. *J. Immunol* **125**, 2539–2543.
77 Wybran, J., Appelboom, T., Famaey, J.P. et al. (1979) Suggestive evidence for receptors for morphine and methionine-encephalin on normal human blood T lymphocytes. *J. Immunol.* **123**, 1068–1070.
78 Sharit, Y., Lewis, J.W., Terman, G.W. et al. (1984) Opiate peptides

mediate the suppressive effect of stress on natural killer cell cytotoxicity. *Science* **223**, 188–190.
79 Brown, S.W., Stimmel, B., Taub, R.N. *et al.* (1974) Immunologic dysfunction in heroin addicts. *Arch. Intern. Med.* **134**, 1001–1006.
80 Hofmann, B., Lindhardt, B.O., Gerstoft, J. *et al.* (1987) Lymphocyte transformation response to pokeweed mitogen as a predictive marker for development of AIDS and AIDS related symptoms in homosexual men with HIV antibodies. *Brit. Med. J.* **295**, 293–296.
81 White, S.C., Brin, S.S. & Janicki, B.W. (1975) Mitogen-induced blastogenic responses of lymphocytes from marijuana smokers. *Science* **188**, 71–72.
82 Abrams, D.I. (1986) The nature of AIDS epidemiology. In: *Acquired Immune Deficiency Syndrome and Chemical Dependency*, p.8. Report of a Symposium. U.S. Dept of Health and Human Services.
83 Stimson, G.V., Alldritt, L., Dolan, K. and Donoghoe, M. (1988) *Injecting Equipment Exchange Schemes: A Preliminary Report on Research.* Goldsmith's College, University of London.
84 *HIV Infection in Scotland.* (1986) Report of the Scottish Committee on HIV infection and Intravenous Drug Misuse. Scottish Home and Health Department. September.
85 *AIDS and Drug Misuse: First Report of the Advisory Council on the Misuse of Drugs.* (1988) London: HMSO. (In Press.)
86 Milne, R.I.G., Keen, S.M. (1988) Are general practitioners ready to prevent the spread of HIV? *Brit. Med. J.* **296**, 533–535.
87 Anderson, P., Mayon-White, R. (1988) General practitioners and management of infection with HIV. *Brit. Med. J.* **296**, 535–537.
88 Boyton, R., Scambler, G. (1988) Survey of general practitioners' attitudes to AIDS in the North West Thames and East Anglian regions. *Brit. Med. J.* **296**, 538–540.
89 Sapira, J.D. (1968) The narcotic addict as a medical patient. *Am. J. Med.* **45**, p.555.
90 Sapira, J.D., Cherubin, C.E. *eds.* (1975) Drug Abuse: A guide for Clinician. p.233. Excerpta Medica, Amsterdam. American Elsever Publishing Co. Inc., New York.
91 Servant, J.B., Dutton, G.N., Ong-Tone, L. *et al.* (1985) Candidal endophthalmitis in Glaswegian heroin addicts: report of an epidemic. *Trans. Ophthalmol. Soc. U.K.:* **104**, 297–308.
92 Suderam, G., McDonald, J. Maniatis, T. *et al.* (1986) Tuberculosis as a manifestation of the acquired immune deficiency syndrome (AIDS). *JAMA* **256**, 362–366.
93 Handwerger, S., Mildvan, D., Senie, R. & McKinley, F.W. (1987) Tuberculosis and the acquired immunodeficiency syndrome at a New York City hospital 1978–1985. *Chest* **91**, 176–180.
94 Reichman, L.B., Felton, C.P. & Edsall, J.R. (1979) Drug dependence, a possible new risk factor for tuberculosis disease. *Arch. Intern. Med.*, **139**, 337–339.

95 Bick, R.L. and Anholt, J.E. (1971) Malaria in drug addicts. *JAMA*, **216**, p.1036.
96 Wetli, C.V., Noto, T.A. & Fernandez-Carol, A. (1974) Immunologic Abnormalities in Heroin Addiction. *South. Med. J.* **67**, (2), 193-195.
97 Brown, S.M., Stimmel, B., Taub, R.N. *et al.* (1974) Immunologic Dysfunction in Heroin Addicts. *Arch. Intern. Med.* **134**, 1001-1004.

Drug use and mortality

98 Ghodse, A.H., Sheehan, M., Taylor, C. *et al.* (1985) Deaths of drug addicts in the United Kingdom 1967-81. *Brit. Med. J.* **290**, 425-428.
99 Ghodse, A.H., Sheehan, M., Stevens, B. *et al.* (1978) Mortality among drug addicts in Greater London. *Brit. Med. J.* **ii**, 1742-1744.
100 Bewley, T.H., Ben Arie, O. & James, I.P. (1968) Morbidity and mortality from heroin dependence. I. Survey of heroin addicts known to the Home Office. *Brit. Med. J.*, 725-732.
101 Bucknall, A.B.V., Robertson, J.R. (1986) Deaths of heroin users in a general practice population. *J. Roy. Coll. Gen. Pract.* **36**, (284), 120-122.

Chapter Five

1 U.K. Home Office. (1984) *Prevention*. Report of the London Advisory Council on the Misuse of Drugs. London: HMSO.
2 London Boroughs Working Party on Drug and Alcohol Problems. (1986) Prevention of alcohol and drug misuse.
3 Hartnoll, R., Lewis, R.S. & Bryer, S. (1984) Recent trends in drug use in Britain. *Druglink*, ISDD, **19**, 22-24.
4 Green, C. & Cromwell, C. (1985) *Heroin and Young Black People (a Discussion Paper)*. London: Drug Indicators Project.
5 Morgan, H. (1984) Do minor affective disorders need medication? *Brit. Med. J.* **289**, p.783.
6 Higgitt, A., Lader, M.H. & Fonagy, P. (1985) Clinical management of benzodiazepine dependence. *Brit. Med. J.* **291**, 688-690.
7 Schuckit, M. & Morrissey, E. (1979) Drug abuse among alcoholic women. *Am. J. Psych.* **136**, 607-611.
8 Blum, R. *et al.* (1969) *Students and Drugs II: College and High School Observations*. San Francisco: Jossey-Bass.
9 Royal College of Psychiatrists. (1986) *Alcohol - Our Favourite Drug*. London: Tavistock.
10 Royal College of General Practitioners. (1986) *Alcohol - a Balanced View*. London: RCGP.
11 Royal College of Physicians. (1987) *Alcohol - a Great and Growing Evil*. London: Tavistock.
12 Stimson, G.V. (1973) *Heroin and Behaviour*. Shannon: Irish University Press.

13 Wille, R. (1981) Ten year follow-up of a representative sample of London heroin addicts: clinic attendance, abstinence and mortality. *Brit. J. Addict.* **76**, 259–266.
14 Chapple, P., Somekh, D.E. & Taylor, M.E. (1972) A five year follow-up of 108 cases of opiate addiction. *Brit. J. Addict.* **67**, 33–38.
15 McBay, A.J. (1986) Problems in testing for abused drugs. *J. Am. Med. Ass.* **255**, (1), 39–40.
16 *The Journal.* 1 April 1987, p. 11.
17 ISDD Research and Development Unit. (1981) *Teaching about a Volatile Situation.* London: ISDD.
18 Anderson, H.R., Dick, B., Macnair, R.S. *et al.* (1982) An investigation of 140 deaths associated with volatile substance abuse in the United Kingdom (1971–1981). *Human Toxicol.* **1**, (3), 207–221.
19 Scottish Home and Health Department. (1986) *Report of the Scottish Committee on HIV Infection and Intravenous Drug Misuse.*
20 Walsh, S.S., Pierce, A.M. & Hart, C.A. (1987). Drug abuse: a new problem. *Brit. Med. J.* **295**, 526–527.

Chapter Six

1 Strang, J. (1986) The generalist's guide to the assessment and treatment of the problem drugtaker. 979–987.
2 Smith, M.D., Kelsey, M.C., Gosling, M. (1987) Guidance for Disinfection of Equipment in General Medical and Dental Practice. Islington Health Authority.
3 Conant, M., Hardy, D., Sernatinger, J., *et al.* (1986) Condoms prevent transmission of AIDS associated retrovirus. *JAMA* **255**, p.1706.
4 Hicks, D.R., Martin, L.S., Getchell, J.P. *et al.* (1985) Inactivation of HTLV-III/LAV-infected cultures of normal human lymphocytes by nonoxyl 9 *in vitro*. *Lancet* **ii**, 1422–1423.
5 Personal communication. Dr. J.R. Robertson.
6 *Mortal. Morbid. Weekly Rep.* Disease Control Centre, Atlanta.
7 Personal communication. Drs. C. Cook and M.S. Lipsedge.
8 Cook, C., Lipsedge, M.S., Henry, J. and Scannell, T.D. (1986) Letter to the Editor. *Brit. Med. J.* **293**, p.506.
9 Personal communication, Dr M. Ross.
10 Brewer, C. (1986) Naltrexone: helping the heroin user to get clean and stay clean. *Brit. J. Hospital. Med.* **36**, (6), p.401.
11 Patterson, M.A. (1984) Treatment of drug, alcohol and nicotine addiction by neuroelectric therapy: analysis of results over seven years. *J. Bioelect.* **3**, (162), 193–221.
12 Gossop, M., Gradley, B., Strang, J. *et al.* (1984) The clinical effectiveness of electro-stimulation *vs* oral methadone in managing opiate withdrawal. *Brit. J. Psychiat.* **144**, 203–208.
13 Personal communication, Dr J. Strang.

14 Ellison, F., Ellison, W., Daulonede, J.P. *et al.* (1987) Opiate withdrawal and electro-stimulation: double-blind experiments. *L'encéphale*, January.
15 Bewley, T. (1975) Conning the general practitioner: how drug abusing patients obtain prescriptions. *J. Royal Coll. Gen. Pract.* **25**, 654–657.
16 Kleber, H.D. & Gawin, F.H. (1984) The spectrum of cocaine abuse and its treatment. *J. Clin. Psychiat.* **45** (12), 18–23.
17 Anker, A.L. & Croley, T.J. (1982) Use of contingency contracts in speciality clinics for cocaine abuse. In: *Problems of Drug Dependence 1981*, 452–459. (ed L.S. Harris) Proceedings of the 43rd Annual Scientific Meeting – the Committee on Problems of Drug Dependence Inc. Rockville, Md: NIDA.
18 Ashton, H. (1984) Benzodiazepine withdrawal: an unfinished story. *Brit. Med. J.* **288**, 1135–1140.
19 O'Connor, D. (1983) *Glue Sniffing and Volatile Substance Abuse: Case Studies of Children and Young Adults.* London: Gower.
20 Merrill, E. (1985) *Sniffing Solvents and other Substances: a New Guide for Parents and Professionals.* Birmingham: PEPAR, 109 pages. (Available from ISDD at £4.80 including p & p.)
21 Black, D. (1982) Misuse of solvents. *Health Trends* **14**, 27–28.

Chapter Seven

1 Lask, B. (1987) Family therapy. *Brit. Med. J.* **294**, 203–204.
2 Raistrick, D. & Davidson, R. (1985) *Alcoholism and Drug Addiction.* Edinburgh: Churchill Livingstone.
3 Wilfred, D.B. (1981) *Drug Abuse for the Primary Care Physician.* Chicago: American Medical Association.

Chapter Eight

1 Skegg, D.C.G., Doll, R. & Perry, J. (1977) Use of medicines in general practice. *Brit. Med. J.* **2**, 1561–1563.
2 Chambers, C.D., Inciardi, J.A. & Siegal, H.A. (1974) *Chemical Coping: the Extent of Non-Addicting Drug Use in the United States.* New York: Spectrum.
3 Horwitz, J.A. The pathways into psychiatric treatment: some differences between men and women. *J. Health Soc. Beh.* **18**, 169–172.
4 Phillips, D.L. & Segal, B.E. (1969) Sexual status and psychiatric symptoms. *Am. Sociol. Rev.* **34**, 58–72.
5 Goldberg, D. & Huxley, P. (1980) *Mental Illness in the Community. The Pathway to Psychiatric Care.* London: Tavistock Publications.
6 Perry, L. (1979) *Women and Drug Use: An Unfeminine Dependency.* ISDD.
7 Parker, H., Chadwick, C. (1987) *Unattractive alternatives. Dilemmas for Drug Services in Wirral: 1987.* Sub Dept. of Social Work Studies. University of Liverpool.

8   Beckman, L.J. (1984) Treatment of women alcoholics. *Alc. Alc. Treat. Q.* **1**, (2) 101–115.
9   Thom, B. (1986) Sex differences in help-seeking for alcohol problems – 1. The barriers to help-seeking. *Brit. J. Addic.* **81**, (6), 777–788.
10 Survey of facilities for women using drugs (including alcohol) in London. *DAWN* (1985).
11 Robertson, J.R. (1985) Drug users in contact with general practice. *Brit. Med. J.* **290**, 34–35.
12 Smithells, R.W., Sheppard, S., Schorah, C.J. et al. (1981) Apparent prevention of neural tube defects by periconceptional vitamin supplementation. *Arch. Dis. Child.* **56**, 911–918.
13 Blinick, G., Wallach, R.C., Jerez, E. et al. (1976) Drug addiction in pregnancy and the neonate. *Am. J. Obstet. Gynec.* **125**, 135–142.
14 Naeye, R.L., Blayne, W., Leblance, W. et al. (1973) Fetal complications of maternal drug addiction: abnormal growth, infections and episodes of stress. *J. Pediat.* **83**, 1055–1061.
15 Fraser, A.C. (1976) Drug addiction in pregnancy. *Lancet* **ii**, 896–899.
16 Rementeria, J.L. & Lontongkhum, L. (1977) Drug abuse in pregnancy in neonatal effects. St. Louis: C.V. Mosby.
17 Davies, J.M., Latto, I.P., Jones, J.G. et al. (1979) Effects of stopping smoking for 48 hours on oxygen available from the blood: a study on pregnant women. *Brit. Med. J.* **ii**, 355–356.
18 Jones, K.L., Smith, D.W., Streissguth, A.P. et al. (1974) Outcome of offspring of chronic alcoholic women. *Lancet* **i**, 1076–1078.
19 Dwyer, L.S., Keller, L.S. & Streissguth, A. (1978) Naturalistic observations of newborns: effects of maternal alcohol intake. *Alcoholism: Clinical and Experimental Research* **2** 171–177.
20 Rementia, J.L. & Nuang, N.N. (1973) Narcotic withdrawal in pregnancy – stillbirth incidence with a case report. *Am. J. Obst. Gynec.* **116**, 1152–1156.
21 Zuspan, F.P., Gumpel, J.A., Mejia-Zelaya, A. et al. (1975) Fetal stress from methadone withdrawal. *Obstet. Gynec.* **122**, 43–46.
22 Connaughton, J.F., Reeser, D., Shut, J. et al. (1977) Perinatal addiction: outcome and management. *Am. J. Obstet. Gynec.* **129**, 679–686.
23 Ploman, L. & Persson, B.H. (1957) On the transfer of barbiturates to the human foetus and their accumulation in some of its vital organs. *J. Obst. Gyn. Brit. Emp.* **64**, p.706.
24 Melchior, J.C., Svensmark, O. & Trolle, D. (1967) Placental transfer of phenobarbitone in epileptic women and elimination in newborns. *Lancet* **ii**, 860–861.
25 Royal College of General Practitioners. (1975) Morbidity and drugs in pregnancy. The influence of illness and drugs on the aetiology of congenital malformations. *J. Roy. Coll. of G.P.* **25**, 631–645.
26 Siep, M. (1976) Growth retardation, dysmorphic facies and minor malformations following massive exposure to phenobarbitone in utero. *Acta Paediat. Scand.* **65**, 617–621.

27 Chasnoff, I.J., Burns, W.J., Schnoll, S.H. & Burns, K.A. (1985) Cocaine use in pregnancy. *N. Engl. J. Med.* **313**, (11) 666–669.
28 Milkovich, L. & Van den Berg, B.J. (1977) Effects of antenatal exposure to anorectic drugs. *Am. J. Obs. Gynec*, **129**, 637–642.
29 Hartz, S.C., Olli, P., Heinonen, O.P. *et al.* (1975) Antenatal exposure to meprobamate and chlordiazepoxide in relation to malformations, mental development and childhood mortality. *New Eng. J. Med.* **292**, p.726.
30 Shannon, R.W., Fraser, G.P. & Aitken, R.G. (1972) Diazepam in pre-eclamptic toxaemia with special reference to its effect on the newborn infant. *Brit. J. Clin. Pract.* **26**, 271–275.
31 Marselli, P.L., Principi, N., Tognoni, G. *et al.* (1973) Diazepam elimination in premature and full-term infants and children. *J. Perin. Med.* **1**, 133–141.
32 Long, S.Y. (1972) Does LSD induce chromosomal damage and malformations? A review of the literature. *Teratology* **6**, 75–90.
33 Jacobson, C.B. & Berlin, C.M. (1972) Possible reproductive detriment in LSD users. *J. Am. Med. Ass.* **222**, 1367–1373.
34 Oats, J.N., Beischer, N.A., Breheny, J.E. & Pepperell, R.J. (1984) The outcome of pregnancies complicated by narcotic drug addiction. *Aust. NZ J. Obstet. Gynaecol.* **24**, 14–16.
35 Desmond, M.M., Schwanecki, R.P., Wilson, G.S. *et al.* (1972) Maternal barbiturate utilisation and neonatal withdrawal symptomatology. *Paediatrics* **80**, 190–197.
36 Sussman, S. (1963) Narcotic and methamphetamine use during pregnancy. *Am. J. Dis. Child.* **106**, p.325.
37 Kendall, S.R., Doberczak, T.M., Mauer, K.R. *et al.* (1983) Opiate versus CNS depressant therapy in neonatal drug abstinence syndrome. *Am. J. Dis. Child.* **137**, (4), 378–382.
38 Chasnoff, I.J., Hatcher, R. & Burns, W.J. (1980) Polydrug and methadone-addicted newborns; a continuum of impairment? *Paediatrics* **70**, 210–213.
39 Tylden, E. (1983) Care of the pregnant drug addict. *MIMS Magazine.* 1 June.

Chapter Nine

1 Glatt, M.M. (1982) *The Alcoholic and the Help he Needs.* 2nd ed. Priory Press.
2 Dorn, N., Ribbens, J. & South, N. (1987) *Coping with a Nightmare.* ISDD.

Index

Abscesses, injection-induced, 114
Accidents, drug-related, 30-1
Acetone, morbidity, 49
ACMD, 5
   AIDS and drug misuse working group, 15
   treatment/rehabilitation report (1982), 9, 11
Addiction, WHO definition, 22, 23
Addicts, notification increase, 7-8
ADFAM, 13
Advice sources, 283-8
   see also Information; Resources
Advice/counselling centres, 12-13
   see also Counselling
Advisory Council on Misuse of Drugs (ACMD), 5
   AIDS and drug misuse working group, 15
   treatment/rehabilitation report (1982), 9, 11
Aetiology, 33-7
AIDS, 5, 123-41, 182
   clinical manifestations, 130-2, 133
   cofactors, 132-5
   and drug misuse, care recommendations, 136-41
   epidemic, 14-15
   epidemiology, 123-7
   heterosexual spread, 123-5
   homosexual spread, 123
   pre-disposing infections, 133
   prevention, counselling, 11
   pyrexia, 104
   transmission routes, 123-7
   see also HIV antibodies; HIV infection
AIDS related complex (ARC), 124, 129-30, 305
Alcohol
   chlormethiazole cross-tolerance, 91
   drug misuse parallel effects, 97-102
   misuse, benzodiazepines, 69

   pregnancy/fetal effects, 257-9
   traffic accidents, 31
   withdrawal syndrome, neonatal, 269-70
Amanita muscaria, 89
Amenorrhoea, 107
   opioid-induced, 64
Amphetamines, 74-9
   action mechanisms, 76-7
   analogues, 96-7
   chronic misuse, treatment, 220-1
   clinical effects, 77-9
   hallucinogenic, 88
   neonatal effects, 268
   pregnancy/fetal effectts, 261
   pyschic effects, 78-9
   psychosis, 78
   sexual activity effects, 108
   tolerance, 77
   withdrawal syndrome, 78-9
   neonatal, 268, 269
Amyl nitrite, 53-4
'Anesthelic' apparatus, 200-1
Angel dust, 89
Anxiety, withdrawal syndrome, 113
Assessment, 176-80
Association of Independent Doctors against Addiction (AIDA), 171
Ataxia, 106

Barbiturates, 65-8
   actions, 66
   injection, 66-7
   misuse, treatment, 221-2, 223
   neonatal effects, 267-8
   pregnancy/fetal effects, 260, 264
   prevalence, 65-6
   sexual effects, 108
   tolerance, 67-8
   withdrawal syndrome, 67-8
   neonatal 267, 269-70
Behaviour therapy, 244

cocaine misusers, 217–18
Benzhexol, 90
Benzodiazepines, 68–74
　action mechanisms, 70
　and alcohol misuse, 69
　dependence, 70
　　drug users, 229–30
　　repeat prescribing, 71–3
　and drug misusers, 69–70
　long-acting, short/medium
　　equivalents, 225
　long-term administration, 71–2, 73–4
　metabolites, 7
　neonatal effects, 268
　NHS prescribable, 73
　organic brain damage, 73
　overprescribing, 69, 71–3
　pregnancy/fetal effects, 261–2, 264–5
　prescribed, dependence, 223–9
　prescribing care, 158
　sexual activity effects, 108
　side effects, 71–2, 73–4
　tolerance, 74
　withdrawal syndrome, 9, 72, 74
　　neonatal, 269–70
Booklets/leaflets, 289
Books, 290
Brain Committee (1961), 6
Breast feeding, 266
Butane, morbidity, 50
Butyl nitrite, 53–4

Caffeine, 93–5
　diuretic effects, 94
Candidal endophthalmitis, 142
Cannabis, 54–8
　AIDS development, 133–4
　carcinogenesis, 55–6
　cultivation/forms/use, 55
　dependence/tolerance, 58
　and heroin use, 37
　immunity effects, 142–3
　legal control, 4
　pregnancy/fetal effects, 262
　prevalence, 54–5
　psychological/clinical effects, 55–6
　psychosis, 57–8
　psychotropic effects, 56–7
　traffic accidents, 30
Carbon tetrachloride, morbidity, 51–2
Cardiovascular complications, 82–3, 105
Care orders, infants, 271–3
Catecholamines, levels, 105

Cerebral atrophy, 106
　benzodiazepine association, 73
'Chasing the dragon', 7–8, 62–3
Children, non-accidental injuries, 31
China, opium smoking, 3–4
Chlormethiazole, 90, 91
　misuse, treatment, 222–3
Chloroform, morbidity, 51–2
Cigarette smoking, pregnancy/fetal
　effects, 256–7
Classification system, 22–6
Clondine
　inpatient regime, 194–5
　naltrexone combination, 195–7
　in opioid detoxification, 192–5
　outpatient regime, 195
　side effects, 193–4
　withdrawal treatment, 9, 192–5
CNS effects, 82, 105–7
　cocaine, 82
Cocaine, 79–84
　action mechanism comparisons, 81
　administration routes, 80
　clinical effects, 81–82
　　high/toxic doses, 82–3
　　low/moderate doses, 81–2
　　repeated use, 83–4
　formulation, 80
　misuse, 79–84
　　medical programmes, 217
　　psychodynamic treatment, 218
　　self-help groups, 217
　　supportive treatment, 218
　　treatment, 216–20
　neonatal effects, 268
　pregnancy/fetal effects, 260–1, 264
　prevalence, 79–80
　sexual activity effects, 108
Cognition, impairment, 110
Cognitive therapy, 244
Colaholism, 95
'Cold Turkey', help, 197–8
Committee on Morphine and Heroin
　Addicts (Rolleston) (1926), 5–11
Community aspects, 27–33
Community drug teams (CDTs), 13,
　167–8
Community responses, 31–3
Community support, primary care
　team, 18–19
Congenital abnormalities, fetal alcohol
　syndrome, 258
Consultation guidelines, 175–6

Contraception, and drug misuse, 253–4
Contracts, detoxification, 209–10, 212
Controlled drugs
  classes A & B, 149
  destruction, 150
  legislation, 145–53
  notification, 150–2
  possession/supply/production, 146
  prescriptions, 146–7
  registers, 147–9
  requisition, 147
  safe custody, 152
  schedules, 293–301
  security, 152–3
Controllers
  external, 35
  internal, 35
Convulsions, 105–6
Counselling
  AIDS prevention, 11
  detoxification, 210–13
  HIV positive patients, 186–8
  pre-conception, 254–5
  pre-HIV testing, 183–6
'Crack', 80
Crime
  and drugs, 27, 28–9, 31
  and maintenance treatment, 29
Crisis intervention service, 238
Cyclizine, 90, 92

D-lysergic acid diethylamide (LSD), see LSD
Dangerous Drugs Act (1920), 4
Day projects, long-term care, 237–8
Degreasing agent, morbidity, 50
Delirium, 113
Delirium tremens, barbiturate withdrawal, 67
Delta agent infection, 120
Dependence
  prescribing care, 158
  syndrome, 25
  WHO definition, 23–4
  see also Withdrawal
Depressant withdrawal syndrome, 99
Depression, 112–13
Designer drugs, 67–8, 95–7
Detoxification, 8–9
  attendance frequency, 213–15
  counselling, 210–13
  long-term, 205–7
  no methadone, 191–201

  pregnant misusers, 263–4
  prescription guidelines, 204–7
  symptomatic prescribing, 192–8
  see also Maintenance treatment
Deviancy, 37
DHSS, management guidelines, 174–90
Diconal, 90
Dihydrocodeine, 207
Disinfection/sterilisation, 181–2
Drug availability, and misuse, 36
Drug misuse
  alcohol parallel effects, 97–102
  and benzodiazepines, 69–70
  chronic, treatment, 247–50
  consequences, family protection, 275
  epidemic, 7–8, 26–7
  family effects, 275
  historical aspects, 3–5
  increase, 6–8
  redefinition, 25–6
Drug slang, 302–3
Drug Trafficking Offences Act (1986), 14
Drug users, innate resources lack, 188
Drugs (Prevention of Misuse) Act (1964), 4
Drycleaning fluid, 50
Dysfunction causation, 26

Economic aspects/criminality, 27
  see also Crime
Electrostimulation, heroin withdrawal, 200–1
Employment, problem drug use relationship, 30
Encephalitis, subacute, HIV infection, 129–30
Endophthalmitis, candidal, 142
Environmental influences, 27
Epidemics, drug misuse, 7–8, 26–7
Ergot, 90
Ethyl acetate, morbidity, 49
Examination, 176

Families Anonymous (FA), 276
Family
  and drugs, 274–80
  GP help, 277–80
  influences, 33
  information needs, 279–80
  persistent misusers, 275
  support, 13, 18
  therapy, 243, 276

Fentanyl, analogues, 95-6
Fetal alcohol syndrome, 257-9
Fetal barbiturate syndrome, 260
Fetus
   drug misuse effects, 256-66
   maternal AIDS, 124, 127
Flashbacks, 88, 113
   treatment, 230-1
Fly agaric, 89

Gangrene, injection-induced, 114-15
Gee's linctus, 90
General psychiatrists, misuser care, 16-17
Genetic influences, 33, 34
Genito-urinary effects, 107-8
Glanz, GP attitudes survey, 22
Glue sniffing, 41
   toluene complications, 47-9
Goal-setting, 245-7
GP care, 15-16
   advantages, 17-20
   continuity, 19-20
   current state, 20-1
   family/friends, 277-80
   initial, 167-8, 172-3
   snags, 215-16
GPs
   AIDS and drug misuse services, 136-41
   attitudes to misusers, 21-2
   drug legislation, 145-53
   and HIV spread limitation, 138-9, 141
   self-awareness, 281-2
   training, 281-2

Habituation, WHO definition, 22, 23
Hallucinogens, 84-90
   misuse, treatment, 230-1
   sexual activity effects, 108
Halons, morbidity, 49
Harm reduction, 163-4
Harmful use, 26
Hazardous use, 26
Help-seeking, non-user coercion, 274-5
Hepatitis, 115-22
   infection prevention, 180-2
   markers, 117-19
   viral, 115-22
Hepatitis A, 115-16
Hepatitis B, 116-17
   acute, 119-20
   fulminant, 119-20
   carriers, 120
   chronic active, 120-1
   immunisation, 121-2
   neonatal, 271
   virus, 181
Hepatitis D, 120
Hepatitis, non-A, non-B, 122
Heroin
   cannabis use effects, 37
   'cutting' adulterants, 63-4
   illicit, 62-3
   immunity effects, 142
   injection practice problems, 63-4
   overdoses, 64
   prevalence, 59, 60
   withdrawal syndrome, 9
n-Hexane, morbidity, 50
History taking, 176
HIV, 123
   supercarriers, 124
HIV antibodies
   positives, advice, 304-12
   testing, 182-8
HIV infection, 211-12
   acute (group 1), 127-8
   CDC classification, 128
   chronic (groups II-IV), 128-30
   harm reduction, 163-4, 304-10
   natural history, 127-32
   neonatal, 271
   neurological complications, 129-30
   PGL, 128-9, 304
   positives, advice, 304-12
   prevention, 180-2
   vertical transmission risks, 186
   see also AIDS; AIDS related complex (ARC)
HIV-II, 123
Hospital care, 169-71
   drawbacks, 170
   long-term, 237
Human immunodeficiency virus (HIV), *see* HIV
Human papillomavirus, 181
Hypomania, 113
Hypothermia, drug-induced, 103-4
Hypoventilation, 104

Illicit heroin, 62-3
Immunity, drug misuse effects, 142-3
Individuals, and drug misuse, 34-40
Infants

care orders, 271-3
  maternal AIDS, 124, 127
Information sources, 279-80, 283-8
  see also Advice; Resources
Initial care, referrals, 173-4
Injecting
  advice on HIV, 184-5
  HIV transmission, 132-3
  medical hazards, 114-42
  problems, 63-4
Intercurrent illness masking, 124-5
Interdepartmental Committee on Drug Addiction (Brain) 1961 report, 6
International Opium Convention (1912), 4
Intoxicating Substances (Supply) Act (1985), 53
IUCDs, drug misusers, 254

Kaposi's sarcoma, 130-1
Khat leaves, 90

Labour
  managment, 265-6
  naloxone contraindication, 266
Lead poisoning, petrol sniffing, 51
Legislation, 145-53
Libido loss, 107
  opioid-induced, 64
Lighter fuel, morbidity, 50
Locus of control, 35
LSD
  action mechanisms, 86
  adverse effects, 87-8
  clinical effects, 86-7
  depression association, 113
  historical background, 85-6
  legal control, 4
  misuse, treatment, 230-1
  pregnancy/fetal effects, 262
  psychic effects, 87
Lymphadenopathy, persistent generalised (PGL), HIV infection, 128-9, 304

Mace, 90
Magic mushrooms, 89
Maintenance treatment
  British (Rolleston) system, 5-11
  contract, 209-10, 212
  and crime, 29
  indications, 250
  methadone failure, 8
  use decline, 9-11
Maladjustment, 37
Malaria, 142
Management, DHSS guidelines, 174-90
Mandrax, 90
Marzine, 90
Marzine RF, 90
Medical care, general, 173
Memory disturbances, 110-11
Mescaline, 88
Methadone, 206-7
  efficacy studies, 10
  HIV infection progression effects, 132-3
  opioid detoxification, 201-16
  stabilisation failure, 8
  see also Maintenance treatment
Methaqualone
  analogues, 97
  legal control, 4
Methyl ethyl ketone, morbidity, 52
Methylene chloride, morbidity, 49-50
Minnesota method, long-term care, 239
Misuse of Drugs Regulations (1973/85), 145, 146-53
Misusers, notification, 21
Morning glory seeds, 90
Mortality, drug misuse, 143-4

Naloxone 61, 103
  contraindication in pregnancy, 266
Naltrexone, clonidine combination, 195-7
National Drugs Intelligence Unit (NDIU), trafficking prevention, 14
Needle exchange schemes, HIV prophylaxis, 135-6
Neonates
  care orders, 271-3
  drug-associated problems, 266-73
  hepatitis B, 271
  HIV infection, 271
  poor bonding, 270-1
  withdrawal syndromes, treatment, 268-70
Neuroadaptation, 24-5
Neuroelectric therapy (NET), 198-201
Nitrites, 53-4
  sexual activity effects, 108
Nomenclature, development, 22-6
Non-accidental injuries, 31
Non-specialist services, long-term care, 239-40

Non-user coercion, help-seeking, 274-5
Notifiable drugs, 150-2
Nutmeg, grated, 90
Nutritional deficiencies, 143
Nystagmus, 106

Opioids, 58-65
  action mechanisms, 59-62
  agonists, 61, 62
  AIDS development, 134-5
  antagonists, 103
  dependence, 63
    methadone, 201-16
    no methadone, 191-201
  injection practice problems, 63-4
  misuse, treatment, 190-216
  neonatal effects, 266-7
  partial agonists, 61
  pregnancy management, 263-4
  pregnancy/fetal effects, 259-60
  prescribing care, 158
  prescription equivalents, 202, 203-4
  prevalence, 59, 60
  receptors, 59-61
  sexual activity effects, 107
  social problems, 64-5
  use problems, 63-5
  withdrawal syndrome, neonatal, 267, 269
Opium smoking, historical aspects/legislation, 3-4
Opportunistic infections, AIDS, 130-2, 133, 305
Overdoses, 103, 144

Paint stripper, morbidity, 49-50
Papillomavirus, human, 181
Parental example, 34
PCP, 89
Pemoline, 90, 92-3
Perception disturbances, 109-10
Peripheral neuropathy, 106
Pernod snorting, 90, 101
Personality factors, 34-5
Pethidine, analogues, 95-96
Petrol, morbidity, 51
Pharmacological effects, 38
Phencyclidine, 89
  analogues, 97
Phensedyl, 90
Phenytoin, 90
Physical dependence, WHO definition, 23, 24

Pneumocystis carinii pneumonia (PCP), 130, 131
Poisoning, treatment, 220
Police/customs operations, Ministerial working group, 13-14
Polydrug users, 101
'Poppers', 53-4
Pre-conception counselling, 254-5
Pregnancy, 255-66
  complications, drug-associated, 255-6
  management, 263-6
Prescriptions/prescribing, repeat, benzodiazepine dependence, 71-3
Prescribed drugs, misuse, 90
Prescriptions/prescribing
  care/security, 159
  detoxification patients, 207-16
  drug misuse prevention, 157-9
  guidelines, 204-7
  pharmacist's role, 208-9
  repeat, 158-9
Prevention, 154-6
  attitudes to misuse, 156-7
  classification, 154
  education, 155-6
  and prescribing, 157-9
  supply restriction, 157-9
Primary care team, community support, 18-19
  see also GPs
Prisons, HIV infection/drug misuse, 140-1
Private care, 171-2
  residential, 238-9
Problem drug use, 25
Propane, morbidity, 50
Psilocybe semilanceata, 89
Psilocybin, 89
Psychedelics, 84-90
  misuse, treatment, 230-1
  sexual effects, 108
Psychiatric morbidity, 111-13
Psychiatrists, misuser care, 16-17
Psychological dependence, WHO definition, 23, 24
Psychological effects, 109-11
Psychomotor function, impairment, 110
Psychosis, drug induced, treatment, 221
Psychosocial effects, 36-40
  alcohol/drug abuse parallels, 98-100
Pulmonary oedema, 104
Pyrexia, withdrawal syndrome, 104

Receptors, opioid, 59-61
Recovery, psychological, 39-40
Rehabilitation, 240-7
  in community, 242-3
  finding, 11
  residential, 9, 240-2
  Scotland, 12
  service provision extent, 11-13
Residential care
  private, 238-9
  rehabilitation, 9, 240-2
Resources list, 289-92
  see also Advice; Information
Respiratory complications, 104
Risk factors, 33-7
Road accidents, drug-related, 30-1
Rolleston Committee, 5-11
Rolleston system, maintenance treatment, 5-11

Salbutamol, 90
  inhaler misuse, 52
Schizoprenia, misdiagnosis, 111-12
Scotland
  HIV infection/drug misuse, 139-40
  rehabilitation, 12
Screening, 159-63
  ethics 161, 162-3
  guidelines, 162-3
  see also Urine testing
Self-aggression, 39
Self-awareness, GPs, 281-2
Self-hatred, 39
Self-help groups, 102
  HIV infection, 187
  long-term care, 238
Septicaemia, injection-induced, 115
Sex hormone effects, 107-8
Sexual activity
  drug effects, 107-8
  safer, advice, 185-6, 307-9
Slang, drug users, 302-3
Smoking, pregnancy/fetal effects, 256-7
'Snappers', 53-4
Social care, 169
Socio-cultural factors, 24, 31, 35-6
  alcohol/drug misuse parallels, 100-102
Spermicides, HIV protection, 185
Subacute bacterial endocarditis (SBE), 104
Subclinical conditional withdrawal, 24
Subcultures, drug misuse, 31

Suicides, 144
Sympathomimetic effects, 105

T helper (T4) lymphocytes
  AIDS, 123
  depression, AIDS development, 133
Temporary residents, initial care, 174-5
Tetanus, 141-2
Tetrachloroethylene, morbidity, 50
Tetrahydrocannabinols, 56
Thrombophlebitis, injection-induced, 114
Tipp-EX thinners, morbidity, 50
Toluene
  cerebellar effects, 48
  complications, 48-9
  morbidity, 47-9
Traffic accidents, drug-related, 30-1
Traffickers, 14
Training, GPs, 281-2
Treatment
  combined, alcohol/drug misuse, 101-2
  and crime rate, 29
  neonatal withdrawal syndrome, 268-70
  specialisation, 6-7
  see also Maintenance treatment; *and various drugs*
Trichloroethane, morbidity, 50
Tricyclic antidepressants, CNS stimulants relationship, 111-12
Tuberculosis, AIDS, 142

UN Single Convention on Narcotic Drugs, 4
Unemployment, problem drug use relationship, 30
Unsanctioned use, 26
Urine testing, 188-90
Uterine growth retardation, alcohol-associated, 257-8

Videos, 291-2
Violence, alcohol/drug association, 31
Vitamin deficiencies, 143
Vitamin supplements, pre-conception, 255
Volatile substance misuse (VSM), 41-52
  clinical signs, 44-5
  compound types, 42
  fetal effects, 259, 264
  incidence, 42-3

344 Index

legislation, 52–3
morbidity, 46–52
mortality, 45–6
treatment, 231–5
user social characteristics, 43
user types, 43–4
Voluntary organisations, 276–7, 283–8
WHO, definitions, 22–4
Withdrawal
 abrupt, help, 197–8
 late experience, 24
 subclinical conditioned, 24
Withdrawal syndrome
 general depressant, 99
 neonatal, treatment, 268–70
Women, and drugs, 251–3
Workplace, drug misuse screening, 161–2